Expertise in
Nursing Practice

Patricia Benner, RN, PhD, FAAN, is professor of nursing in the Department of Physiological Nursing at the University of California, San Francisco and an Honorary Fellow in the Royal College of Nursing, United Kingdom. Dr. Benner is the author of *From Novice to Expert: Excellence and Power in Clinical Nursing Practice* which has been translated into 8 languages and provides the background for this research; co-authored with Judith Wrubel *The Primacy of Caring, Stress and Coping in Health and Illness;* is editor of the book *Interpretive Phenomenology: Caring, Ethics and Embodiment in Health and Illness,* and co-edited with Susan Phillips *The Crisis of Care: Affirming and Restoring Caring Practices in the Helping Professions.* She is currently directing a research and development project funded by the Helene Fuld Foundation entitled "Teaching Critical Thinking and Clinical Judgment in Nursing: A Thinking-in-Action Approach" at the University of California, San Francisco, which addresses the pedagogical issues raised in this work.

Christine A. Tanner, RN, PhD, FAAN, is professor of nursing, Community Health Care Systems, School of Nursing, Oregon Health Science University in Portland, Oregon. She has conducted research on clinical judgment in nursing for over two decades, resulting in the publication of numerous journal articles and books. She co-authored with Carnevali, Woods, and Mitchell *Diagnostic Reasoning in Nursing;* and with Lindeman, *Using Nursing Research.* Formerly Director of the School of Nursing Office of Research Development and Utilization, Dr. Tanner has served as consultant on numerous research projects, and her work has challenged contemporary notions of the relationship between research and practice. She has provided leadership in nursing education reform, serving on several task forces and committees for the National League for Nursing, and has consulted with schools of nursing in the U.S., Canada, and abroad. She is currently Editor of the *Journal of Nursing Education.*

Catherine A. Chesla, RN, DNSc, is assistant professor in the Department of Family Health Care Nursing, University of California, San Francisco. She teaches family theory, family intervention and family research methods to graduate nursing students. In her research, she examines family responses over time to the chronic illness of a member, using an interpretive phenomenologic approach. She has published research articles in journals such as *Family Relations, Journal of Community Health Nursing, Journal of Family Nursing,* and *Image; A Journal of Nursing Scholarship.* Currently, she is working with a multi-disciplinary research team to examine family patterns of responses to examine the personal, family, and provider characteristics and processes that influence well-being in persons with non-insulin-dependent diabetes and their families.

Expertise in Nursing Practice

Caring, Clinical Judgment, and Ethics

Patricia Benner, RN, PhD, FAAN

Christine A. Tanner, RN, PhD, FAAN

Catherine A. Chesla, RN, DNSc

with contributions by

Hubert L. Dreyfus, PhD

Stuart E. Dreyfus, PhD

Jane Rubin, PhD

SPRINGER PUBLISHING COMPANY

Springer Publishing Company, Inc.
536 Broadway
New York, NY 10012-3955

Cover design by Tom Yabut
Production Editor: Pam Lankas

96 97 98 99 00 / 5 4

Library of Congress Cataloging-in-Publication Data

Benner, Patricia
    Expertise in nursing practice : caring, clinical judgment and
ethics / Patricia Benner, Christine A. Tanner, Catherine A. Chesla.
        p.   cm.
    Includes bibliographical references and index.
    ISBN 0-8261-8700-5
    1. Nursing—Decision making.   2. Clinical competence.   3. Nursing—
Study and teaching.   4. Nursing—Study and teaching (Continuing
education)   5. Nursing ethics.   I. Tanner, Christine A., 1947–   .
II. Chesla, Catherine A.   III. Title.
    [DNLM: 1. Nursing.   2. Clinical Competence.   3. Ethics, Nursing.
WY 16 B469e 1995]
RT73.B365   1995
610.73—dc20
DNLM/DLC
for Library of Congress   95-31425
                                                                         CIP

Printed in the United States of America

CONTENTS

FOREWORD

Benner's earlier book, *From Novice to Expert: Excellence and Power in Clinical Nursing Practice* was received enthusiastically by nurse clinicians who recognized their work in the descriptions of nursing knowledge and skill. The book adapted and enriched the Dreyfus Model of Skill Acquisition for nursing. It was one of the first works to demonstrate the power of using narrative descriptions to capture clinical and ethical judgment. The earlier book challenged some of our most cherished myths, such as: "skill is the mere application of knowledge"; "clinical judgment can be replaced by breaking tasks down into small units and passed off to narrowly trained personnel"; "formal education is sufficient to produce clinical expertise," and more. Others in fields such as social work, physical therapy, and teaching also responded to the work, recognizing similar complexities in their own professions.

However, *From Novice to Expert*, rich as it was, was unable to play out all the many implications of the Dreyfus Model for nursing administration, practice, and education. That left completing the task to the reader. Many of us finished the book thinking, "that means we should do . . . instead of . . ." Some of us enjoy the armchair exercise of searching for implications, of looking for the changes that should be made accordingly. Others prefer to be provided the pathway through the woods or at least a map.

This new book, *Expertise in Nursing Practice*, although not giving all the answers, provides lots of paths and numerous maps, as well as raising many new issues. This work continues to challenge our traditional understanding of what it means to know, to be, and to act skillfully and ethically in nursing practice. Equally important, the book enables the reader to see how we might begin to shape our systems to better accommodate expert caring work. One of the truths of learning made clear by the work is that clinical learning is a dialogue between principles and practices. To truly grasp a principle, to learn it functionally, requires many practical experiences in which the principle is embedded. Numerous examples of experiential learning and the working out of principles in practice are presented. These multiple examples offer new challenges and open new possibilities for innovation in practice and education.

This new Benner, Tanner, and Chesla book is powerful in its implications. It allows the reader to see the complexity of clinical judgment and caring practices. Like the earlier book, this one uses a research approach that is compelling. Because of its careful documentation, readers will have a hard time ignoring the message. Because the implications are multifold, the book cannot be faulted for only beginning the mammoth task of explicating them.

For me, however, the book had a more personal message and appeal. I realize that all readers will come away with their own unique perspectives, but here are some of the thoughts that were ringing in my head as I put down the book.

It made me think of how the reality of different levels of skill acquisition conflicts with our professional stances, for example, with the notion that a graduate of an accredited school is somehow a finished product, that he or she is ready to perform as a nurse. The book underlines the fallacy of the notion that "a nurse is a nurse is a nurse." True, our nurse administrators have been fighting that image with non-nurse managers for as long as I can remember. Yet, here is the book that can be given to those other managers to explain and validate that perception.

The interweaving of all professionals, especially nurses and physicians, was re-emphasized for me in this book. It was clear that, in many cases, only the presence of one expert level profesional was the life-saving factor. And the expert might just as easily be the nurse or the physician. One expert of either profession might make the critical difference; one nurse who insisted that the physician respond—now and in this way, for example. I thought not only of the expertise required on that nurse's part, but of the bravery, the need to resist the presses of the system to sit down, be quiet, let others decide.

And although the book speaks to the glory of achievements by the expert nurse, one cannot ignore the shadow side. The absence of one expert professional may spell a death or permanent injury for a patient. This is the side we don't want to admit or talk about. When we tell a patient's family, "We did everything we could" that statement may be accurate. But we fail to say, "A more expert team might have been able to do more." To glory in the successes of the experts requires that we recognize the vulnerabilities of those at lower levels of development, and that we look at the potential impact on their patients.

In earlier eras, head nurses instinctively balanced case assignments on knowledge of the capabilities (developmental levels) of staff nurses. And it was possible to do this because some patients were more critically ill than others. Today, at least in the hospital situation, that is not so easy: every patient is very ill. The only solution seems to be continuous teaming of nurses over the long time required to acquire expertise. Ironically at a time when this model forces us to look at the need for dialogue, and mentoring, and even (yes, I'll say it) apprenticeship, our applied models have carried us in other directions. Primary nursing, for example, is essentially a one-on-one model, and economically driven staffing systems leave little time for the mentoring required. Remember, I'm not telling you about the book here so much as the sort of pondering it sets off in the reader's head. At least that's what it did for me.

Mostly I was left thinking of outcomes, of patients who were saved because there happened to be an expert nurse at hand, of patients who weren't saved because a less-experienced nurse (or physician) failed to pick up on clues in time. It made me think of the messiness of life, of the fact that our notions of scientific control are mostly sops to give us the courage to face a scary situation every day. Life is scary, and thinking that nursing "science" can change all that is scary, ignores life's realities. Still, I could not ignore the fact that accepting the ideas presented here would give us a better handle on the situation and better outcomes, too. Still in my arm-chair mood, I wondered, could we continue to hide behind our scientific masks after reading this book? This work points to the kind of wisdom, knowledge, and skill required by all clinicians to make our science useful and safe. And it points to a broader understanding of rationality than mere mechanistic calculation. These are just some of the thoughts that spun through my head after finishing the manuscript. And, if we really accepted the implications of this new book, would we be brave enough to act on them?

I would personally like to thank these colleagues for bringing to me the wealth of knowledge and perceptions presented in their book, these clues to the paths we should take. Will nursing follow the right paths? That has always been the question.

BARBARA STEVENS BARNUM, RN, PhD, FAAN

CONTRIBUTORS

Hubert L. Dreyfus, PhD, is professor of philosophy at the University of California, Berkeley. He is internationally known for his writing and teaching on the limits of Artificial Intelligence, and the relationship between everyday social practices, theory, and science. His published books include: *What Computers Still Can't Do* (3rd ed., 1992); *Being-in-the-World: A Commentary on Heidegger's Being and Time, Division I* (1991); *Mind over Machine* (with Stuart Dreyfus) (1988); *Michel Foucault: Beyond Structuralism and Hermeneutics* (with Paul Rabinow, 1982); and numerous articles including "You Can't Get Something for Nothing: Kierkegaard and Heidegger on How Not to Overcome Nihilism" with Jane Rubin, *Inquiry, Vol. 30* (1–2), March, 1987.

Stuart E. Dreyfus, PhD, has researched skill acquisition in order to assess the compatibility of various mathematical modeling and artificial intelligence efforts with uniquely human skills. Besides teaching mathematical modeling in the Industrial Engineering and Operations Research Department at the University of California, Berkeley, he has taught Cognitive Ergonomics, exploring the implications of various theories of skill acquisition for the design of human-computer systems. He has written several mathematical texts as well as co-authoring the book, *Mind Over Machine,* with his brother, Hubert Dreyfus.

Jane Rubin, PhD, has doctoral degrees in Philosophy and Psychology and is a practicing psychotherapist and teacher in San Francisco, California. She has taught courses on Kierkegaard, Michel Foucault, and Charles Taylor at the University of California, Berkeley, and the University of California, San Francisco, School of Nursing. Her teaching has greatly influenced the thinking of this work. She is author of "Narcissism and Nihilism: Kohut and Kierkegaard on the Modern Self" in Douglas Detrick and Susan Detrick (Eds.), *Self Psychology: Comparisons and Contrasts* (1989); and with Hubert Dreyfus wrote "Kierkegaard, Division II, and Later Heidegger" in *Being-in-the-World: A Commentary on Heidegger's Being and Time, Division I.*

x

ACKNOWLEDGMENTS

This is the first large-scale effort to articulate the nature of clinical and ethical expertise in nursing. This project was truly a community effort. We are especially grateful to Alan Trench and his colleagues at the Helene Fuld Trust for catching our vision for this project and funding it for 4 years. Many doctoral and master's students contributed to the work at both the University of California, San Francisco and the Oregon Health Sciences University.

At the University of California, San Francisco, students and colleagues were integral to the completion of this work. Barbara Habermann, Patricia Hooper, Gina Long, and Susan Thollaug assisted with data collection. Data analysis was also assisted by master's student Karen Reese. Data marking and interpretation engaged many who were at the time doctoral nursing students, including Elena Bosque, Lisa Day, Nancy Doolittle, Barbara Haberman, Patricia Hooper, Margaret Kearney, Annemarie Kesselring, Victoria Leonard, Joan Liaschenko, Ruth Malone, Karen Plager, Lee SmithBattle, Hopkins Stanley, and Daphne Stannard. Daphne Stannard and Ruth Malone helped produce the video that documented some of the central study findings, entitled "From Beginner to Expert", which was produced by the Fuld Institute for Technology. Daphne Stannard deserves special recognition for her consistent contributions in helping the project cohere and stay organized during the latter phases of writing and manuscript preparation. Kathy Horvath and Janet A. Secatore also have our thanks for contributing to long-distance data-collection efforts. We also had able staff assistance from Karen Allen, J. J. Hollingsworth, Julie Richards, Belinda Young and Julie Alden.

Several faculty and graduate students at Oregon Health Sciences University worked with the research team. Sheila Kodadek, Associate Professor of Family Nursing at Oregon Health Sciences University, and Peggy Wros, then doctoral student and now assistant professor of nursing at Linfield College, and Martha Haylor former doctoral student and now assistant professor of nursing at the University of Victoria School of Nursing, in Victoria, British Columbia were instrumental in the conduct of the study at the Portland site. They assisted in interviews and observations, data entry, verification, coding and overall management, interpretation of data, and preparation of early manuscript drafts. Many other faculty and graduate students participated in data interpretation. Caroline White, professor of nursing, and Margaret Imle, associate professor of nursing, both at OHSU, and Monical Dostal, Linda Budan, Yoko Nakayama, and Dawn Doutrich, all graduate students at the time of the study, were also very helpful in data coding and interpretation. Patricia Archbold, professor of nursing, Lisa Chickadonz, assistant professor of nursing, and Caroline White provided wonderful critiques of earlier drafts of manuscripts.

We are grateful to the hospitals that supported the effort by donating staff time for interviews. And most of all, we are grateful to the 130 nurses who told their clinical stories and the 48 of these who allowed us to observe and interview them while they were working.

The core research team, Patricia Benner, Christine Tanner, and Catherine Chesla to this day enjoy working together. Catherine Chesla did a masterful job directing the first 2 years of the project and then became a full-fledged Coinvestigator. Jane Rubin, Hubert L. Dreyfus, and Stuart E. Dreyfus gave ably and generously of their expertise as consultants. We have chosen to present their chapters as the separately authored works they are, and not to present these consultants as authors of the whole book, in part to relieve them of the responsibility and task of working on the whole manuscript. The book was written collaboratively, with each author signing off on each chapter. We did, however, have primary responsibility for the first drafts of the chapters. Therefore questions should be directed to the author of the first draft. Patricia Benner wrote first drafts for the introduction, Chapters 4, 5, 8, 9, and 13; Christine Tanner wrote first drafts for Chapters 1, 6, 10, and 12; Catherine Chesla wrote first drafts for Chapter 3 and the "Background and Methods" in Appendix A.

Our families were steadfast in their support: Special thanks to Richard, John and Lindsay Benner; to Lisa Chickadonz, Jacob, Katie, and Spencer; and to Jeff, William, and Andreis Vanderbilt.

INTRODUCTION

This book extends the research presented in the book *From Novice to Expert: Excellence and Power in Clinical Nursing Practice*, published by Addison-Wesley in 1984. No one could have predicted the response of practicing nurses all over the world to that account of gaining clinical expertise, and the articulation of the domains of nursing practice. *From Novice to Expert* has been translated into Finnish, German, Japanese, Spanish, French, and Swedish, and a limited number of copies were translated for Russian nurse educators. It has been the source of many conferences and nursing curricula, and the basis for clinical promotion programs in many hospitals in many parts of the world. Nurses commented that *From Novice to Expert* put into words what they had always known about their clinical nursing expertise, but had difficulty articulating.

We believe that this book illuminates the project begun in *From Novice to Expert* with a few changes and many additional nuances. This work provides a much thicker description of the acquisition of clinical expertise and a much more extended examination of the nature of clinical knowledge, clinical inquiry, clinical judgment, and expert ethical comportment. This book is based on a 6-year study of 130 hospital nurses, most of them critical care nurses. In this study we found that examining the nature of the nurse's agency, by which we mean the sense and possibilities for acting in particular clinical situations, gave new insights about how perception and action are both shaped by a practice community. We came to more clearly understand the distinctions between *engagement with a problem or situation* and the requisite nursing *skills of involvement* with patients and families. These existential skills of involvement, knowing how close or distant to be with patients and families in critical times of threat and recovery, are learned over time experientially. Indeed, we will make the claim that the skill of involvement with patients and families seem to be central in gaining nursing expertise, because promoting the well-being of vulnerable others requires both problem engagement and the existential skills of personal involvement. In this study we came to see the interlinkage of clinical and ethical decision making—how one's notions of good and poor outcomes and visions of excellence shape clinical judgments and actions.

We discovered new aspects of each stage of skill acquisition, but we came to see the competent stage as particularly pivotal in clinical learning because it is at this stage that the learner must begin to recognize patterns and, to become proficient, must allow the situation to guide responses. We came to understand the proficiency stage as a transition into expertise. This study points to the importance of active teaching and learning in the competent stage in order to coach nurses in making the transition from competency to proficiency.

Through this study, the role of sharing narratives, or storytelling, in understanding a practice, demonstrating reasoning in transitions, in communicating intentions, meanings, and concerns, and in creating a community of dialogue and memory has come into sharper focus. Narrative accounts of actual clinical examples reveal everyday clinical and caring knowledge central to the practice of nursing. The concerns, fears, hopes, conversations, and issues of nurses are disclosed and preserved in telling and discussing the stories. A story allows for less linearity, more parentheses or asides, and better captures both forward and retrospective thinking, because the end of the story is known by the storyteller. Thus, a narrative can better capture practical clinical reasoning as it occurs in transition. We have learned that practitioners, through experience within a socially based practice, build narratives and memories of salient clinical situations as they move from novice to skillful practitioner. With experience, concrete situations become coherent and help the practitioner develop a sense of doing better or worse, of recognizing similarities and differences, and of participating in common meanings and practices. Others' practice narratives allow practitioners to recognize reoccurring distinctions and common clinical entities and issues.

The context of nursing practice has changed dramatically in the 11 years since *From Novice to Expert* was published. The caring practices central to nursing were articulated in 1984 in the midst of nursing shortages and in the budding awareness that caring practices were far more than sentiment or attitudes, but were skilled relational and practical know-how. It is these caring practices that render high-tech cures and instantaneous therapies safe. In 1995, in the midst of a very uncertain health care reform, where cost savings are sought primarily in the care provided rather than the cures and diagnostic tests offered, we believe that this work offers a crucial guidepost for quality care. There is a growing trend to train less educated workers to do many of the tasks nurses have done in order to cut health care costs. In this context, this work calls for an examination of reliability as well as efficiency. Where constant monitoring and astute clinical judgment are required to manage highly unstable patients, fewer tasks can be delegated without losing the nurses' ability to "know the patient" (Tanner, Benner, Chesla, & Gordon, 1993) and recognize early crucial warnings of patient change.

We believe that this work demonstrates what we tend to cover over in the Western tradition: that skilled know-how is a form of knowledge in its own right, and not a mere application of knowledge. Experienced clinicians have mastered a kind of knowledge not available from the classroom. We hope that this work brings out of hiding clinical knowing and clinical inquiry that get eclipsed by our anxiety to teach science and technology. We do not seek to devalue science and technology, only to make room for the disciplined inquiry and ethical comportment that render our science and technology safe in the practice of caring for individual patients and families. We want a larger, legitimate space for teaching practical reasoning in transitions, the hallmark of any clinical practice. We look forward to the new dialogues within and outside the discipline that this work will create.

Like *From Novice to Expert*, this is both a study of skill acquisition and a research-based articulation of the nature of clinical nursing knowledge. We believe that the work will have relevance for other practice disciplines, such as medicine, social work, teaching, occupational therapy, physical therapy, and others. And though all the examples are nursing examples, the progression from principle-based practice, guided by science, technology and ethics, to response-based practice, guided by practical knowledge accumulated through engaged reasoning, will be relevant and recognizable by all practitioners.

DESCRIPTION OF THE STUDY

This book is based upon an interpretive study of nursing practice in critical care units that was conducted between 1988 and 1994. The study was conceived by Patricia Benner and Christine Tanner and proposed to the Helene Fuld Foundation for funding. Coinvestigators who were involved from the proposal phase were Hubert L. Dreyfus and Stuart E. Dreyfus. We here present a brief overview of our approach to the study of nursing practice. A detailed discussion of our concerns and actions in design and conduct of the study can be found in Appendix A.

Four key aims that structured the study were:

1. To delineate the practical knowledge embedded in expert practice;
2. To describe the nature of skill acquisition in critical care nursing practice;
3. To identify institutional impediments and resources for the development of expertise in nursing practice; and
4. To begin to identify educational strategies that encourage the development of expertise.

As in all interpretive work, the project was initially structured, but not constrained, by these guiding aims. In the following pages we illustrate our findings regarding these central questions, and demonstrate as well the central themes and narratives that went beyond the original aim of the inquiry.

The design of the study was influenced by a concern to access practice of nurses in ways that allowed the practice to become visible in all of its aspects. The study design additionally extended what we had learned from previous interpretive study of nursing practice (Benner, 1984a; Benner & Wrubel, 1989) and clinical judgement (Benner & Tanner, 1987; Tanner, 1989, 1993). Additional concerns were to access practice that was carried out in various types of institutions, in different geographic locations, by nurses of varying skill levels practicing with persons with divergent illness processes across the lifespan.

Interpretive phenomenology (see Appendix A for a more detailed explanation of term) was used to access the everyday practice and skill of critical care nurses. The aim of this approach is to explain particular and distinct patterns of meaning and action in the practice of nurses studied, taking into account the context in which they worked, their history, and their particular concerns. Rather than try to characterize a modal or general practice, we attempt to articulate particular and distinct patterns of meaning and action in the nurse-informants. The approach is (a) systematic in its use of tested modes of gathering narrative on practice, (b) disciplined in its focus on the meanings and concerns that can be interpreted from direct text from informants, as opposed to a focus on theoretical abstractions from that text, (c) self-critical and self-corrective in its continual return to the text for arbitrating disputes in interpretation, and (d) produces a consensually validated interpretation that is agreed upon by multiple readers (Benner, 1994b; Packer & Addison, 1989; Van Manen, 1990).

One hundred and thirty nurses practicing in intensive care units and general floor units from eight hospitals, seven of which are located in two far Western and one in the Eastern region of the country, comprised the group of informants. Nurses were drawn from neonatal, pediatric, and adult intensive care units; those practicing in adult units were distributed evenly across surgical, medical, cardiac, and general intensive care units. Because we sampled for a relatively homogenous group, 98% of the nurses held a minimum of a bachelor's degree. The hospitals from which the informants were drawn included predominantly tertiary care teaching hospitals as well as a community hospital and a Veterans Administration hospital.

Nurses were selected for their expected level of practice (advanced beginner through expert) by supervisors who were asked to consider years of experience, and, for the nurses who were in practice more than 5 years, the quality of their practice. We anticipated that variability of practice would be captured naturalistically in the beginning and intermediate nurses, but with the experienced nurses, we set out to capture variability by asking supervisors or head nurses to name nurses who had been in practice 5 or more years and were considered superb nurses, and nurses who had been in practice the same amount of time but provided safe but less than exemplary care. The final sample was comprised of 25 nurses with less than 1 year of experience; 35 nurses with at least 2 but less than 5 years experience; 44 nurses with 5 or more years of experience and identified as expert, and 26 nurses with 5 or more years of experience and identified as experienced but not expert in their practice. (See Appendix B for detailed description of informants.)

Two central approaches were used to access the everyday experience and skill of nurses caring for patients in critical care: narrative interviews and observation. Small group interviews with four to six nurses who had the same amount of practice experience were conducted repeatedly for three sessions. Nurses were asked to present narratives of recent practice with particular patients and to help assist with obtaining a complete narrative from each informant by actively contributing questions and clarifying uncertainties. A second approach to understanding practice was direct observation of 48 nurses who were observed for three periods of 2–4 hours while they were engaged in direct care of patients in their units. All interviews and any direct discussion during observation periods were audio-recorded and transcribed verbatim to produce a text for interpretation.

Interpretation of text was comprised of initial interpretations of each interview by a subset of the research team prior to the following interview with each group; small group interpretation of portions of text that addressed particular questions; and large group interpretations, in which the full team gathered to examine interpretive accounts that had been worked out on initial questions. The process of interpretation included repeated examination of the text for understanding it as a whole, for understanding its most salient points, and for understanding the complete, if detailed aspects of the text. Several units of analysis were considered in the ongoing interpretation: individual narrative about each patient, the individual nurse's practice as a whole, the practice of nurses who practiced at the same level, the practice of nurses who practiced at the same institution, and groups of narratives that clustered around a particular theme. Subsets of the research team who were concerned about particular units of study concentrated on the interpretation of that particular text.

We hope that we have put into words once again what nurses and all clinicians know in their practice and that the marginalized caring practices presented here compel the reader to consider the societal worth and knowledge inherent in the caring, diagnostic, and therapeutic work that nurses do. We hope that practitioners from other fields will join us in this conversation so that together we can design better institutions of public caring—in our schools, families, social work, courtrooms—in all places where protection of vulnerability, sponsorship of growth, and the promotion of better citizenship occurs.

Chapter 1

CLINICAL JUDGMENT

The interpretive study of nursing practice provides new insights into how skilled clinicians make judgments in their everyday practice. In this chapter we will show, through interpretation of narrative interviews, that the clinical judgment of expert nurses differs greatly from the usual understanding that has dominated the academic nursing culture for the last 30 years. Specifically, we will show that:

- The clinical judgment of experienced nurses resembles much more the engaged, practical reasoning first described by Aristotle, than the disengaged, scientific, or theoretical reasoning promoted by cognitive theorists and represented in the nursing process.
- Experienced nurses reach an understanding of a person's experience with an illness, and hence their response to it, not through abstract labeling such as nursing diagnoses, but rather through knowing the particular patient, his typical pattern of responses, his story and the way in which illness has constituted his story, and through advanced clinical knowledge, which is gained from experience with many persons in similar situations. This experientially gained clinical knowledge sensitizes the nurse to possible issues and concerns in particular situations.

The vast majority of research on clinical judgment, and on educational approaches to improve it, has focused on that which is deliberative, conscious and analytic; and some would, no doubt, argue that clinical judgment is not judgment at all unless it has these characteristics. In nursing, we have used "clinical decision making," "nursing process," "clinical problem solving," and, more recently, "critical thinking" as interchangeable terms all referring to roughly the same phenomenon. This language both reflects and shapes our

1

understanding, orienting us toward seeing clinical judgment as rational, and directed only toward resolution of problems and clearly defined ends. To those conversant with the literature, some terms are also theory-laden. For example, in the decision-theory literature, "decision making" is taken to mean the rational selection of alternatives from a set of mutually exclusive possibilities; the selection is based on values associated with each possible outcome, and the probability of each outcome given the possible course of action. The continuing use of this language, and the characteristic focus on conscious analysis, often results in an inappropriately broad generalization: that all expert judgment is deliberative and analytic and if not, it could be improved by making it more analytical.

However, Dewey (1904, 1916/1973), Dreyfus (1979), Dreyfus and Dreyfus (1986) among others have called attention to the notion of "thoughtless mastery of the everyday"; for example, we can get to and from work, walk, have a social conversation responding to another's needs, and ride an elevator, maintaining appropriate social distance, all without conscious deliberation. Similarly much of expert performance in nursing, being attuned to subtle changes in the clinical situation, attending to salient information, and understanding and responding to patients' issues or concerns also often takes place without any conscious deliberation at all. In this chapter, our intent is to open up new possibilities about clinical judgment in the practice of expert nurses by attending to these nonconscious, non-analytic aspects of judgment.

We use the term "clinical judgment" to refer to the ways in which nurses come to understand the problems, issues, or concerns of clients/patients, to attend to salient information, and to respond in concerned and involved ways; included in our understanding of the term is both the deliberate, conscious decision-making characteristic of competent performance and the holistic discrimination and intuitive response typical of proficient and expert performance (Dreyfus & Dreyfus with Athanasiou, 1986).

We will develop the arguments advanced above by introducing a typical exemplar from a nurse practicing at the expert level, highlighting several aspects of her clinical judgment and describing how these same aspects have either been neglected or misrepresented by technical rationality models of clinical judgment. Then we will examine in more detail the meaning of practical reasoning as it relates to clinical judgment in nursing, and explore alternatives to a diagnostic-treatment model of nursing practice. We do not intend to offer a complete theory or model of clinical judgment, but rather wish to call attention to significant aspects of expert practice. We believe that uncovering the assumptions of the technical rationality model and revealing even a few aspects of clinical judgment will set up new possibilities for our educational practices.

ASPECTS OF CLINICAL JUDGMENT UNCOVERED IN NARRATIVE ACCOUNTS

In this section we will use an exemplar from a nurse practicing at the expert level to explore aspects of clinical judgment. We will illustrate how assumptions and typical research methods of cognitive models have obscured each of these aspects of judgment.

The following account is very typical of nurses practicing at the expert level, both in the nurse's clinical grasp of the situation and in her action as a moral agent; it also captures the several dimensions of family care explicated by Chesla (1990).

Nurse: We had a patient who had been in the OR having a CABG (coronary artery bypass graft). I'd gotten word that he had been hospitalized before, had a very poor heart, multiple MIs, poor ejection fraction. As I was coming to work that evening, I had also gotten word that his family was sitting and waiting in our waiting room. The patient wasn't back from surgery yet, and I heard they were there, so I thought I'll go out and meet them, which I try to do when it works out that way. They were stressed to the max; the minute I walked out they jumped off the chair, they knew I was coming to talk with them. I introduced myself, explained that we really don't hear much until they actually get up to the unit and just talked about what to expect and that they could come in after an hour or so. They proceeded to tell me this whole story about what this poor man had gone through and how it was so rough on him, and so on.

So the patient returned from surgery, and sure enough, was sick as everything, on every drip known to man, ballooned, had had a real hard time coming off bypass, the whole thing. As I listened to the report and I went into the room, I looked at him, and it was clear that it's going to be a miracle if this man leaves this hospital alive. That was the sense I had. So I got settled. I went out and had the family come and just tried to give them a sense of what to expect . . . And we just hit it off or something. They needed—it was like they were just looking for this release valve and I gave it to them. At that point we just kind of clicked.

A few days went by and the patient was really sick, but eventually, amazingly he kind of turned the corner and we were able to start weaning drips. We got him de-ballooned. We got him extubated. And we were all astounded that this man was alive, he was extubated, he was lucid, and he was talking to me. His grandson came in and visited, and his grandson was his pride and joy. The two of them were going at it. He told me how he got his nickname, what he did with his grandson, went to this ballgame, to that ballgame. But it was still obvious, even though he looked better, it was really obvious that he was very, very fragile and any little thing was going to tip him over the edge. And another day or so went by, and it came time to pull his chest tubes and unfortunately he got a pneumothorax and that was all he needed. I knew that any little thing was just going to be his demise, and sure enough he ended up having to get reintubated, chest tubes put in. It was decided at that point that what he needed was medical management and he was sent back to CCU.

A few days later, his family came up looking for me. H. had gotten to the point where he was in end-stage cardiac disease and there was nothing else they could do and they finally decided to make him a DNR. I said to the family, "Do you mind if I just go in and see him?" At that point he was ventilated and sedated and paralyzed and he had the tropical IVAC forest behind the bed. I had seen him that sick but it bothered me to go down there and see him that sick again. He had gotten better and my last image of him was this man sitting up in bed raving about his grandson.

I went out to the family; they were obviously preparing themselves for his death, and I just felt awful 'cause here I see this man getting better then right back to being as sick as he could possibly be. They were beside themselves. I think they felt guilty about making him DNR and they had this insatiable need to know that they had done everything they could. They felt like, well, maybe there's more.

Int: Were they asking you that?

Nurse: Not in those words, but that was the sense I was getting from what they were saying. Finally, it hit me. I just got this image of him sitting up in bed talking to his grandson and I said, you did do everything. Look how sick he was when he first came into the unit. He got better. We helped him get as better as his heart would let him get. But his heart was too sick. They were kind of able to say, "Yeah, I guess we did." He did get better, but he was just too fragile.

At that point, all of us are sitting in the room, tears are coming down the eyes, and at that point they were able to just kind of loosen up and talk about him. And talk, it was like they were preparing themselves for his death. And you know it just seemed like someone sort of took them off the hook. You don't have to feel guilty anymore. At this point, making him a DNR was the kindest thing you could do for him. I feel like in that situation, even though the outcome for the patient was bad, I was able to make a difference with them, because they were going through a lot. It was kind of hard for me, because it's always stressful when someone dies, and you have to go and tell the family. You know, it's always "What do I say," you know, where do the words come from. For him, I drew on the situation of him, being sick, getting better, look at these milestones he's gone through just in the past few weeks. It's especially hard in those situations where I have to tell the family. I don't mind so much if I know them, but if they don't know me and know what I've been through with their family member, I don't like that. Sometimes I feel like I really know them and that they would appreciate hearing it from someone they know and that someone they know cares and has worked really hard with them and with the patient.

In this situation, the nurse's central concern was her involvement with the family of a dying patient. The nurse seeks out the family, is solicited by their story of the patient's illness and suffering, and recognizes their preeminent position in the patient's world. The nurse, solicited by the patient and family, "just sort of clicks" with them. She provides perspective for the family through her experience with similar patients, orienting the family to the patient's current status and possible outcomes, while being sensitive to the family's ability to hear and understand her explanations. The nurse's clinical judgments in attending to, and understanding the family's concerns, the ways in which she responded to their concerns, supporting them in their grief, and working through their decisions about no heroic measures were the central themes of the narrative. It should be apparent from this exemplar how little of this practice could be captured by a diagnosis-treatment model. She immediately understood how on edge the family was, and responded to their need for a "release valve." No theory can capture the meaning of this experience for the family; the labels characteristically used in the nursing diagnosis literature simply do not convey sufficient meaning for this nurse to know how to respond to this particular family's concerns.

Also significant in this account are the clinical judgments involved in getting a good clinical grasp, the skill of seeing. The nurse, through having heard about the case from other nurses in the unit, had a prior understanding of the severity of the particular patient's condition and practical knowledge of what would ordinarily be expected of patients in similar circumstances, setting up what would stand out in the particular situation as relevant. She recognized the patient's fragility, saying it was "really obvious that any little thing might tip him over."

What is transparent in the practice is the skill of managing rapidly changing situations—understanding the patient's fragile state, managing the ventilator, chest tubes, drips—these simply do not show up as an issue for the nurse, although clearly she was responsible for this aspect of the patient's care. This nonconscious holistic discrimination of the patient's state and fluid, skillful response, with little evidence of rational calculation, is characteristic of expert clinical judgment. In this situation, at least five interrelated aspects of clinical judgment stand out.

First, the nurse comes to the situation with a fundamental disposition toward what is good and right. It is clear to her that an important part of her practice is noticing and attending to the family's concerns, and to that end, she seeks out the family. Her sense of what is an important end set up what she noticed in the particular situation. What is ordinarily viewed as the main ethical concern in a situation like this—that is, whether continuing life support is in the best interest of the patient—shows up in the narrative, but it is not the central issue for this nurse in this particular situation. Although obviously troubled and saddened by the patient's decline, she recognizes that death is likely imminent and she turns to supporting the family in being with the patient, and in beginning to work through their guilt and grief. In the technical-rationality model of practice (Schon, 1983, 1987) the work of the practitioner is an instrumental means-ends analysis, with the major decision being which interventions will result in the desired outcomes. The ends, or the "good" in Aristotelian terms, cannot be evaluated through this instrumental reasoning. In nursing, as in medicine, when the goal comes into question, it is a matter of ethics and at least in modern times, ethical and clinical decision making have been viewed as distinct domains in both research and practice (Gortner, 1985; Katefian, 1988).

We argue that even in clinical situations, where the ends are not in question, there is an underlying moral dimension: the fundamental disposition of the nurse toward what is good and right and action toward what the nurse recognizes or believes to be the best good in a particular situation. In the above exemplar, the good that is evident in the nurse's actions in this particular situation is comforting the family. This is not a private, subjectively held "value," nor one that necessarily generalizes across all situations. While the moral dimension of everyday judgment is beginning to receive some attention (Ackerlund & Norberg, 1985; Bishop & Scudder, 1990, 1991; Gadow, 1988; Wros, 1994), it has typically been ignored in the decision-making literature.

Second, the nurse in this situation relies on extensive practical knowledge from working with many, many patients after coronary artery surgery, and with many families of acutely ill persons; and during the course of her care she comes to know H. and his family, both their pattern of responses and who they are as a people. As she describes her actions, recognizing the patient's downhill course, supporting and facilitating the grandson's participation, and responding to the particular concerns of the family, it is evident that no theory could prescribe how she should respond in this particular situation. Rather, it is the tacit knowing (Polanyi, 1958), skilled know-how (Benner, 1983), or knowing in action (Schon, 1983) and knowing the particular patient (Jenks, 1993; Jenny & Logan, 1992; MacLeod, 1993; Tanner, Benner, Chesla, & Gordon, 1993) that sets up the possibility for the nurse to recognize and respond in this particular situation.

In the technical-rationality model of professional practice, the only knowledge that counts is theoretical knowledge. Theory as an abstraction gives the practitioner insight into a broad range of particular, clinical situations. It is presumed that the competent practitioner is able to see a particular situation as an instance of some abstraction; for example, that a particular family situation is an instance of ineffective coping. The theory also prescribes appropriate nursing responses. In this view, then, professional practice is the instrumental application of scientifically derived knowledge and theory to the problems of practice (Schon, 1983, 1987).

Most studies of clinical judgment in both medicine and nursing are founded on the technical-rationality model of professional practice. Most, including those investigating "processes of judgment," its measurement and correlates of skill in judgment, have relied on the use of simulations and some variation of thinking aloud, during or after the simulation [see Tanner (1987) and Fonteyn (1991) for reviews of this literature; and Grobe, Drew, & Fonteyn (1991), Henry (1991), and Jones (1989) as particular examples of this approach to study]. Simulations are used as a way to present the same stimuli to subjects, so that variation due to experience, training, personality traits, etc. can be examined; moreover, simulations are used to reduce extraneous "noise" so that the performance of the subject in relation to controlled features of the "task" can be objectively evaluated.

Generally, these studies tell us that there are differences in how beginners and experts "process information" in problem-solving tasks, but that there is a huge problem of "task specificity," i.e., that performance and approach vary greatly according to the so-called "demands of the task environment." In some studies, there is almost as much variation within the same individual across "tasks" as there is between experience groups. (See, for example, Corcoran, 1986; Tanner, Padrick, Westfall, & Putzier, 1987.) Moreover, most studies exploring the relationship between years of experience and performance on simulation have found improved performance for the first 6–8 years, then a decline. (See, for example, Davis, 1972, 1974; del Bueno, 1990; Verhonick, Nichols, Glor, & McCarthy, 1968.) But what counts as good performance in these studies is, in part, the ability to make explicit what for experts may necessarily be tacit. Additionally, experts are likely to rely on context and whole patterns, knowing the particular patient and family for their judgments; these aspects simply cannot be portrayed meaningfully through simulation, because they require involvement in the situation.

A third aspect of clinical judgment that shows up in the exemplar and which is typically unaccounted for in technical-rationality models of judgment is the context of the particular situation and the nurse's own emotional responses. In the situation above, the nurse was solicited by the family's concerns. Standing outside of the situation was not even a possibility for her. She understood the past for this patient, had an immediate clinical grasp of the present crisis, and could project the future. Because of this understanding, the nurse could help the family anticipate what lay ahead for H., drawing on their story of his past, and understanding of the current situation and a projection of the likely future. The nurse describes her emotional involvement, and how it bothered her to see H. so sick. She referred to coming to understand his world: "My last image of him was this man sitting up in bed raving about his grandson." For this nurse, the patient is no longer a medical case, but a person with a life full of meaning. She is engaged emotionally in a part of his life world, and "feels awful" to see his decline. This emotional involvement made it possible for her to respond to the family in a sensitive and meaningful way.

Neither context nor emotion have typically been accounted for in most studies of clinical judgment. The reliance on models and methods that control for or ignore context, emotion and the individual's experience has eliminated the possibility of seeing these as important in clinical judgment. As Gardner (1985) summarized:

> A feature of the cognitive science is the deliberate attempt to deemphasize certain factors which may be important for cognitive functioning but whose inclusion at this point would unnecessarily complicate the cognitive-science enterprise. These factors include the influence of affective factors or emotion, the contribution of historical or cultural factors and the role of the background context in which the particular actions or thoughts occurred. (p. 6)

According to rational-technical models, the clinician is a private subject, standing outside the situation, touching reality only through mental representations. The common sense of our discipline and of the Western tradition is that in order to perceive and relate to things, we have some content in our minds that corresponds to our knowledge of them. This assumption of representation shows up in much of our literature aimed toward theories and concepts as guides for action—assuming that underlying every human action, most notably expert human action, is a theory in some form of mental representation. Within this philosophical tradition, emotions usually have been considered as subversive to knowledge. Reason, rather than emotion, has been regarded as the indispensable faculty in acquiring knowledge. The rational is typically contrasted with the emotional. In cognitivist accounts, emotion has been considered to have two components: an affective, or feeling, component and a cognitive component that appraises the feelings. We see this division show up in our educational practices, with cognitive and affective behaviors, and the recurring struggles of educators to assert what feelings are appropriate. What is missing in these accounts is the recognition that emotions are to some extent socially constructed and that knowledge and emotion are mutually constitutive; judgment occurs in the context of a particular situation, when the nurse is emotionally attuned to the situation, and meaningful aspects simply stand out as important and the choice of responses is guided by the nurse's interpretation of the particular situation.

A fourth aspect of clinical judgment that shows up in the exemplar is intuition. By intuition, we mean a judgment without a rationale, a direct apprehension and response without recourse to calculative rationality. On this view, intuition is born of experience and is not a magical, mystical quality belonging exclusively to women. In the exemplar above, the nurse recognized a pattern of likely demise. She commented, "It was really obvious that he was very, very fragile and that any little thing was going to tip him over the edge."

Intuition has been a hotly debated topic for hundreds of years. Westcott (1968) has summarized the many positions on intuition in western philosophy:

> There is considerable diversity in the consideration of intuition . . . The principal issues in the great conflict between empiricism and intuitionism remain concerned with whether there are alternative ways of knowing alternative truths and realities. If so, is one higher, more perfect or more absolute than another? do we act within the confines of reason and evidences, as we usually do, deprive ourselves of vast realms of knowledge—perhaps incommunicable, and entirely personal, but powerful and satisfying? (p. 27)

Contemporary debates in psychology center on the extent to which intuition is a special case of inference, that is, a rational process which is unconscious and inaccessible, or is an altogether different road to a "special kind of knowing" (Westcott, 1968, p. 27). Cognitivists claim that we touch the world through internal representations; recognizing a pattern is an intellectual process of matching these internal representations with external events (English, 1993). In the above example, a cognitivist would claim that the nurse carried around in her head internal representations of "fragileness," and simply matched the cues present in the external situation with the features of the internal representation. But this interpretation does not account for what shows up as salient in the particular situation, how the nurse even notices relevant aspects. Fundamental to this argument is a different understanding of what it means to be human. For cognitivists, the metaphor for human action is the computer. This view overlooks the possibility that humans inhabit their worlds in an involved way, rather than through mental representations or schema; salient aspects, nuances, and meanings simply show up. The cognitivist view also fails to recognize the ways in which clinicians become socialized into their professional culture, developing habitual ways of seeing and responding to patients.

Despite the claims of cognitivists such as English (1993), intuition has gained increasing recognition in the nursing literature as a legitimate aspect of clinical judgment. Historical studies, like that by Rew and Barrows (1987), illustrate the influence of the dominant rational perspective on a developing discipline like nursing. They conclude that intuition has received little serious attention in the research literature, and more commonly is denigrated as inappropriate in a scientific discipline. Yet discourse among practitioners about intuition is lively (Burnard, 1989) and naturalistic studies of nursing practice have revealed its important role in clinical judgment

(Benner & Tanner, 1987; Leners, 1993; Pyles & Stern, 1983; Rew, 1988; Schraeder & Fischer, 1987; Young, 1987).

In virtually all of these studies, intuition is characterized by immediate apprehension of a clinical situation and is a function of acquaintance with similar experiences. In most, this apprehension is often a recognition of a pattern, as we described the phenomena from our preliminary studies (Benner & Tanner, 1987). For example, in her study of experienced nurse informants, Leners (1993) most recently described initial "cues" which she described as contextual and relational in nature; Schraeder and Fischer (1987) also describe the "cues" nurses use in their intuitions about neonates as "physiologically based but not easy to quantitate," (p. 48) pointing to patterns such as movement, posture, and tone. Based on her study findings, Rew (1988) identified three aspects of intuition—knowledge that is received in an immediate way, perceived as a whole, and not arrived at through a conscious, linear analytic process.

In most of these studies, nurse informants provided particular accounts of intuition in which the informant anticipated a patient's decline before there was any objective evidence. We also found in our early work (Benner, 1984; Benner & Tanner, 1987) that early warnings of a patient's demise are a memorable if not frequent occurrence in the practice of experienced nurses and that pattern recognition and holistic similarity recognition allow for this early warning. But we have found that intuition constitutes a significant part of the everyday practice of expert nurses; it is at the heart of the skillful fluid performance so characteristic of expert practice. Conscious, rational calculation is typically required by the new graduate, where experience is absent, and the nurse is left to consciously "figure it out." New graduates often require at least a mental checklist to know what to watch for in particular patient situations; the more experienced nurse has a sense of salience, where important aspects of the case simply stand out because of her prior knowledge of the particular situation and because of her experience with similar situations. Rational calculation is not required for her to notice relevant details.

To respond by intuition is not the same as thoughtless and automatic responses—quite the contrary. We have found that while intuition is clearly possible when nurses don't know the patient, based on experiences with similar patients, knowing the patient and involvement with him supports the direct apprehension and understanding that we describe as intuition. Moreover, we have found, like the Dreyfuses, that expert nurses also use a kind of deliberative rationality to check out their whole intuitions.

The conscious use of calculative rationality produces regression to the skill of the novice or at best, the competent performer. To think rationally in that sense is to forsake know-how and is not usually desirable. If decisions are important and time is available, a more basic form of rationality than that of the beginner is useful. This kind of deliberative rationality does not seek to analyze the situation into context-free elements, but seeks to test and improve whole intuitions. (Dreyfus & Dreyfus with Athanasiou, 1986, p. 36)

We have evidence in numerous other exemplars of experienced nurses employing this strategy. It is particularly apparent when nurses are preparing to make a case with a physician for different treatment options than those currently prescribed; they want to assure themselves that their grasp of the situation is the best one available, and they purposefully test out other possible understandings of the situation. Other approaches include (1) considering the relevance and adequacy of past experiences that may underlie a current intuition and (2) consideration of possible consequences if the intuition is wrong.

A final aspect of clinical judgment that is illustrated in the exemplar above is the role of narrative in understanding the patient's story, meanings, intents and concerns. Early in the episode, the family told H.'s story, a story of extreme illness and suffering. Running throughout the nurse's account is a sense of her becoming increasingly involved with both the patient and family by understanding his story, how his illness has disrupted it, and the meaning of his relationships with family, particularly his grandson.

Kleinman, Eisenberg, and Good (1978) have called attention to the narrative component of illness, claiming that patients' narratives may help clinicians direct their attention not only to the biological world of disease but to the human world of meanings, values, and concerns. Bruner (1986) claims that human motives, intents and meanings are understood through narrative thinking, which he contrasts with paradigmatic thinking that conforms to the rules of logic. In this exemplar the nurse's understanding of the patient's situation and her connection with the family was made possible by hearing their account of their experience with the illness. Further, this understanding set up the nurse's ordering of priorities—seeing the patient first, then meeting again with the family. Ultimately this understanding also created the possibility for her to respond to the family's grief and feelings of guilt in an involved, meaningful way; this would not have been accomplished had she stood outside the situation, or not engaged in hearing the human dimensions of their experience. In short, narratives communicate aspects of the human experience with illness that cannot be conveyed through decontextualized abstract labels, or through disengaged, analytical reasoning.

SUMMARY

The study of clinical judgment using cognitive models and methods has limited the possibility of seeing other important aspects of clinical judgment. By highlighting these aspects, we do not mean to say that rationality has no place. Calculative reasoning, requiring analysis of particular situations, consulting research and theoretical literature for possible interpretations and solutions, and explicit weighing of the possible outcomes and consequences of each potential action, does and should figure prominently in the practice of experienced clinicians. Our claim is that this is not the only form of reasoning, nor necessarily the best. Rather, the reasoning that is a significant part of the everyday practice of expert clinicians is one that relies also on intuition, including deliberative rationality, on a disposition toward what is good and right, on practical wisdom gained from experience, on involvement in the situation, and on knowing the particular patient through being attuned to his usual pattern of responses and through hearing narrative accounts of his illness experiences.

THE APPEAL OF RATIONAL MODELS

In Chapter 2, Dreyfus and Dreyfus trace the roots of the western tradition of rationalism to ancient Greece. The possibility of categorizing, explaining, and predicting human responses based on scientific knowledge and generalizable theory is indeed appealing, and has captured the imagination of nursing academics for the last several decades. While clearly scientific knowledge and theory are important to clinical judgment in nursing, they are not the whole story. The nursing literature is replete with admonishments to clinicians to replace their intuitions with reason, to explain their particular case studies with scientific theory, and to analyze or justify ethical positions by recourse to principles. By these accounts, practical engaged reasoning has been relegated to the margins of professional discourse.

The most extreme forms of disengaged reasoning can be illustrated by use of prognostic scoring systems in individual patient care decisions. Systems such as APACHE III have been developed (Hall, Schmidt, & Wood, 1993) to evaluate the outcomes of various critical care interventions, given the seriousness and complexities of the patient's condition. Such prognostic systems aim to develop models that will foster wise decisions about when to use heroic measures, and predict when those measures are likely to be futile. Knaus et al. (1988), for example, suggests four benefits derived from accurate predictive models:

1. They allow the physician to focus efforts on patients most likely to benefit.
2. They assist in the decision to limit or withdraw therapy.
3. They facilitate the comparison of performance between ICUs.
4. They facilitate the assessment of new technologies and allow for comparative analysis with standard therapy (Guest, 1993, p. 1).

Such scoring systems can be refined over time with outcome measures associated with various treatments. They can guide the clinical and ethical decision making regarding treatment for particular patients, offering a clinical moral compass to prevent excessive optimism or pessimism. However, they can offer reliable treatment guidelines in the situations with extremely low (<20) or high (>140) scores. The range of the score is 0–254. Scores in the middle range require additional disease-specific and patient/treatment considerations to be helpful (Guest, 1993). Such systems should not be reduced to objective visions of administering a clinical prognostic scoring system at designated points and "justly or fairly" continuing or discontinuing treatment based on the score. While useful, such guidelines can never replace clinical and ethical judgment in the particular situation, because added clinical and ethical assessment of the patient's response to treatment and changes in condition over time is required for wise and compassionate decisions.

Four major societal forces support continued reliance on rational models as the source for both ethical and clinical decision making:

1. the quest to develop generalizable fair and just rules that can be applied impartially to all persons and clinical situations;
2. the desire to develop justifiable rationing systems based on large data sets that yield cost/benefit ratios in order to achieve distributive justice and curtail the excessive spending of disproportionate amounts of money on ineffective treatments or the last 30 days of life;
3. an epistemological understanding of rationality, where oppositional choices are made between right and wrong decisions, based upon criteria developed to judge two complete explicit positions, and the adequacy or inadequacy of those decisions in relation to the criteria (Taylor, 1993); and
4. the movement toward understanding health care as commodity, so that treatments are commercially evaluated and paid for while care, attentiveness, and recovery are only marginally considered in the accounting systems *and* in the public policy discourse about health care.

Abstract reasoning based on criteria alone fails to consider transitions in patients' conditions, and transitions in the understanding of the clinical situation as it unfolds. The argument for taking into consideration transition and experiential learning gains made, as a clinical situation unfolds for patients, families and health care workers is drawn from the argument that Charles Taylor has made in relation to cross-cultural comparisons and historical understanding (Taylor, 1989, 1993). Taylor (1993) has argued that we lose sight of the articulating function of reason when we adopt the purely foundationalist model of reasoning in the epistemological tradition.

> This understands rational justification as (a) effected on the basis of crite-
> ria, (b) judging between fully explicit positions, and (c) yielding in the first
> instance absolute judgment of adequacy or inadequacy, and comparative
> assessments only mediately from these. But we have just seen an important
> role in our reasoning is played by irreducibly comparative judgements—
> judgements about transitions—in articulating the implicit, and in the direct
> characterization of transitional moves which make no appeal to criteria at
> all. To block all this from view through an apodeictic model of reasoning is
> to make most moral discussion incomprehensible. Nor does it leave unim-
> paired our understanding of science and its history, as we have amply seen.
> The connections between scientific explanation and practical reason are, in
> fact close; to lose sight of one is to fall into confusion about the other. (Tay-
> lor, 1993, p. 230)

PRACTICAL REASONING
AND CLINICAL JUDGMENT

Let us return now to the arguments we set forth at the beginning of this chapter. We claimed that the clinical judgment of expert nurses resembles Aristotelian practical reasoning far more than means-ends rational reasoning represented by models such as the nursing process. We showed through interpretation of one exemplar how aspects of practical reasoning are evident in the judgment of expert nurses, and examined the ways in which these aspects are obscured when clinical judgment is viewed through the lens of the technical rationality model. Now we will explore further the nature of practical reasoning, illustrating through further exemplars how both the notion of the good and practical wisdom are prominent aspects of clinical judgment of experienced nurses.

Rational models of clinical judgment assume that recognition of clinical states requires systematic assessment of a context-free list of parameters, the ability to distinguish normal from abnormal findings, and analysis of assessment data to derive a diagnosis. This pattern is, of course, one way in which skilled clinicians begin to get a clinical grasp; it is necessary when they don't know the patient, when no particular aspects of the situation claim their attention, or when aspects of the clinical picture don't add up and the clinician is struggling to figure out the nature of the situation. But skillful practice in seeing and understanding a whole clinical situation requires much more than analysis of elements from a context-free checklist. The clinician's fundamental disposition toward what is good and right sets up what will be noticed in particular situations. Caring practices which create the possibility for the nurse to know the patient as a person also open new horizons for seeing and understanding what is most important to the patient and family. Knowing the patient's typical pattern of responses also sets up the possibility to notice subtle qualitative changes. And finally, practical knowledge born of experience creates expectations for particular populations of patients (for example, the anticipated trajectory for recovery from coronary artery bypass graft surgery) and allows for informal technology assessment.

Rational models of decision making, in the most extreme case, also suggest that treatment choices may be made on the basis of informal probability assessment. On this view, once a diagnosis is made, the clinician generates a list of treatment options. Each option is associated with several possible outcomes. The outcomes are weighted in terms of desirability, and in terms of likelihood given the treatment choice. These probabilities then can be combined to derive the best treatment choice. Approaches have been described which encourage patient participation in treatment decision making—i.e., in assigning values to possible outcomes. These models, of course, don't account for transitions and changing relevance in real clinical situations. What we have found instead is that nurses' actions are continuously adjudicated and modified on the basis of the particular patient's responses, rather than an abstract theoretical model of probability assessment (see Chapter 6).

Notions of the Good

The nurse's disposition toward what is good and right is not a matter of individual ethics, but is rather socially constructed and embedded within the discipline as well as within the norms and mores of the particular unit on which she practices (see Chapter 8). It is in the background of her practice and sets up what she notices and how she responds in particular situations. Moreover, it is not principle based, in the sense of rules or precepts which the nurse can make explicit and which are generalizable across situations. Rather, it is a good that becomes apparent in the actions of the nurse in the particular situation. But it is also not totally particularistic, subjective, and private. There are common goods that show up across exemplars in nursing; for example, the intention to humanize and personalize care, the ethic for disclosure to patients and families, and the importance of comfort in the face of extreme suffering or impending death, all of which set up what will be noticed in the particular clinical situation and which shape the nurse's particular responses.

In this section, we will explore, as an example, the prevalent ethic for comfort measures, the primacy of alleviation of suffering as a moral good, and the ways in which this ethic shapes nurses' perceptions of and responses to particular clinical situations.

In the following discussion, a group of neonatal nurses are talking about the complications of disruptive and painful procedures for premature infants without adequate comfort measures, and the possibility of substituting comfort measures for sedation in many instances if a person has expert ability in comforting and handling the infant. They express their distress with nurses and physicians who do not see this as an important goal in their response to babies:

Nurse 1:   It really bugs me. A lot of times, too, people don't try comfort measures. I think they're a little too fast with the sedations sometimes and they don't do basic things like when people go to start IV's on these kids. They just sort of throw them over on their backs, grab an extremity, start sticking and the screaming even if they're intubated. And there are things that you can do to prepare the baby and get it comfortable, get it sucking on something, bundle it up so it doesn't flail around when you first stick it. You know they tolerate it so much better. And it drives me crazy because they say "Well, this kid's desaturating horribly" and he needs a spaghetti line.

Nurse 2:   I wonder why?

Nurse 1:   You didn't have to get this kid into this state, you know. If you had taken it a little more slowly, and done a little preparation, the kid would have tolerated it fine. People aren't really conscious of comfort measures.

Nurse 2:   It takes time before you get past that kind of tunnel vision, where the task is what's paramount and not the kid. Where getting IV in is really the only thing on your mind.

Nurse 1:   Or they just don't think it's important. They just figure the kid's going to cry and there's nothing you can do and it's . . . getting it over with.

These nurses have a strong sense that caring practices, particularly comforting practices, are not rule based, and require more than an intellectual understanding:

Ten years ago I probably never thought that much about a baby's comfort. You get into this high-tech taking-care-of-critical-patients mode. But now even with a really critical baby, I still find myself thinking a lot about the comfort throughout. The critical care aspects get to be second nature after a while, and you don't have to think about them so much, and you have more time to think about other things. . . . I think a lot of people know about the importance of comfort care with premature infants intellectually, but they don't do it. It isn't a part of their practice.

In their discussion, they point to the tunnel vision that is created when comfort is not important, when it is assumed that suffering is unavoidable. But for these nurses, because comfort is an important end, they have learned new possibilities for helping babies to be comfortable even during painful procedures. It is clear from this excerpt that the ethic of comfort can only be located in the activity itself, and that the capacity to deftly comfort is hard-won in an intensive care nurse. Also the excerpt illustrates that the caring practice is shaped by the possibilities inherent in the situation and in the sensitivities and skill levels of the nurses.

In yet another exemplar, a nurse talks about the clinical blindness created by not seeing prevention or alleviation of pain as a primary end:

I was taking care of a 39-year-old Samoan lady who had had a renal transplant, then rejected it, and then got a huge necrotizing fasciitis in her wound. She was on the ventilator and developed pneumos and had chest tubes. The residents came in one afternoon and wanted to pull the chest tubes on one side and proceeded to get ready to do it without any warning, didn't allow me to give her any pain medicine. And then because it was early July, I don't remember exactly, they were teaching. They were doing it because there were new residents there, they were describing it in the most graphic terms. They might as well have said they were going to pull the garden hose out of this lady's chest, because that's what it sounded like. It made *me* squeamish, and I've seen hundreds of tubes pulled out. So I finally interrupted them and said, "When can I give her some pain medication? When are you going to do this; she really needs it." "Oh, she doesn't need any pain medication." It really irritated me; they were both young, probably younger than me and probably never had a chest tube pulled out. They probably had no idea that it hurt, and it was like, why don't you realize this is a *person* laying in this bed. You shouldn't be standing beside her bed and describing in graphic detail how what you're going to do to pull this chest tube out, much less not give her any pain medicine.

This nurse was outraged by the young residents' inability to see the patient, to understand the likelihood that this procedure was going to be painful, to know who this person was and what her typical response to pain was, to place comfort above their wish to learn and get through the procedure. The sense of frustration and anguish at not being able to prevent needless suffering is a common theme in these nurses' narratives.

In the following narrative, a nurse's honest appraisal of breakdown and a patient's excessive suffering because of it clearly illustrates the notion of the good, as well as practical moral reasoning in transition.

Nurse 1:   We had a transfer during the night and I was coming on to the day shift and this gentleman was transferred because of poor ABS', he had vascularities and he was basically bleeding into his lungs. He was a Do Not Resuscitate by his wishes and his family's wishes. He came to us because they wanted to full go, you know, everything they could up to intubation. So basically he'd been fairly stable overnight. I mean it was pretty tenuous but just before I came on at 6:00 AM, his PO_2 dropped to 40. He was wearing a 100% nonrebreather at 6 liters and the nurse that was taking care of him during the night had tried to get a morphine order for him just for comfort's sake because he was starting to get a little restless. The intern was very, very reluctant, but he did finally agree to a subcutaneous morphine order, which the night nurse gave and it seemed to settle him down for a little bit. By the time I got into the room, he was starting to become more restless again, but we were also doing everything under the sun for him. It was a very busy time, hanging bloods and medicines. I watched this man just deteriorate before my eyes. He became so restless and tachypneic. He started to become incoherent and I found myself going out of the room three or four times to talk to the team about increasing his medication or putting him on an IV morphine drip, and they were very reluctant. They sort of agreed with me, but they were waiting for his attending to come in to see him to make some decision about him. They were waiting for the family to come in to see him. They felt that they wanted him to be awake for the family. They did increase the order for the subcutaneous morphine which I gave him. It didn't really make a bit of difference. So I sort of had to deal with each member of the team as they came on. It was early in the morning before rounds, and the resident came on and she agreed, "Yes, he should be on a morphine drip," but they weren't ready to do that. And then finally, our attending came in at the same time I'd drawn another gas, which showed that he hadn't improved at all. Indeed, he was dying. He was a dying man, and I was really torn, because I knew that my priority was to make him comfortable. At the same time, I had all these orders that I had to do, so hanging his bloods and blood products and what have you. They finally wrote the IV morphine order and I already had it made up. I had one of the nurses make it up for me and when I went to bolus the IV morphine, I looked up at the monitor and he started to brady down to about 30 and it was just, it was less than two hours from the time I started, but it felt like 15 minutes, it just went by so fast, I was, it was just a very, very upsetting experience. I started to cry and I bolused it anyway. I hung the morphine, I knew it wasn't going to make a bit of difference, but I just felt very helpless, I felt as though I didn't do enough for him. I wished that I had made the team come into the room with me and watch him, because I was watching him and I was . . . what he was going through. Bleeding continuously out of his mouth, and he was just so uncomfortable.

This nurse went on to describe her moral anguish, ways in which she might have prevented this patient's suffering in his final moments of life. She felt that the medical staff were unwilling or unable to see that the patient was likely to die:

Nurse 1: He had been in the unit for a few hours. That's the whole problem with an ICU—the focus is on keeping someone alive, regardless. Especially when they first arrive . . . It took that second blood gas before they—I don't know if they thought he was going to miraculously have a better gas the second time around. There was nothing really that was done in between that would have made a difference . . . As things continued to progress on nights and he needed to get blood, and he needed to get plasma, and we were giving him Lasix and he was not making urine, it was sort of to the point where he was beyond—he was in that stage of pulmonary edema where you're just not going to get someone out of it. His blood pressure was dropping. We were trying to give him blood to increase his hemoglobin so that he could breathe better, and were just filling up his lungs. We weren't helping him, we were hurting him. So then as the night wore on, the importance of the morphine or sensation became more important.

This nurse experiences moral anguish because her patient suffered a needlessly horrendous death. She feels responsible for not being free enough to ensure that the physicians understood the patient's suffering. This is a narrative of ethical learning. One can imagine that this nurse will recognize a similar situation in the future and be able to act more effectively to get what is needed for the patient. This is also an example of a gray zone. The nurse is clear that comfort should have been primary. She does not defend her actions, though she understands how emergency treatment demands clouded her thinking and action. In retrospect, she wishes that she had marshalled her colleagues more effectively and had insisted on the physicians directly observing the patient. The patient and family had agreed that intubation and extremely heroic measures were not in order, but if it gained additional time, treating with IV medications would be acceptable. A transition occurred, and the patient's suffering increased, while the chances for his survival diminished. The moral situation changed and the nurse is now filled with frustration and regret over not preventing an agonizing death.

In each of the above exemplars, the nurses saw as a primary end the prevention or alleviation of suffering and the provision of comfort, in doing everyday procedures that may cause discomfort, in the extreme suffering and anxiety during the final moments of life. When provision of comfort is a moral good, nurses are open to seeing patient suffering in new ways. They see new possibilities for balancing competing claims; the possibility of comfort is always considered together with other concerns and issues—the need to do repetitive and painful diagnostic procedures, for example, or helping a patient maintain consciousness until his family arrives. Hence what they see and how they respond in particular situations are shaped by this moral good. They are open to learning new comfort measures, and have a wealth of clinical knowledge about ways in which pain and suffering can be alleviated or prevented.

Caring Practices that Reveal and Preserve Personhood

Central to the clinical judgment of expert nurses is what they describe in their everyday discourse as "knowing the patient." In our pilot work and in the present study, we found that nurses frequently talk about "knowing the patient," by which they mean both knowing the patient's typical patterns of responses and knowing the patient as a person (Tanner et al., 1993). The way in which a nurse's clinical judgment is shaped by knowing the patient as a person, and the caring practices that allow a person to reveal himself to the nurse, are illustrated in the following paradigm case.

The nurse describes caring for a 60-year-old black man who is quadriplegic from a motorcycle accident many years ago and who is disfigured by a past radical neck surgery for cancer. He is admitted to the critical care unit for a respiratory failure due to infection and the health care team makes the agonizing decision of placing him on a respirator, knowing that it might be impossible to wean him:

Nurse 1: I think we could have made a decision on not treating him fully, based on what he looked like and what we thought he was. And I really stood up for him. I don't think some people ever got beyond just looking at him and just saying: "This man is disfigured and not able to take care of himself, and whatever." As far as prioritizing the beds, if we were really strapped for beds, they would think about putting him on general care and taking him off the ventilator. But no one thought it was an easy decision.

Int: It sounded like you had a strong feeling that he wanted to live. How did that come about and do you know when it came about?

Nurse 1: I think he always had it. He was an incredible fighter. I mean I would see him angry or I would see him withdrawn. But even withdrawn, he was actively withdrawn. He wouldn't look at you. He would follow you, track you in the room and everything but then would look at you . . . At one point in time the physicians were asking him: "You want to die, don't you?" They weren't trying to do him any harm. No one ever didn't take care of him. He just gravitated towards these excellent physicians. I don't know how.

Int: What do you think was different about the way you saw him versus the way the doctors saw him when they thought that he wanted to die?

Nurse 1: I don't think they stood with him and looked at him or gave him a Pepsi, or saw him watch the ball game. He really derived a lot of pleasure from living . . . I think it was more of a case of their perception of quality of life versus our perceptions of George's quality of life and as we got to know him more, and what he was like at the skilled nursing facility, [we concluded] that the quality of life for him was really very good . . . They didn't see him as a social director on his unit. He was a spokesperson for the patients, he helped people who had alcohol and drug problems. He had a girlfriend there who was also wheelchair-bound and they used public transportation together. They were the Valentine King and Queen. I think the doctors just looked at him and saw "This is as good as it gets, and this is really depressing, and he is really depressed and so why continue? This is torture." He was really a big baseball fan and wanted to watch the ball games . . . to me that is not someone who has given up. [Later in the same interview after describing his active measures to control his day, she comments] Somebody who is that manipulative or that active in planning my day is really not somebody who doesn't want to have to deal with living or doesn't have the strength to go on.

This is a story of engaged practical reasoning, where knowing and preserving personhood was central. As the nurse got to know George and what was important to him, it set up the possibility to see him in new ways, to challenge the prevailing view of George's quality of life, to notice indications of what life meant to him. This is particularly noteworthy in this situation and countless others like it, where possibilities for verbal communication are virtually nonexistent, so other ways of knowing and understanding the person must be relied on. At one point in the story the nurse tells how hard it was at first to learn to read George's lips, to understand what he was saying. She said: "He would be saying, 'Ballgame, ballgame, ballgame,' and I would ask: 'You need to have a bowel movement?' Finally I understood 'ballgame.'" She describes connection through fighting, through peacemaking, through turning on the ballgame, through giving him Pepsi-Cola (as opposed to tea, or Coca-Cola, or orange juice), through listening to and reporting the phone calls from the skilled nursing facility asking about his progress, through getting his story of how he used to drive a Cadillac and that was when he had his accident. Through narrative accounts of George's life, the nurse came to understand who he was as a person, what was important to him, and what his concerns might be. Through these stories, nurses come to know the patient in a way that is essential for advocating for them, for making appropriate judgments about therapy, for caring and curing. It is essential to person- and world-preserving.

When one is critically ill, one's world collapses, and one's notion of self as agent, member, and participant is threatened. In the midst of all the technology, expert nurses find ways to let the world in and push back the assaults on personhood. This is illustrated in the following interview excerpts.

I think in a critical care setting that we have to help re-personalize a patient because a family comes in and they see alarms, tubes, teams, and beds and all this paraphernalia and this body that does not look like their loved one. They are not used to seeing them laid flat out with a blue gown over them. I think that if you re-personalize the patient through talking to the family that it helps us to understand the human being who is in the bed . . . One of the biggest things that you deal with in that situation is, what would he want or what would she want, or what are they like? I always ask questions about my patients because often we greet them when they have totally succumbed to anesthesia. And when they become more long term, I ask the family to bring pictures that *we* can see. It doesn't only help the patient . . . (a bit later, referring to pictures of a patient with dogs) When he woke up and I asked him about his dogs, it did make him feel good to see them again, and it made me know a little bit about him.

This nurse echoes a common theme in this study of expert clinical nursing practice in intensive care units. The nurse works with the patients' and families' world, humanizing the technology and domesticating the alien environment. These nurses actively try to preserve and conserve the dignity and personhood of their patients:

> . . . The patient would not like to know that he had something drooling out of his mouth, so wipe his mouth . . . We look at the monitors and look at the drips and figure everything out, but their appearance makes a big difference to families and how this person is.

Knowing the Patient's Patterns of Responses[1]

Nurses, in the context of particular clinical episodes, describe their detailed knowledge about the patient's patterns: how she moves, what positions are comfortable, how her wounds look, how the patient eats, how she tolerates being off a ventilator, how infants tolerate feedings and respond to comfort measures, what rituals soothe and reassure, what timing of care works best—all very local, specific knowledge about particular patients' responses, physical functioning, and body topology. Within this broad category are several particular aspects of knowing the patient: (1) responses to therapeutic measures; (2) routines and habits; (3) coping resources; (4) physical capacities and endurance; and (5) body topology and characteristics.

Here is an example of one such description:

Nurse: I took care of a baby who was about 26 or 27 weeks who was about 900 grams who had been doing well for about 2 weeks. He had an open ductus. The difference between the way he looked at 9:00 and the way he looked at

11:00 was very dramatic. I was at that point really concerned about what was going to happen next. There are a lot of complications of patent ductus, not just in itself but the fact that it causes a lot of other things. I was really concerned that the baby was starting to show symptoms of all of them. You look at this kid, because you know this kid and you know what he looked like 2 hours ago. It is a dramatic difference to you but is hard to describe that to someone in words. You go to the resident and say "Look, I'm really worried about X, Y, and Z," and they go OK, then you wait one half hour, 40 minutes, then you go to the fellow and you say "You know I'm really worried about X, Y, Z." They say "We'll talk about it on rounds."

Int: What is the X,Y,Z you are worried about?

Nurse: The fact that the kid is more lethargic, paler, his stomach is bigger, he's not tolerating his feedings. His chem strip might be a little strange. All these kinds of things . . . there are clusters of things that go wrong. At this time, I had been in the unit I think a couple or three years. I was really starting to feel like I knew what was going on, but I wasn't as good at throwing my weight into a situation like that.

Here the nurse is talking about particularizing her theoretical knowledge of the complications of patent ductus to this particular child. Because she knows the child, she is able to recognize changes in the way he responds—being more lethargic, paler, not tolerating feedings—qualitative distinctions which require prior local, specific, and ineffable knowledge about how this child usually responds. This nurse describes a situation that is not at all uncommon—having a grasp on the patient situation, but not being able to describe the specifics sufficiently in order to make a case with the physicians.

In this case, the nurse sought assistance from a second nurse who was more experienced:

Rounds started shortly after that and she walked up to the attending very quietly, sidled up and said "You know, Sara is really worried about this kid." She told him the story and said "He reminds me of this child we had 3 weeks ago." Everything stopped. He got out his stethoscope and listened to the child, examined the child and said, "Call the surgeons."

The more experienced nurse "made the case" not by recourse to calculative reasoning and elemental bits of information, but by pointing out the resemblance of this child's particular situation to a prior shared experience. She made the case by knowing how to approach this particular physician, one who reportedly practiced "anecdotal medicine," by having shared understanding and experiences, and by having won his respect through several years of working together.

As we have described elsewhere (Tanner et al., 1993; Benner, 1994d) nurses also talked about an uneasiness when not "following the body's lead" and about "not knowing the patient," and about "making decisions from a distance." In these practical maxims they are arguing for an engaged moral and clinical reasoning based on understanding the patient and family and the patient's responsiveness to treatment:

> The resident wanted to let this man go, but residents oftentimes don't make the decisions. Dr. L. (the attending physician) has come around once, because I remember a man in the old ICU in bed 1 . . . he was dying. The resident was saying: "You know we should probably let this man, his wishes are to be DNR. We should probably let this man go." And the attending said something like: "Well, in some percent of the time, this kind of patient responds." And the resident said: "Well, maybe you are right." And I looked, and I said, "Now wait a minute. You've been here all night long, you know exactly what's going on. Dr. L., you haven't been here at all. The resident knows what's been going on with this man (the patient) all night long. Maybe you might want to listen to what he says about what's going on." and Dr. L. said, "Well, well." and eventually they made him a DNR.

Repeatedly nurses expressed their confidence in clinical and moral decisions that come from those who have been actively engaged with the patient and family and understand the transitions in the situations as they have occurred. In the above excerpt, the nurse had no confidence that the attending understood the particular patient's situation; in fact, the attending's response was characteristic of disengaged clinical reasoning. The nurse's distrust stemmed from her awareness that the attending did not have a grasp of the particular clinical history that would be essential for wise clinical and moral decision making.

Knowing the patient, as these nurses describe it, goes beyond formal assessments in several ways. First, because the nurse knows the typical patterns of responses, certain aspects of the situation stand out as salient, while others recede in importance. Second, making qualitative distinctions and comparing the current picture to this patient's typical picture are made possible by knowing the patient. And third, it allows for particularizing prescriptions and abstract principles. The rational model of clinical judgment holds that deciding on a course of action is simply a matter of instrumental application of scientifically based knowledge. The limitations of this model have been well described by Dreyfus, Dreyfus with Athanasiou (1986) and Schon (1983). Nurses in their narrative accounts in this study show repeatedly how clinical judgment requires particularizing formal prescriptions and abstractions, through understanding how *this* patient responds under *these* circumstances. Knowing the patient is the nurse's basis for particularizing care. The following nurse describes knowing a premature infant and how that influences her care and judgment of the infant:

The baby I'm taking care of now is a twitty little preemie. She is the ultimate preemie. All you have to do is walk in front of her isolette and have a shadow fall across her face and she desaturates. She cannot stand knowing there is anyone else in the world, but I found that I was able to suction her by myself and keep her saturation in the 90's just by being slow and careful. This baby usually has terrible bradycardia and desaturations when she is suctioned. She developed a reputation for being a real little nerd, but I haven't had any problem with her for the first couple of hours.

Knowing the preemie is personalized and particularistic even though this baby's responses are typical of premature babies; as the nurse notes, "she is the ultimate preemie." Knowing the particular baby and her responses is at the heart of clinical judgment about the source of the baby's oxygen desaturation and bradycardia, and directs the nurse's care for the baby. The practical discourse about knowing a patient spans extremely deprived situations in critical care and the more communicative situations of general care, as illustrated by the following negative example in the pilot study on a general medical unit:

Nurse: This patient was acting weird but no one knew her baseline. I spent a lot of time with her, walking her down the hall, doing her care, because I didn't know her and couldn't figure her out. She had been confused and goofy, but now she was mellowing out, but we didn't know if that was her baseline . . . I felt so frustrated all day long . . . I had read her chart, but I still didn't get a feel for this patient, although I was doing all these things. I went into report and gave a much more comprehensive report than on any of the other patients, because I think my anxiety level was higher, because I don't feel I know this person. It may be that I took care of a patient two weeks ago, but two weeks later, I still don't know *that* patient. It makes me feel very uncomfortable.

Int: What do you mean by really knowing a patient?

Nurse: It is getting an idea of what they look like, how they talk, how they eat their breakfast. It is stupid stuff, it is not even medical.

This interview illustrates that despite its centrality to practice, the informal discourse on knowing patients is underdeveloped without the legitimacy and status of technical-procedural discourse. Nevertheless, nurses describe knowing their patients as central to good clinical judgment and practice. In the above excerpt, the patient is on chemotherapy and at risk for sepsis due to immunosuppression; therefore, knowing the patient is essential for early detection of changes. The excerpt also illustrates that "knowing a patient" discourse is current, situational, particularistic, and contains the immediate history of the patient's condition.

Practical Knowledge About Particular Patient Populations

As in Benner's prior work (1983, 1984a), narrative accounts by nurses in the present study revealed the wealth of practical knowledge that supports clinical judgment. The skills of noticing and responding rest on practical knowledge, such as qualitative distinctions (see Chapters 6 & 7), and informal technology assessment (see Chapter 8). While many aspects of practical knowledge are described in this text and elsewhere, here we will take up the way in which practical knowledge about patient populations sets up the possibility for a perceptual grasp and for responding to rapidly changing situations.

In the following exemplar, the nurse described a 70-year-old woman who is first day post-op for an abdominal aortic aneurysm repair. The clinical understanding of the situation by the house staff, and hence by the new nurse taking care of her, was that the patient is "taking her time to warm." She had labile blood pressure and metabolic acidosis and had remained unresponsive since surgery. The new nurse had spent much of the shift trying to keep up with the "Nipride game" being played by the house staff managing her care. The expert nurse "could see" that help was needed, that "there was a flurry of activity," that the new nurse was in desperate need for help.

> I had a sense of what was going on and I looked at the patient and there were two things that I noticed right off. One that her abdomen was very large and very firm, and the other thing was that her knees were mottled, and I said, "She has a dead bowel." And they said, "She doesn't have a dead bowel." And I said, "She has a dead bowel." All right, trying to back off a little bit, I said, "Would we consider that maybe she has an ischemic bowel."

The expert recognized a pattern, knew that she had the correct grasp, coached others to see the situation in the same way, and in other ways made a case for a different treatment plan. Her confidence in her understanding of the situation set up the possibility for advocacy and for making a case. The story unfolds that the expert nurse made the case that the patient needed to return to surgery, but the attending could not be reached. Still the house staff did not pick up on the urgency, and thought it could wait until the attending arrived. The patient quickly decompensated, and once again the expert told the physicians that the woman was going to code:

> I said, "This woman is going to die." And as I'm saying this, the family needs to know. Someone better go talk to this family now. . . . The poor nurse taking care of the patient was devastated . . . because she had been trying to manage this all morning and not having the experience. She's kind of going along with what they're doing, which is, which is fine. If you don't know, how can you, you just don't know. I was very sad, very angry because I felt

that I was giving them every clue that they could have to make a decision about this woman. . . . I really think at times they see with different eyes than we do. And the attending had come in and said it—they were thinking that it was just part of the patient's recovery and they were having a rocky recovery course.

In this exemplar, the nurse had extensive experience working with patients recovering from this kind of surgery. She expected that the patient should be responsive; moreover, she recognized immediately clinical signs that were out of the ordinary, and concluded, without recourse to rational calculation, that the patient was suffering from dead bowel. This nurse was a connoisseur (Polanyi, 1958); the clinical signs she noted were significant only in light of the patient's history and current situation. As the situation continued to progress without intervention, the nurse recognized the onset of a downhill trajectory, and sought to convince others of the urgency of the situation. While she understood the beginner's lack of clinical knowledge which would help her understand the situation, she was distraught at her inability to get appropriate medical intervention.

SUMMARY AND CONCLUSIONS

In this chapter we have illustrated how the clinical judgment of expert nurses is simply not captured by models depicting it as instrumental means-ends analysis. We have shown through several exemplars the way in which the nurses' fundamental disposition toward the good, her underlying notion of the good, sets up what she notices in any clinical situation and how she responds. We have illustrated the moral dimension of the everyday judgments in critical care, using as an illustration the ethic of care in providing for comfort.

Over the last two decades, the prevailing diagnosis-treatment model of nursing clinical judgment has been heralded for its utility in describing nursing practice. As a process, it presumably describes the way in which nurses go about making judgments—first they assess and diagnose, then they treat those diagnoses. Nursing diagnosis as a general concept has been viewed as the perceptual lens through which nurses see and understand their patients. As an effort directed toward developing a taxonomic structure, it is viewed as a way to classify the phenomena of concern to nurses; and ultimately such a taxonomy is intended to serve as a guide for theory development and research, as a mechanism for improved intra- and interprofessional communication through using labels that convey commonly understood meanings, as a method for record-keeping, and accounting for the costs of nursing services. Obviously no single dimension of a professional practice can achieve all that nursing diagnosis as a concept and as a taxonomic effort was intended to do. Our data point to limitations in two of its purported contributions to nursing practice.

As a process, the diagnosis-treatment model was simply not apparent in the narrative accounts provided by nurses at any level, but clearly not in those by nurses practicing at the expert level. The judgments were rather characterized by immediate apprehension of the clinical situation, progressive understanding of the patient's story through his narrative accounts, and the capacity to notice qualitative changes by knowing the patient's pattern of responses; nursing actions were typically response-based, relying on whole intuitions of what had worked in past similar situations, and modified in accordance with this particular patient's responses to it. In this kind of fluid, skillful response, there was virtually no evidence of "treatment" based on explicit nursing diagnoses.

Secondly, in the hundreds of narrative accounts provided by nurses in this study, there was absolutely no reference to a nursing diagnosis as either a taxonomic label or as a perceptual lens through which nurses saw and understood their patients. Although most nurses in our study had been schooled in nursing diagnosis and worked in institutions that had adopted one of the existing taxonomies for record-keeping, none of our informants had apparently adopted it as a central feature of their clinical judgments.

This is not to say that we are ready to recommend abandoning the movement to identify and classify the phenomena of concern to nurses. We believe this effort has served the discipline well in clarifying what phenomena are uniquely the concern of nurses. Rather, we wish to pose questions about the utility of the diagnosis-treatment model and its limitations in capturing significant aspects of nursing practice. Bishop and Scudder (1990, 1991) provide an excellent accounting of why the use of standard labels may fail to capture the meaning of human experiences in illness, and hence be useful in guiding nursing responses. And the Dreyfus and Dreyfus analysis of theory in a practice discipline, in this text, offers additional insights into the limitations of abstractions, like nursing diagnosis, in serving as a useful guide to nursing actions.

NOTE

1. This analysis is drawn largely from Tanner et al. (1993). "The phenomenology of knowing the patient." *Image: The Journal of Nursing Scholarship*, 25(4), p. 273–280. Used with permission.

Chapter 2

THE RELATIONSHIP OF THEORY AND PRACTICE IN THE ACQUISITION OF SKILL

Hubert L. Dreyfus and Stuart E. Dreyfus

The theory of nursing, as we shall use this phrase, encompasses both the medical and nursing *scientific knowledge* that has been imparted to the trainee, mostly in nursing school, and the "*rules of thumb*" that are largely acquired during on-the-job training and experience. The term "medical scientific knowledge" is rather self-explanatory. Such knowledge draws primarily upon the sciences of chemistry and biology and predicts, among other things, changes in chemical concentrations and biological events that various invasive actions will produce. Typical rules of thumb are of the form: if you observe the following phenomenon, then you should take the following action. These are rules of good nursing practice that have been developed, over time, based on experience, but which generally deal with whole situations too complex for analysis in purely scientific terms.

The practice of nursing refers to the actual on-the-job behavior of experienced nurses considered to be experts by their peers and supervisors. Is this skilled coping behavior the result of the application of theory? Or is what is taught by experience something more than an increasingly refined and subtle theory? If so, what is it? How does it come about? How can it be encouraged and rewarded? These are the issues that this and other chapters in this book will address.

Briefly summarized, we shall argue that while practice, without theory, cannot alone produce fully skilled behavior in complex coping domains such as nursing, theory without practice has even less chance of success. In short, theory and practice intertwine in a mutually supportive bootstrapping process as the nursing graduate develops his or her skill. Only if both are cultivated and appreciated can full expertise be realized.

The relation between theory and practice, between reason and intuition, has concerned our culture since our western way of being human was first defined in ancient Greece. And although it has not been often noted, the supposed science of medicine which arose in Greece played a crucial role at the beginning of this cultural self-determination. It also turns out that 2000 years later in our modern world the practice of nursing has a double aspect which gives it a unique place in our understanding of what western man has become. Now that medicine has in fact become a theoretical science, nursing has the task of applying medical theory, thereby revealing both the power and limits of this theory and of any theory. Moreover, nursing, as a caring practice, goes beyond theory altogether and shows that, where human meaning is at stake, one needs a kind of intuition that can never be captured by rational theory. Thus the practice of nursing reveals what 2000 years of western thinking has tended to deny: that theory is dependent on practice and reason requires intuition.

To understand the complicated relation between theory and practice and between reason and intuition illustrated in the practice of nursing, we have to go back to the time when Hippocrates was trying to move medicine from folk wisdom to a scientific art of healing, while, at the same time, Socrates, born 9 years after Hippocrates in 469 B.C., was trying to understand this new intellectual achievement, of which medicine was only one example. Physics, astronomy, and geometry had, around 400 B.C., taken off from everyday, practical, measuring and counting and thinkers were asking: What is special about these new disciplines? The answer, proposed by Socrates and refined by the philosophical tradition, was that these new disciplines were based on theory. Theory has five essential characteristics. The first three were identified by Socrates. (1) *Explicitness.* Ideally a theory should not be based on intuition and interpretation but should be spelled out so completely that it can be understood by any rational being. (2) *Universality.* Theory should hold true for all places at all times. (3) *Abstractedness.* A theory must not require reference to particular examples. In the *Euthyphro* Socrates presupposes these requirements when he assumes that moral behavior must be based on abstract, universal principles and so asks the prophet Euthyphro to justify his behavior by providing an explicit, universal and abstract definition of piety—angrily rejecting Euthyphro's appeal to examples and his own special intuition.

Descartes (1641/1960) and Kant (1963) completed the Socratic account of theory by adding two more requirements: (4) *Discreteness.* A theory must be stated in terms of context-free elements, that we now call features, factors, attributes, data points, cues, etc.—isolable elements that make no reference to human interests, traditions, institutions, etc. (5) *Systematicity.* A theory must be a new whole in which decontextualized elements are related to each other by rules or laws.

Plato expressed all five characteristics in the myth of the cave: the theorist must remove his object of knowledge from the everyday, perceptual, social world in order to see the universal relations between the explicit and abstract elements, in this case, the ideas. Freed from all context, the elements form a system of their own—all Plato's ideas are organized by the idea of the Good. Plato saw that while everyday understanding is implicit, concrete, local, holistic, and partial, theories, by contrast, are explicit, abstract, universal, and range over elements organized into a new total whole.

The next question was, what do these new theoretical disciplines have to do with everyday practice? And in answering this question, the favorite example was medicine. Unlike physics, astronomy, and geometry which were purely abstract, Hippocrates claimed to have a theory which told physicians what to do. For this reason Socrates admired Hippocrates and held up the new medicine as a model of knowledge for philosophers to study. [Hippocrates returned the compliment by remarking that "a philosophical physician resembles a god."] The question for Socrates thus became: How is a theory-based craft like medicine different from skills based on rules of thumb, like stone-cutting and cooking? His answer, that still has serious consequences for our current lives, grew out of two observations. Both were true observations about medicine, but, like a good philosopher, Socrates overgeneralized them. He saw that physicians claimed to be able to explain why they did what they did, and that their explanations were based on principles from which the behavior in question could be seen to follow rationally. Generalizing these observations, Socrates claims in the *Gorgias* that any craft must have "principles of action and reason"(Gorgias, 501a).

The claim that a craft or *techne* must be based on a theory that could be articulated by the practitioners led Socrates to rule out of account all forms of intuitive expertise which do not seem to be based on any principles at all. Cooking, for example, unlike medicine, is "unable to render any account of the nature of the methods it applies" (Gorgias, 465a). It "goes straight to its end, and never considers or calculates anything" (Gorgias, 465a). Socrates holds that such intuitive abilities are not crafts at all and that experts in these domain have no knowledge but a mere knack. This would apply to intuitive experts from basketball players to chess masters and virtuoso musicians, all of whom are unable to articulate rational principles based on a theory to explain what they do.

Socrates thought that these sorts of experts were really not experts at all but just clever crowd pleasers operating on hunches and lucky guesses. Only experts like doctors, who could explain why they did what they did, had solid, reliable knowledge. According to Plato, cooks have a knack for making food taste good, but only doctors know what is good for you and why. But this troubled Socrates, since skilled statesmen, heroes, and religious prophets did not claim to be acting on principles like doctors, and so seemed to be on the same level as cooks. Socrates set out to check whether such experts were, in fact, basing their actions on theories. He hoped to show that morality and statesmanship were, indeed, crafts by eliciting rules or principles from experts in these domains. For example, Socrates assumes in his dialogue, *Euthyphro,* that Euthyphro, a religious prophet, is an expert at recognizing piety, and so asks Euthyphro for his piety recognizing rule: "I want to know what is characteristic of piety . . . to use as a standard whereby to judge your actions and those of other men" (*Euthyphro,* 6e3-6). He wants a principle which would ground piety in theory and so make it knowledge.

Euthyphro's response to this demand is like that of any expert. He gives Socrates examples from his field of expertise, in this case, mythical situations in the past in which men and gods have done things which everyone considers pious. Socrates faces the same problem in the *Laches* where he asks Laches, presumably an expert on courage, "What is that common quality, which is the same in all cases, and which is called courage?"(Laches, 191e), but gets no rules. This leads Socrates to the famous conclusion that since prophets and heroes could not state the consistent, context-free principles which provide the rationale for their actions the way doctors could explain their prescriptions, all their skills were mere knacks. And even doctors could not produce the finished and tested medical theory that they were just beginning to establish. So Socrates found that no one could meet his test for knowledge and he reluctantly concluded that no one knew anything at all—not a promising start for Western philosophy.

This is where Plato came to the aid of Socrates. Perhaps experts were operating on principles they could not articulate, Plato suggested. Experts, at least in areas involving nonempirical knowledge such as morality and mathematics had, in another life, Plato claimed, learned the principles involved, but they had forgotten them. The role of the philosopher was to help such moral and mathematical experts recall the principles on which they were acting. These principles would ground the skill. Knowledge must be "fastened by the reasoning of cause and effect" and "this is done by 'recollection'" (*Meno,* 98a).

A generation after Plato, Aristotle already suspected that something crucial had been left out of Plato's medical model of knowledge. Rather than seeing the ability to give reasons for their actions—like doctors—as the test of expertise, Aristotle sees precisely the immediate, unreasoned, intuitive response as characteristic of an expert craftsman. "Art (*techne*) does not deliberate" he says in *Physics,* Bk. II, Ch 8. Moreover, Aristotle was clear that even if there were universal principles based on a theory, intuitive skill was needed to see how the principles applied in each particular case. He derives an illustration from ethics, which Plato thought must be based on universal rules: "[I]t is not easy to find a formula by which we may determine how far and up to what point a man may go wrong before he incurs blame," Aristotle notes. He then adds, "But this difficulty of definition is inherent in every object of perception: such questions of degree are bound up with the circumstances of the individual case, where our only criterion *is* the perception" (Aristotle, *Physics*, Book II, Chp. 8).

The same would, of course, apply to medicine. The two areas where theory impinges on the concrete case, diagnosis, and treatment, are areas which would require experience and intuition. Aristotle was right. Expert diagnostic systems such as the computer programs MYCIN and INTERNIST based on principles but without intuition and judgment, do better than the nonexpert but have failed to capture the specialist's expertise.

A systematic evaluation of MYCIN was reported in *The Journal of the American Medical Association* (Yu et al., 1979). MYCIN was given data concerning ten actual meningitis cases and asked to prescribe drug therapy. Its prescriptions were evaluated by a panel of eight infectious disease specialists who had published clinical reports dealing with the management of meningitis. These experts rated as acceptable 70% of MYCIN'S recommended therapies (Yu et al., 1979).

The evidence concerning INTERNIST-1 is even more detailed. In fact, according to *The New England Journal of Medicine*, which published an evaluation of the program, "[the] systematic evaluation of the model's performance is virtually unique in the field of medical applications of artificial intelligence" (Miller, Harry, Pople, & Myers, 1982). The evaluators found that:

> The experienced clinician is vastly superior to INTERNIST-1 in the ability to consider the relative severity and independence of the different manifestations of disease and to understand the temporal evolution of the disease process. (Miller et al., 1987, p. 494)

Dr. G. O. Barnett, in his editorial comment on the evaluation, wisely concludes:

> Perhaps the most exciting experimental evaluation of INTERNIST-1 would be the demonstration that a productive collaboration is possible between man and computer—that clinical diagnosis in real situations can be improved by combining the medical judgment of the clinician with the statistical and computational power of a computer model and a large base of stored medical information. (Barnett, 1982, p. 5)

Nurses who have to turn the conclusions of theory into treatment have to supply this clinical judgment. As Patricia Benner (1984) points out, clinical judgments, such as maintaining a patient within specified physiological parameters with medications, requires experience-based intuition.

The Platonic rationalist tradition, however, would support the expert systems builders. There must be a theory underlying all expertise, they claim, so one should be able to find and articulate the principles underlying even diagnosis and treatment. We will formulate these principles, program them, teach them, and even test for expertise by examining students on how well they know them. But Aristotle's argument that one must at some point use judgment to decide how to apply the rules, plus the general failure of expert systems using rules without judgment, suggests that even a discipline that has a theory must ultimately rely on practical intuition when it needs to touch reality.

To understand the role of intuition, even in a theoretical discipline like medicine, and the implication of this relationship for nursing, we must take a fresh look at what a skill is and what the expert acquires when he achieves expertise. We must be prepared to abandon the Greek view that a beginner starts with specific cases and, as he becomes more proficient, abstracts and interiorizes more and more sophisticated rules. It might turn out that skill acquisition moves in just the opposite direction: from abstract principles to particular cases.

We have mentioned above the belief, all too prevalent in our highly rationalistic, scientific western culture, that the role of experience is merely to refine theory. We reject the view that, presumably unconsciously, subtle theory produces skilled performance, not because we can prove that it is wrong, but, in part, because no plausible arguments have been offered (beyond the assertion that no other explanation exists) that it is right. As we shall see later, this assertion is being called into question as understanding slowly emerges about how the brain's neuronal activity accompanied by synaptic modifications during learning can produce improved performance based on experience—a process that cannot be adequately explained as the acquisition of theoretical knowledge.

Furthermore, it certainly does not look reasonable to say that the application of principles and rules of thumb produce skilled human coping, given the effortlessness and speed with which skilled drivers, for example, cope with changing situations or with which skilled carpenters, say, carry out their activities. Even highly skilled chess players, coping with what appear to be difficult situations requiring planning, reasoning, and careful assessment of various trade-offs, can play chess at the rate of one second or less per move and still produce games of very high quality. And, what's more, they can do this even if they are required simultaneously to do simple computational tasks that seem to leave little, if any, room for theoretical thinking about chess.

Add to this the fact that computer scientists have been striving unsuccessfully for more than 30 years to produce artificial intelligence by programming vast numbers of facts, various principles of logical inference, and rules of thumb into computers. Even though computers can store far more facts than any human can remember and can apply inferential rules thousands of times more rapidly and with more accuracy than can human beings, programs optimistically called "expert systems" consistently fail to perform at the level of human experts in areas such as nursing, in which people learn with experience to make rapid, effective decisions. Through these intense efforts toward artificial intelligence, the hypothesis that intelligence consists of nothing more than rules and principles has been put to an empirical test, and has been found wanting.

It seems to us that it is more plausible to believe that sufficient experience, accompanied by no theoretical knowledge, could produce skilled coping behavior. After all, animals cope skillfully with their environments through trial-and-error learning, in addition, of course, to innate behavior, without benefit of theoretical knowledge or reasoning abilities. But a skill like nursing is far more complex than foraging for food or avoiding enemies. It is probably impossible to learn to excel in a skill like nursing drawing exclusively from trial-and-error and from imitation without acquiring and using articulatable scientific knowledge or rules of thumb. As we develop our explanation of the acquisition of complex skills, we shall delineate what are probably the necessary contributions of both theory and of practice to the process.

In developing our description of skill acquisition, we, and various colleagues, have observed, and in some cases experimentally studied, the learning process not only of nurses—which, of course, is the focus of this book—but also of chess players, airplane pilots, and automobile drivers. We have, furthermore, unashamedly relied heavily on the recollection of some of our own learning experiences. We urge the reader, while tracking with us the evolution of skillful coping behavior, to recall his or her own learning experiences, in nursing but also in other areas, to see if they fit with our description.

The careful study of the skill-acquisition phenomenon has shown us that a person usually passes through at least five stages of qualitatively different perceptions of their task as skill improves. Hence, we call what follows a five-stage model of skill acquisition. A closer examination of some of these five stages would probably allow their decomposition into their own stages, so our choice of five should not be regarded as definitive, only as sufficient for our purposes. As we examine in detail how a novice, if he or she possesses innate ability and has the opportunity to acquire sufficient experience, gradually becomes an expert, we shall focus upon the most common kind of skill, sometimes called "unstructured." The domains in which such skills develop admit of a potentially unlimited number of relevant facts and features. The ways that these elements interrelate to produce later events is often unclear and not capable of being captured by precise rules. Nursing is certainly carried on in such an environment, although the nursing student, learning facts and procedures, may be unaware of this. Managers, teachers, and even economic forecasters live in such an unstructured world. Chess, on the other hand, is a structured domain, with a well-defined set of relevant facts (the position of the pieces on the board) and of legal moves and their effect upon the position. While it is this structured property of chess that makes it possible for computers, using primarily brute-force enumeration of a huge number of possibilities, to come very close to the best human performance, human players, lacking the computational speed, accuracy, and memory capacity of computers, must treat chess as an unstructured domain and rely on other abilities such as pattern discrimination and learned associative behavior to master the game.

Because a high level of skill in an unstructured domain seems to require considerable concrete experience with real situations, and because any individual will have had more experience with some types of situations than with others, a person can simultaneously be an expert with respect to certain types of situations while being less skilled with respect to others. Hence, expertise, as we shall use the term, does not necessarily apply to a whole skill domain, but to at least some significant part of one. There are, perhaps, no expert nurses, but certainly many nurses achieve expertise in the area of their specialization.

Not all people achieve expertise, even with considerable concrete experience in their domain of specialization. Chess is so designed that only a few can achieve expertise, and therein lies its attraction. Automobile controls are so designed that almost any driver can become what we call expert, although some will always be more expert than others. Nursing seems to lie somewhere in between. We have uncovered, happily, a great many rewarding examples of true expertise, but at the same time we have found that, despite considerable experience, some nurses never seem to achieve this level, even in their specialized area. Why this is so, and what might be done about it, is one issue we shall discuss further in a subsequent chapter.

Being an expert, or being at any particular stage in our skill-acquisition model, does not necessarily mean performing as well as everyone else or exhibiting the same type of thought process.

We refer to "stages" because (1) each individual, when confronting a particular type of situation in his or her skill domain, will usually approach it in the manner of our first stage, "novice," then as described in our stage two, "advanced beginner," and so on through our five stages, and (2) the most talented individuals employing the kind of cognitive processes that characterize a certain stage will perform more skillfully than the most talented individuals who are at an earlier stage in our model. The five stages that we shall now lay out are called novice, advanced beginner, competent, proficient, and expert.

STAGE 1: NOVICE

Normally, the instruction process begins with the instructor decomposing the task environment into context-free features which the beginner can recognize without benefit of experience. The beginner is then given rules for determining actions on the basis of these features, like a computer following a program. Through instruction, the novice acquires rules for drawing conclusions or for determining actions, based upon facts and features of the situation that are recognizable without experience in the skill domain being learned. These elements are either objective ones, such as instrument readings, or subjective ones, of which the novice can reasonably be expected to have acquired a recognitional ability based on prior experience in other domains. Any adult beginning nursing school, can identify, for example, a state of high agitation, even though no formula applied to objective features such as heart rate can consistently do this job.

The knowledge imparted to the novice is what we have called theoretical knowledge, yet, even at this first level, it can require, for its application, assessments, such as that of extreme agitation, that admit of no theoretical description. We have already at this initial stage an example of the superiority of combining theory and experience-taught capabilities.

To make our skill description more accessible, we shall illustrate our distinctions with examples chosen from automobile driving, since almost all readers will have acquired this skill. In later chapters, using actual words of nurses as well as descriptions of their behavior, we shall follow the skill-acquisition process as it relates to nursing.

The novice driver is given, among many other rules, a formula for the safe distance at which to follow another car as a function of objectively determined speed as indicated by the speedometer. Of course, the novice is not told how to recognize a car as opposed to an elephant (which probably should not be followed as closely), since this ability is assumed to have been already acquired. Interestingly, no strict rules have ever been found that would allow a computer, using only objective data such as a digitized video image, consistently and correctly to distinguish a member of the class of cars from all other objects, demonstrating the inadequacy of depending upon theory alone. It seems that our car-recognition ability comes from experience through a brain-modification process that neurophysiologists and mathematicians studying artificial neural networks are beginning to understand in terms of synaptic reinforcement and inhibition based on outcomes of behaviors. The ability to discriminate between different sensory inputs and to learn to respond differently to different classes of input almost certainly does not depend on rules and principles, even unconscious ones, of the type given novices during their theoretical training.

The ability to recognize an agitated individual or to distinguish cars from other moving objects on a road, as we have said, seems explainable in terms of brain processes, but not in terms of rule-based reasoning. In what follows we shall use the term "intuition" when writing about this ability. Intuition, as we understand it and use it, is neither wild guessing nor supernatural inspiration, but the sort of ability, explainable in physiological terms, that we use all the time as we go about our everyday tasks.

STAGE 2: ADVANCED BEGINNER

Performance improves to a marginally acceptable level only after the novice has considerable experience coping with real situations. While this encourages the advanced beginner to consider more objective facts and to use more sophisticated rules, it also teaches the learner an enlarged conception of what is relevant to the skill. Through practical experience in concrete situations with meaningful elements which neither the instructor nor student can define in terms of objective features, the advanced beginner starts intuitively to recognize these elements when they are present. We call these newly recognized elements "situational" to distinguish them from the objective elements of the skill domain that the beginner can recognize prior to seeing concrete examples. Just as the beginning driver could bring an ability to recognize a car to the driving domain because he or she had seen many examples of cars prior to learning to drive, the advanced beginner, after seeing many examples of elements unique to the domain of study, begins to recognize them. Rules for behavior may now refer to these newly learned elements as well as to objectively recognizable ones and to elements recognizable due to experiences prior to studying the new domain of skill. With the addition of many new elements now known by the learner to be relevant to the skill, the task appears to become more difficult, and the advanced beginner often feels overwhelmed by the complexity of the skill and exhausted by the effort required to notice all relevant elements and to remember an increasing number of more and more complicated rules.

The advanced beginner driver, having been taught as a beginner to shift gears at certain speeds regardless of the traffic and terrain, learns to anticipate speed and hence gear changes necessitated by traffic. Simultaneously the advanced beginner begins to recognize the engine sounds that indicate the need to change gears and uses these situational aspects in addition to speed to decide when to shift.

STAGE 3: COMPETENCE

With more experience, the number of potentially relevant elements of a real-world situation that the learner is able to recognize becomes overwhelming. At this point, since a sense of what is important in any particular situation is missing, performance becomes nerve-wracking and exhausting, and the student might wonder how anybody ever masters the skill.

To cope with this problem and to achieve competence, people learn through instruction or experience to adopt a hierarchical perspective. First they must devise a plan, or choose a perspective, which then determines which elements of the situation are to be treated as important and which ones can be ignored. By restricting themselves to only a few of the vast number of possibly relevant facts and features, decision making becomes easier.

The competent performer must devise new rules and reasoning procedures for a plan or perspective determination, so that already learned rules for actions based on relevant facts can then be applied. These rules are not as easily come by as the rules given beginners in texts and lectures. The problem is that there are a vast number of different situations that the learner may encounter, many differing from each other in subtle, nuanced ways, and in each a plan or perspective must be determined. There are, in fact, more situations than can be named or precisely defined, so no one can prepare for the learner a list of what to do in each possible situation. Thus competent performers have to decide for themselves what plan to choose without being sure that it will be appropriate in the particular situation. Now coping becomes frightening rather than exhausting, and the learner feels great responsibility for his or her actions. Prior to this stage, if the learned rules didn't work out, the performer could rationalize that he or she hadn't been given good enough rules rather than feel remorse because of a mistake. Of course, often at this stage things work out well and a kind of elation unknown to the beginner is experienced, so learners find themselves on an emotional roller coaster.

This combination of necessity and uncertainty introduces an important new type of relationship between the performer and his or her environment. The novice and the advanced beginner, applying rules and maxims, feel little or no responsibility for the outcome of their acts. If they have made no mistakes, an unfortunate outcome is viewed as the result of inadequately specified elements or principles. The competent performer, on the other hand, after wrestling with the question of a choice of perspective or goal, feels responsible for, and thus emotionally involved in, the result of his choice. An outcome that is clearly successful is deeply satisfying and leaves a vivid memory of the situation encountered as seen from the goal or perspective finally chosen. Disasters, likewise, are not easily forgotten.

As the competent performer becomes more and more emotionally involved in his or her tasks, it becomes increasingly difficult to draw back and to adopt the detached rule-following stance of the beginner. While it might seem that this involvement-caused interference with detached rule-testing and improving would inhibit further skill development, in fact, just the opposite seems to be the case. As we shall soon see, the replacement of the detached rule-following stance of the novice and advanced beginner by involvement, should it occur, sets the stage for further advancement, while resistance to the frightening acceptance of risk and responsibility can lead to stagnation and ultimately to boredom and regression or withdrawal.

For example, a competent driver is no longer merely following rules designed to enable him or her to operate a vehicle safely and courteously. Instead, he begins a trip by selecting a goal. If, for example, a driver wishes to get somewhere very quickly, comfort and courtesy play a diminished role in the selection of maneuvers and slightly greater risks might be accepted. Driving in this manner, pride might be felt if the trip is completed quickly and uneventfully, and remorse generally follows arrest or near-collision. Should the trip involve, say, an incident in which the driver passes another car dangerously, so that only quick action by the other driver prevents an accident, the competent driver can respond to this experience in one of two qualitatively different ways. One response would be for the driver to consciously *decide* that one should hardly ever rush, and modify the rule used to decide to hurry. Or, perhaps, the rule for conditions for safe passing might be modified so that the driver only passes under exceedingly safe circumstances. These would be the approaches of the driver doomed to timidity and fear, and, by our definition, to competence. Or, responding quite differently, one could accept the deeply felt consequences of the act without detachedly asking oneself what went wrong and, especially, why. If one does this, it is likely that one won't be quite so likely to hurry in the future or to pass in similar situations, but one has a much better chance of ultimately becoming, with enough frightening or, preferably, rewarding experiences, a relaxed and expert driver. As we indicated when we discussed the advanced beginner's recognitional abilities, it is innate and natural for driving behavior to be unconsciously enhanced through experience by synaptic brain changes without these changes taking the form of conscious or even unconscious rule-modification.

STAGE 4: PROFICIENT

Suppose, as characterized above as the second of the two qualitatively different ways of learning from experience, that events are experienced with involvement as the learner practices his or her skill, and that as the result of both positive and negative experiences responses are either strengthened or inhibited due to synaptic brain changes rather than rules of behavior being modified. Should this happen, the performer's theory of the skill, as represented by rules and principles will gradually be replaced by brain-synapse-produced, situational discriminations accompanied by associated responses. Proficiency seems to develop if, and only if, experience is assimilated in this atheoretical way, then intuitive behavior replaces reasoned responses.

As the brain of the performer acquires the ability to discriminate between a variety of situations entered into with concern and involvement, plans are intuitively evoked and certain aspects stand out as important without the learner standing back and choosing those plans or deciding to adopt that perspective. Action becomes easier and less stressful as the learner simply sees what needs to be achieved rather than deciding, by a calculative procedure, which of several possible alternatives should be selected. There is less doubt that what one is trying to accomplish is appropriate when the goal is simply obvious rather than the winner of a complex competition. In fact, at the moment of involved intuitive response there can be no doubt, since doubt comes only with detached evaluation of performance.

Notice that we have stressed how the involved, experienced performer sees goals and salient facts, but not how he or she sees immediately what to do to achieve these goals. This is because there are far fewer ways of seeing what is going on than ways of intervening through actions. The proficient performer simply has not yet had enough experience with the wide variety of possible actions in each of the situations he or she can now discriminate to have rendered the best response automatic. For this reason, the proficient performer, seeing the goal and the important features of the situation, still must *decide* what to do. To do this, he or she falls back on detached, rule-based determination of actions.

The proficient driver, approaching a curve on a rainy day, may intuitively realize, due to brain activity induced by synaptic modifications produced during prior experiences, that he or she is going dangerously fast.

He or she then consciously decides whether to apply the brakes or merely to reduce pressure by some selected amount on the accelerator. We call this driver proficient, rather than expert, because valuable moments may be lost while an action is consciously chosen, or time pressure may lead to a less than optimal choice. But this driver is certainly more likely to safely negotiate the curve than is the competent driver, who spends additional time *deciding,* based on speed, angle of bank, and felt gravitational forces, that the car's speed is excessive.

STAGE 5: EXPERT

The expert not only knows what needs to be achieved, based on mature and practiced situational discrimination, but also knows how to achieve the goal. A more subtle and refined discrimination ability is what distinguishes the expert from the proficient performer. This ability allows the expert to discriminate among situations all seen as similar with respect to the plan or perspective, distinguishing those situations requiring one action from those demanding another. As with the proficient performer, synaptic modifications caused by actions experienced with involvement account for responses that turn out to be appropriate being reinforced, while those that do not work out well are inhibited. In short, the expert not only sees what needs to be achieved, but also how to achieve it. When things are proceeding normally, experts don't solve problems and don't make decisions; they simply do what experience has shown normally works, and it normally works.

The expert driver at all times, except during exceptional moments, experiences himself or herself as simply going somewhere, not as manipulating a complex piece of machinery called a car, just as a normal walking person somehow experiences himself or herself as approaching the destination and not, as a small child might, as consciously and deliberately propelling the body forward. Approaching a curve under wet conditions at a high speed, the expert not only feels that he or she is going too fast, but simply does, with the brake or accelerator pedal, whatever is appropriate. The unconscious, involved relation of the driver to the road is never broken by detached, conscious thought.

In this idealized picture of skillful coping it might seem that experts needn't think and are always right. Such, of course, is not the case. While most expert performance is ongoing and nonreflective, the best of experts, when time permits, think before they act. Normally, however, they don't think about their rules for choosing goals or their reasons for choosing possible actions, since if they did they would regress to the competent level. Rather, they reflect upon the goal or perspective that seems evident to them and upon the action that seems appropriate to achieving their goal. We call this reflection "deliberative rationality" and discuss it below.

It seems that a beginner makes inferences using strict rules and features just like a computer, but that with talent and a great deal of involved experience the beginner develops into an expert who sees intuitively what to do without applying rules and making inferences at all. Philosophers have given an accurate description of the beginner and of the expert facing an unfamiliar situation, but as we have seen, normally experts do not *solve problems*. They do not reason. They do what in experience has normally worked, and naturally, it normally works.

Likewise in nursing (Benner, 1984a), the beginner follows rules and the expert trusts intuition. But it is important to add that nursing, unlike chess and driving, is a skill which relies on theoretical understanding. Thus, although the expert nurse will find that he or she relies on fewer and fewer rules in applying theory to practice, practice will be improved not just by experience, but by a deeper and deeper understanding of medical theory.

When one sees the importance of practice and intuition, so long neglected in the West, one is tempted to invert the traditional hierarchies in which theory is superior to practice and rationality is superior to intuition, but to invert these terms is to stay within the traditional system of thought. The relations between these important human capacities are much too complex to be captured in any hierarchy. Nursing, like all medical practice and the practice of scientific disciplines in general, is a special combination of theory and practice in which it is clear that theory guides practice and practice grounds theory in a way which undercuts any philosophical attempt to say which is superior to the other. Likewise, in cases of breakdown or in new areas where intuition is not developed, reasoning is a necessary guide, but reasoning always presupposes a background of intuitions that can never be replaced by rationality, thus the necessity of intuitively guided practice. Nursing, then, turns out to be an especially illuminating craft in which one can see both the power and the limits of theoretical rationality.

We call the kind of inferential reasoning exhibited by the novice, advanced beginner, and competent performer as they apply and improve their theories and rules "calculative rationality." By "deliberative rationality," on the other hand, we mean the kind of detached, meditative reflection exhibited by the expert when time permits thought. We shall only briefly touch upon this process here, partly because we have discussed it in more detail elsewhere, and partly because nursing skill, unlike, say, long-range planning, rarely allows much time for meditative deliberation.

Sometimes, due to a sequence of events, one is led into seeing a situation from an appropriate perspective. Seeing an event in one way rather than some other almost as reasonable way can lead to seeing a subsequent event in a way quite different from how that event would have been interpreted had a second perspective been chosen. After several such interpretations one can have a totally different view of the situation than one would have had if, at the start, a different, reasonable perspective had been chosen. Getting locked into a particular perspective when another one is equally or more reasonable is called "tunnel vision." An expert will try to protect against it by trying to see the situation in alternative ways, sometimes through introspection and sometimes by consulting others and trying to be sympathetic to their perhaps differing views. For example, a nurse who sees a certain unpleasant patient's behavior as malingering might see subsequent behavior as confirming evidence and thereby miss a developing medical crisis until it is almost too late. If the nurse had time to stand back and rethink the evolving pattern of behaviors or to talk it over with another nurse, he or she might suddenly realize the true meaning of the present and past events. Deliberative rationality stands at the intersection of theory and practice. It is detached, reasoned observation of one's intuitive, practice-based behavior with an eye to challenging, and perhaps improving, intuition without replacing it by the purely theory-based action of the novice, advanced beginner, or competent performer.

Another example of where theory interacts with practice occurs when an expert intuitively feels that a situation is so novel as to preclude intuitive response. The first reaction of the expert will be to seek the advice of someone for whom the current situation is not novel, due to their differing experiences. If that is impossible, recognizing intuitively the need for theory, the expert will try to recall the rules and scientific knowledge he or she learned as a beginner in order to cope with the novel situation. Not only novel medical conditions can elicit competent, calculated behavior, but also changes in working environment. If a nurse has been assigned to a new ward or transferred to a new hospital with a different working culture, it might be better to calculate out a competent response to a familiar situation than to intuitively respond in a way that was considered expert under previous circumstances.

We have seen now how theory interacts with practice in surprisingly interesting and important ways. Anyone seeing skill as merely theoretical knowledge or as only practiced response will miss much of this intriguing picture. The very rules and principles so highly valued by the theoretician almost always, when closely examined, are seen to require for their application facts and features, some of which are recognized thanks to practice but undefinable by theory. Practice, on the other hand, would probably be of little avail were it not preceded by training concerning the relevant features in various situations and some theoretical understanding of relationships and correlations among these features. With these learned conceptual and theoretical ideas to start from, the learner can safely begin to take responsibility and acquire experience. More importantly, it is quite possibly the brain-instantiation of this conceptual knowledge that experience will eventually override, as these rule-based procedures are replaced by the synaptic modifications that make possible an intuitive response. Without theory as a starting point, no two observers, given the same experiences, would be likely to see things in remotely similar ways. A new set of circumstances would likely be responded to by these observers in radically different ways rather than in the consensually accepted way evinced by similarly trained experts. Without consensual agreement concerning good practice, no meaningful after-the-fact discussion could occur, and little progress in improving the overall skill level of the group could transpire.

To see why, we must first distinguish illness from disease. According to Benner and Wrubel (1989) *disease* is an organic dysfunction, of which modern medicine has a theory, whereas *illness* is the experience of the breakdown of one's body and thus of one's everyday world. As they note:

> As long as one has no symptoms or other disruption of usual functioning, there is no experience of illness, even though disease may be present and the body may be suffering damage at the cellular, tissue or organ level. . . . Nurses are in the unique position of being able to understand both the disease experience and the meanings that the patient brings to that experience. As a result, nurses can help shape the illness experience for the patient by guiding, interpreting, and coaching. (Benner & Wrubel, 1989, pp. 8–9)

Nursing, because it treats both disease and illness, is at the same time a paradigm case of applied theory and an outstanding example of a practice that is in principle beyond the reach of theory and analytical reason.

Disease is a dysfunction of the body, a physical object governed by physical laws, so it should come as no surprise that Hippocrates' vision of the physician as scientist is finally being achieved. But it would be a mistake characteristic of our rationalistic culture to think that the success of medicine in any way suggests that there can be a theory of nursing as a caring practice. Caring in the context of nursing consists in keeping open the possibilities that can be saved in the world of the sick person, while aiding the person in letting go of possibilities that are no longer realistic. If man were simply a rational animal, as the Greeks thought, then there might be a theory of having a world and how to keep it. But a school of philosophy, developed in the beginning of this century, and based on the existential thought of Soren Kierkegaard, denies that man can be understood as some combination of body and mind. Human beings, Martin Heidegger (1926/1962), the most famous philosopher in this school, said, are defined by the stand they take upon themselves, which in turn sets up the range of possibilities open to them. In this view, human being is a unique way of being in that everything human beings do follows from their individual self-interpretation. The meaning of a whole life is basic and determines what possibilities show up and how they make sense to a person. Moreover, we are not objective, theoretical spectators of our lives and of the world, but involved participants. Things show up as mattering to us. Heidegger sums this up by saying that the human being does not have fixed properties like an object or animal, but that man's basic way of being is care. It is this way of being that must be understood, preserved, and enhanced by nursing as a caring profession. As Benner and Wrubel (1989) put it:

> Nurses promote healing through assisting the patient in maintaining the human ties and concerns. And it is this human connection that gives people the courage to weather their illness (p. 87).

Since the human way of being is involved and holistic, there can be no abstract, analytical theory of it. Caring is what one might call an existential skill. It is, indeed, what Socrates would have called a knack, but since, unlike cooking, it is a matter of life and death and involves the whole person, that term hardly seems appropriate. It shows the power of a tradition based on the theory of disease that the existential skills have no traditional name that does honor to their importance and uniqueness, and we seem to have no appropriate word for them in our vocabulary. The best we can come up with is that caring, as a way of helping people by entering their world, is a higher kind of knowledge which we can call understanding.

Psychotherapy, which claims to have a theory of mental disease, i.e., a scientific account of the mind and of its normal and abnormal functioning, might seem to belie our claim that there can be no theory of tact. But if the existential thinkers are right, and we think they are, a psychology such as psychoanalytical theory (modeled on medical theory) with its handbook of psychopathology (modeled on bodily pathology) is a dream that can never be realized. It is interesting in this connection to note that as psychotherapists gain experience in caring for patients, in spite of their intense theoretical disagreements, they come more and more to resemble each other in their practice. This suggests that psychotherapists make less and less use of theory as they gain expertise. Nurses, on the other hand, insofar as their work consists in applying medical theory, learn and apply more and more theory as they increase in experience and expertise. Their understanding of where theory is appropriate should help nurses resist any temptation to formulate the principles of their existential skills. The current theories of caring in nursing are typically interpretive perspectives on care, but this should not undermine their legitimacy (Benner, 1994a; Morse, Bottorff, Neander, & Solberg, 1991).

This does not mean that there is nothing one can say about the tact involved in world preserving. We have already said a good deal. One can describe the general structure of human beings, the way care consists of mattering, possibilities and inhabiting a shared world. This is what Heidegger (1926/1962) calls an existential account of the human being. One can also describe in detail how specific cultures, families, and individuals structure their worlds. Since meanings are shared, one can also select and describe typical cases, laying out what matters and what possibilities are opened and closed in typical situations. One can then make qualitative distinctions between more and less successful interventions. One can also look at the stages through which caring skills develop, and formulate maxims to aid beginners. But the nurse, who is an expert in caring, knows that he or she cannot be guided by principles or any pseudosciences of the psyche, but must enter into the situation of the patient and be guided by participation and intuition.

In this domain there can be no clinical *knowledge*, as Plato would define it, but there can and must be clinical *understanding*. Thus, in caring, as in the case of the *application* of medical theory, one finds a practice requiring involvement for which there can be no theory. But there is an important difference between the treatment of disease and the care of illness. In the case of applying the general principles of medicine the nurse must be involved in the activity of using the technology and must learn to read the bodily signs of disease, not, of course, as cues for the application of rules, but as patterns which solicit the appropriate intuitive response. The nurse, however, is not only involved in the activity of beginning to bear the science and technology of medicine on a specific body with a specific disease, but also in caring. In caring the nurse must be able to take on the perspective of the patient, and make his or her peace with the situation and its suffering in order to be touched by the situation of a fellow human being and have the tact to enable that person to surmount his or her illness. Only by combining both technological and existential skills in their unique practice is the nurse able to heal both the body and the person.

Thus, nursing has an even more privileged place among western skills than that of providing an outstanding example of the essential place of practice and intuition in a theoretical discipline. Nursing is also—and this constitutes its total uniqueness—a domain which shows forth clearly that in some human areas there is no place at all for abstract, objective, universal theory, nor for analytic rationality. Besides being the perfect model of a craft (*techne*), the caring practices of nursing provide a paradigm case of skills that have no theoretical component at all.

Chapter **3**

ENTERING THE FIELD:
ADVANCED BEGINNER PRACTICE

Although transition from nursing schools to professional practice has received considerable attention (Fisher & Connelly, 1989; Kramer, 1974) the actual practice and clinical learning of new nurses has been studied less (Benner, 1984; Benner & Benner, 1979). In this chapter, the practice of new graduates who had worked as professional nurses for 6 months or less was examined through their narratives of direct patient care, through their spontaneous discussions of their professional issues and dilemmas, and through observations of their practice. This explication of new graduates' practice supports and extends the Dreyfus model of advanced beginner practice (Dreyfus & Dreyfus with Athanasiou, 1986) and further articulates Benner's earlier descriptions of new graduates' practical skills and dilemmas.

Two central aspects of advanced beginner practice will be explored. First, the clinical world of advanced beginners, the particular ways in which clinical situations show up for advanced beginners, and the aspects of those situations that stand out for them are discussed. Advanced beginners enter unstructured clinical situations in an open, yet apprehensive way. Clinical situations present to advanced beginners as a set of tasks that must be accomplished. The task requirements are central, and all other aspects of the clinical situation, such as the patient's changing status or the family's concerns and distress, form the background for their focus. Clinical situations also present to advanced beginners as opportunities for learning from practical realities, particularly in relation to their theoretical training. In a similar vein, clinical realities appear to be somewhat ordered, requiring the appropriate application of appropriate knowledge. A fourth prominent aspect of the advanced beginners' clinical world is that the situation shows

48

up as a test of their personal capabilities. Each of these facets of advanced beginner practice is taken up in detail in the following section.

A second major aspect of practice is the advanced beginner's clinical agency. "Agency" is defined as the way in which responsibility for care is taken up and includes how nurses influence clinical situations, given their particular clinical world. Advanced beginners demonstrate clinical agency that is unique to their skill level. They care for patients in ways that are largely guided by factors that are external to the immediate patient care situation. Standards of care and unit procedures, as well as physicians' and nurses' orders, provide this external guidance. Additionally, patient records of past nursing care and the requirements to complete such records further direct practice. In their role vis-à-vis the larger health care team, advanced beginners demonstrate extraordinary dependence on the expertise of others, a striving to assert their own independent practice, and a continual questioning about their capacity to contribute.

CLINICAL WORLD OF ADVANCED BEGINNERS

Requirements for Action

Clinical situations present to the advanced beginner as a set of requirements for action. Seen through the perceptual net of norms and procedures of care, patients actually appear to advanced beginners as perplexing collections of problems and conditions for action. Particularly when the clinical situation is complex, beginners have minimal capacity to attend to the patient as a person. Rather, what absorbs their attention and energies are the complex inventories of things to be done, all of which appear to be equally relevant.

Nurse 1: We had Mr. M., this guy who was in liver failure and he was essentially a one-to-one patient. I had him and I had two other patients. And I was like oh, there's that panic thing when I come in and they're saying all about the different labs and this IV and that IV, this tube and that tube.
Nurse 2: You get a major rush.
Nurse 1: "WHAT!" The first thing that happens, I feel myself going (takes a big loud breath) like this, my whole body is just tensing.
Nurse 2: And you haven't even opened the cardex yet.
Nurse 1: Just tensing. And they opened the cardex and there was so much written on there, you can't even decipher what's what and I was like this (all tensed up).

The emotional overlay of this and many advanced beginners' narratives is one of temporarily incapacitating anxiety. Concern over their own competence intrudes on advanced beginners' capacities to read and cope with clinical situations. As in this instance, advanced beginners' anxieties and their early grasp of the patient's condition preclude them from ordering in any meaningful way the information presented by other nurses. Similarly, the treatments ordered in the cardex appear at first to be a meaningless jumble of information. Advanced beginners' grasp of the clinical situation is comprised of a basic ordering of what is wrong with the patient in the moment, and what must be done for the patient in the time that he or she is in the nurse's care. Bringing the information presented into some meaningful order and sketching out a plan of action totally engrosses advanced beginners, particularly with new or unfamiliar patients. They cannot readily expand their vision to the patient's past experiences or future expectations. For example, in the exemplar above, the nurse reported having a successful shift with the patient, primarily because she was able to get her anxiety in check, structure her care in a step-by-step fashion, and complete everything ordered by the conclusion of her shift.

> And I just talked to myself and I had a great night because this was the first time I did it. . . . I was (saying to myself) "Okay. Just take it one step at a time. You're only human, do one thing then go onto the next thing. It will all get done, it will get done easier if you're calm and because you think better that way". . . . And the shift went great.

Throughout their narratives, advanced beginners attend, as this nurse does, to the details of the patient's physical and technologic support. Most evident to these nurses are the multiple and competing tasks that must be accomplished in the patient's care. Their work is shaped by a concern to organize, prioritize, and complete those tasks. Advanced beginners' narratives are replete with descriptions of their efforts to handle the numerous and competing demands for their time and energies. They construct elaborate strategies to organize their days by creating lists of things to be done and schedules to complete them. Patient stories are memorable because they challenge the advanced beginners' capacity to organize and prioritize tasks. This is in marked contrast to more experienced nurses who are concerned with the content of care, with patients' complex and changing conditions, and with meeting the particular needs of the patients and families they serve. After they leave the patient bedside, advanced beginners' lists, more so than the patients' status, continue to haunt them.

> (At the end of a day), I feel tired and I feel maybe a sense of worry or concern. Did I get everything, did I do everything I was supposed to do? Did I notice changes fast enough? So there's this kind of checking and rechecking.

Certainly advanced beginners express deep concern about patients' well-being, but at this level, concern for taking good care of patients is translated almost exclusively into concern for completing all the ordered treatments and procedures.

Further evidence that the clinical situation reveals itself to advanced beginners as an inventory of tasks comes from their narratives of success. For advanced beginners, success is defined as the completion of many tasks in a short amount of time. They also feel a sense of accomplishment when they leave the patient in "good shape," that is, with few, if any, tasks undone. For example, one nurse was elated when she was able to arrange home oxygen equipment and complete patient teaching prior to the gentleman's sudden and unexpected discharge. Increasing clinical skill is valued because it contributes to the smooth flow of the nurse's day. For example, in the following scenario, an advanced beginner describes the satisfaction she derives from her improving her skill in monitoring telemetry patients and in preparing them to be digitalized. The skill is valued because it prevents her from being derailed from the schedule of activities she had mapped out for the patient.

> That's a good feeling when you can kind of key into these things (changes in the patient picked up on telemetry) before they happen, 'cause once they happen they usually screw your whole day up and you don't know which way to turn. And it always happens at the most inopportune moment.

It is typical of advanced beginners that highest priority be given the maintenance of planned schedules and that patient improvement becomes a welcome side effect of this effort.

Clinical Situation as Source of Learning

Much of the perceptual work of advanced beginners is recognizing the concrete manifestations of clinical signs and symptoms. They strive to "see" and recognize clinical entities that they have studied only theoretically. The concrete reality of conditions like dyspnea, blood reactions, and hypotensive crises become apparent, but recognizing these conditions requires effort of the advanced beginner, particularly when first encountered. Engaged as they are by this work of recognition, beginners have less attention available for understanding the ways in which these states vary in their presentation or change over time. Additionally, although advanced beginners recognize new conditions, they do not always immediately recognize how to manage those conditions and therefore need coaching about what interventions are needed. Their narratives evidence a clinical understanding that is partial, abstract, and divided into fairly broad categories of understanding like the "lady with all the tubes," the "psych patient," and "the classic case of blood reaction."

The quality of learning is quite different for new as opposed to more experienced nurses. Beginners have a level of trust in the environment and in the legitimacy of co-workers' knowledge which allows them to absorb information as fact. This trust sets up qualities of freedom and exhilaration in learning that are probably only available to those who do not yet comprehend the contingent nature of both the situation and what is known about it. This freedom in learning is furthered because advanced beginners do not yet feel responsible for managing clinical situations with which they are unfamiliar.

In what follows, an advanced beginner evidences this "lightness of being" about learning as he describes a postoperative patient who had undergone complex GI surgery. His entire statement was delivered in an excited, enthusiastic tone.

> I had learned so much. There are two clinical nurse specialists involved right now. There are people on the unit who are CNIIs and CNIIIs who are just really knowledgeable on major GI surgery on infants. I talked to all these people and pediatric surgery were really helpful, and our attendings and fellows were . . . I mean, I just learned so much in the last three days, I couldn't even tell you.

Probably only the beginner can have this kind of pure pleasure in learning about a new clinical disease or problem. His comment (and the exemplar that surrounds it) demonstrated an innocence that we observe only in advanced beginners and only in situations where adequate institutional support for learning is provided. Beginners' innocent and unqualified learning contrasts well with the complex puzzle solving evident in more experienced nurses. Intermediate and advanced nurses must always weigh the tensions and the competing risks involved in managing any clinical situation. The risk fields don't yet seem to be set up for the advanced beginner, so learning seems more straightforward and enabling. It may be developmental, because once beginners develop a fuller grasp of clinical implications and personal responsibilities, this lightness of being will evaporate. Then their learning will be tempered by the competing concerns that the more advanced clinician can predictably feel in almost any clinical situation.

Because of their limited practical experience, clinical situations are temporally delimited for advanced beginners. They focus most clearly on the immediate moment and day, while larger aspects of the patient's condition do not come into their field of vision. They have limited experience working with patients through different phases of an illness trajectory and therefore have not seen how patients fare at different phases of their illness. They cannot place into perspective a patient's experience on a particular day. Any new symptom or response is seen in isolation and thus raises greater concern than it would if seen as part of the normal course of disease and recovery. Even if nurses learned in their formal training what an illness trajectory might encompass, they need to experience several patients' recoveries first hand to recognize and eventually anticipate stages in recovery.

The following incident illustrates how a nurse learned about illness trajectories in bone marrow transplant patients through her extended experience with one child. She had cared for the patient consistently after he had received his graft and knew from experience that the child turned to his family for support when stressed. Nonetheless, she became concerned when the child became more and more withdrawn, refusing to speak or interact. At that time the child was quite ill with either a medication reaction or graft-versus-host disease. He spiked temperatures of 40 and 41 degrees, was receiving amphotericin, and had tremors, shaking, and diarrhea.

> I was real concerned about what was happening psychosocially. Here we have this kid in this isolated room and he was just turning inward more and more and more, and what we were doing was making him pull more and more inward. And what were we going to do so we didn't have this psychotic kid on our hands that we created? So that's what I was trying to figure out.

Five days later, when the child's fever subsided and he was much less ill, she noted a remarkable improvement in his pattern of relating to staff. From this, the nurse learned that physiologic as well as psychologic issues must be taken into account when examining a child's status, and that these can change dramatically in a matter of days. She acquired a broader perspective on the illness trajectories of children with bone marrow transplants and a capacity to place in context the varied responses of children undergoing this procedure.

Advanced beginners' grasp is also limited to aspects of the situation that they can see and understand. They comment that they cannot see the "big picture," meaning the interrelatedness of the patient's multiple physiologic systems. They seem frustrated by this lack of grasp and look forward to the day when they can practice like more experienced nurses around them. For the moment, the ability to understand how the pieces fit the whole picture, is beyond most advanced beginners' skill. For example, during an observation, a nurse reported that he had to obtain a 24-hour urine for creatine clearance. When asked why the test was needed, he responded factually that the test was devised to determine how much creatine the patient excreted in his urine in 24 hours. With continued probing, the nurse realized the question was about the relevance of the test to the patient's status. The nurse then admitted, somewhat embarrassedly, that he didn't know which physiologic system the test evaluated, and he'd have to "look it up," when he had a chance.

Similar incidents evidencing a fragmented or partial grasp of the patient's condition were common in advanced beginner narratives and practice. Their eagerness to learn and to absorb information was palpable, but their capacity to order that information into a meaningful whole was seldom apparent in this group. We observed nurses who could provide adequate wound care for patients but could not name the type of surgery the patient received, despite the fact that this information is given in report and listed prominently on the cardex and in the patient's chart. We talked with nurses who listed correctly the steps to a fine-tuned neurological assessment, yet could not identify the significance of particular positive signs in the assessment for the immediate patient condition. While these practitioners had passed many exams on the relevant signs and symptoms for diseases and surgeries, they still had difficulty translating this theoretical learning into the practical implications for particular patients with multiple problems. Their partial grasp of clinical situations points up the difficulties beginners have mastering the complex demands of critically ill patients. The safety of patients is protected by advanced beginners' awareness of their partial grasp and their respect for and reliance on the judgments of expert nurses around them.

> I think it's hard sometimes because you don't recognize the obvious answer. Just intubate the child. But then there's so many other parts of it that other people who have more knowledge are able to look at and say "yes but this might happen and that might happen." Then you have to really weigh the differences. And I'm not real comfortable with it. It's really easy to think you know what's best and in reality there's a whole realm of things that are going on that you're not really understanding.

Clinical Situations as Ordered and Regulated

Advanced beginners exhibit a reliance on nursing theory and principles of practice that they've learned in their basic education, or from practicing nurses. They trust that clinical situations have a discernable order that might be grasped if they could recall sufficient knowledge of the body and of procedures of care. They experience breakdowns in their ability to care as problems of insufficient knowledge or poor organizational skills. A conversation between two advanced beginners exemplifies this perception:

Nurse 1: I think what's stressful is the expectations on us to be good all the time, and to have that knowledge right now.

Nurse 2: Right, because it's not just one system that is failing, it's all the systems that are failing. And those patients get real real critical when everything's going on, and you have to think about everything that could possibly go wrong. And everything is going wrong, and you just, it's like the knowledge should be there and where is it? And it's not.

And if it is there, yes, it's in the notes, but you've still got to read it, and you don't have time right now to get out that piece of paper and say, "Okay, dig toxicity, this is what I should look for and this is what I should do."

These advanced beginners trust that if they can call to mind the appropriate knowledge, their task is to systematically "apply" that knowledge to the problem at hand. Most can not yet appreciate the undetermined, changing nature of clinical problems, nor can they notice the many aspects of nursing practice that are not contained in unit protocols or procedures. The clinical situation simply shows up for them as a puzzle requiring the application of the "right" knowledge and the "right" procedures and techniques of care. They suggest that part of their work is in recognizing which situation calls for what knowledge or procedures.

It is not surprising that advanced beginners perceive clinical situations as procedural or theoretical puzzles. Prevailing educational practices in basic nursing education suggest that theoretical knowledge should underpin and support all nursing practice and that basic nursing education should prepare nurses theoretically so that they can apply this knowledge in the field. Advanced beginners are simply working out this educational philosophy in their early practice as they search their fund of "knowledge" derived from their basic education and from orientation, to guide them through unfamiliar clinical situations.

The following exemplar illustrates how advanced beginners strive to rely on familiar knowledge and care procedures, even in ambiguous clinical situations. The nurse took over the care of a critically ill liver transplant patient who was thought to be septic. She entered the rapidly evolving situation without a clear report of what was wrong with the patient. Her clues that something was wrong were that the physician told her to return to the bedside and monitor her patient, and that there was a high level of medical staff activity around the patient.

Nurse: So I kind of felt bad at the start that I didn't know what was going on with this patient. I felt that something must be going on with her, and I didn't know about that. . . .

They came in and about three doctors started giving the orders. And I was trying to assimilate all the things that they wanted me to do and prioritize the best I could in the situation. . . . And I just felt real irritated because I wasn't doing a good job and nothing I did pleased them even though I was working really hard. And my nursing supervisor was in there working too. And when I arrived, the person before me had had a horrible day, the room was not supplied or restocked and I didn't know where anything was and it was dirty, which drives me really crazy.

My supervisor would make comments like: "Now remember, your main concern tonight is the respiratory system." It was just like, I think that's pretty basic and I think that I knew that her oxygen saturations are dropping and that that's a concern of mine. In nursing school, we have drilled into us the fact that respiratory system [*laughs*] is the most important thing. . . .

Int: She was in septic shock and you didn't know it at the time.

Nurse: Well they suspected maybe, but I think that it turned out that she wasn't. She just had some biliary sludging.

Int: So at the time, did you feel you understood why you were doing the things you had to do?

Nurse: No, not at all. Not at all. Had no idea. I made a comment to one of the doctors, "It'd sure be nice for me to know what I am doing all this stuff for." And then the doctor would give me orders and obviously I hadn't prioritized the way that she had prioritized and I really resented her for days. . . . And so I feel like just one night can really destroy my ego for a week. . . . It just seemed like nothing went right, basically, except that the patient lived and she was fine.

This exemplar demonstrates how advanced beginners must at times work in situations when they lack even a minimal grasp of the patient's condition. In critical moments, they have few options except to follow the directives of more experienced clinicians. This nurse focused her efforts on trying to prioritize and complete the multiple orders given her, and to "please" the physicians supplying the orders. Her frustrations and injured ego resulted from working at her maximum capacity and still not understanding the logic of the clinical situation.

In the midst of this incredibly stressful and disordered scene, the nursing supervisor attempted to focus the advanced beginner on the patient's respiratory status. The advanced beginner heard this suggestion as a repetition of a familiar "rule" that she had heard repeatedly in nursing school, "Attend to the respiratory system first." The particular importance of respiratory monitoring in the care of this patient at this moment did not seem to strike home. Rather, the focusing suggestion was dismissed and the beginner's attention remained on responding to orders.

Monitoring and managing this patient was probably beyond the beginner's capacities. What seems unfortunate is the lack of opportunity for the advanced beginner to process the event with the team involved, in an effort to gain some perspective on her accomplishments. Team members involved may have felt that her functioning in the situation was completely adequate, given her skill level. Further discussion might have helped this new practitioner to take less personally the sharpness and intensity with which the experts in the room asked things of her. Lacking this reflection and feedback from others once the crisis for the patient had passed, the new practitioner found the experience "destroyed (her) ego for a week." Even if her actions were less than satisfactory, further discussion of her actions in the situation might have guided this nurse to act differently in the future, and to reflect in a new way on the care she provided.

Clinical Situations as a Test of Personal Capabilities

A fourth aspect of advanced beginner practice also highlighted by the previous exemplar is that clinical situations are perceived as a test of advanced beginners' personal knowledge and abilities. Much of the anxiety is about personal insufficiencies in the face of clinical demands. The narratives evidence continuous self-awareness and monitoring. Advanced beginners are so concerned about themselves that they sometimes interfere with their own abilities to read clinical situations and act safely. Their anxieties cause them to distance themselves from the patient situation, concerned equally about their own abilities and the patient's status. This is in marked contrast with more advanced clinicians, who often focus on the clinical situation with little focus on their abilities in their narratives or their clinical work.

In critical situations encountered unexpectedly or for the first time, the anxiety often disables advanced beginners. There is a period of stark terror in which they recognize they are in over their heads, and lose all capacity to plan or act. Then, once help is summoned, they experience an almost magical resolution to the situation. The details of what happens to the patient and his treatment drop out of the narrative, as nurses focus on their own "adrenalin rush" and how they survive the situation. For example, in the following situation, a preoperative patient who was considered healthy and stable suddenly slumped forward onto his bed, unconscious. The advanced beginner, who was called to the room by the unconscious man's roommate, initially froze.

> At the time I just wanted to get someone in there because I was thinking— my first thought was blank—I don't know what to do. First of all, I don't know what's going on with him, and second of all, I don't know what I should do. For a split second I just sort of lost every piece of knowledge that I ever gathered; any bit of common sense is gone.

This nurse first tried to reason with the fainting patient: "Please, you're having surgery tomorrow!" She then tried to reason with herself that the situation wasn't so bad, she just needed to get a blood pressure reading on the gentleman. Quickly realizing the impossibility of simultaneously holding the gentleman up and getting his blood pressure, she summoned help. Once help arrived, the nurse seemed to lose track of details of the patient's condition and treatment. Rather, she relates her sense of relief and pride at being a part of the saving team.

> And it's like, "Oh my God," you get swept up in it. And I don't know, it seems like it went really well. It sounds corny but you do have this feeling where it makes everything worth it when everyone pulls together like that, everyone's doing something. And it turned out he was ok and he ended up going for his surgery the next day.

This nurse never filled out the story of what happened to the patient and in fact, did not seem to know. Rather, she was satisfied that he had survived, and that she had survived the episode. In a separate incident, an advanced beginner expressed the same relief at her own survival, rather than that of the patient, when her patient experienced a serious drug reaction.

Int: How did you feel when it was all over?
Nurse: I felt relieved that I had made it through it and I had made the right decisions. . . . I think the major thing was that I had survived it, so if it happens again, I'll know what to do.

Although the critical moments in patient care present the most dramatic challenges to the beginner's sense of self-competence, even routine patient care can make the beginner quite anxious. In the following group discussion, several nurses suggest that they live on the edge of panic most of the time they are practicing.

Nurse 1: I got CHEST TUBES one day. AAAAHH! Oh no. I can't. Panic. I mean, I have this button that says, "prone to sudden fun attacks," and I should cross it out and write panic on it. Because that's what I do all day long. I'm like AAAH all up and down the hallway. And (the nursing preceptor) said, "Don't worry about it. We'll go in, we'll take the dressing off. I'll show you what it looks like." And then after she showed me that, it was fine. . . . She went in and took it off and "Oh, is that it?" She's like "That's it." OK, I can deal with this now.
Nurse 2: That panic stuff—you said that panic button . . . I have that too when it's like . . .
Nurse 1: I'm like that button all day long.

Advanced beginners' concerns for themselves in the situation reflect their relative newness and discomfort with the nursing role. In critical care practice they are often asked to operate at the edges of their knowledge and abilities and to manage situations that are beyond their actual skill level. Consequently, they have pressing concerns for how challenging the clinical situation will be for them and how effectively they will manage the patient needs, as well as how well they present themselves as competent nurses in the situation. Concerns for the patient's well-being are always threaded through their narratives, but the concerns for self are also very evident.

The pervasive anxiety present in advanced beginners' practice is probably unavoidable, and yet may serve important purposes. First, it helps them to notice themselves in the situation, and thus consciously and reflectively take on the role of the nurse. In their self-consciousness, beginners notice power relations and their personal impact on the situation. Through trial and error, they may learn new ways to affect situations, which will aid them in their future practice. As they become more expert, and can work more skillfully with a variety of situations, they will become less of an obstacle to the smooth flow of care. However, this early phase of nursing, where beginners "act like" a nurse but don't "feel it inside," may be important to their development in that it allows them to enter the role cognizant of their own limitations. Only when advanced beginners embody the nursing role and understand it very well, can they begin to test or stretch the role in artful ways. Going through the critical, objective level probably helps them understand the role and its boundaries.

The anxieties of advanced beginners also serve to make them more vigilant in their care and monitoring of patients. Most have a healthy respect for what they don't know, and this uneasiness about unknown clinical problems causes them to watch attentively for any change in a patient's status. Early in their practice they primarily worry that at any moment, their patient might die. As they gain more experience, additional concerns surface.

Nurse 1: Before, I was worried that every time I'd leave my patients, they would drop dead on me or something, and now I feel real comfortable that I can leave them.
Nurse 2: I think it's a different fear from when you first started.
Nurse 1: Yes, because you know what can go wrong more so now. Before it was just the fear of the unknown.

With more experience, their worries become more refined. They learn to distinguish when patients are stable enough to survive intermittent as opposed to continuous monitoring. As they learn more about clinical situations, their worries become more focused, but also more complex. For example, in the following an advanced beginner traces how her emotions have changed about patients' elevated temperatures.

I thought then that when they spike a temp, it was always in their lungs. It did not occur to me that, for some reason, it (the bowel resection) could leak. But now I think of all the different reasons why the temp could occur, where before I kind of shrugged it off and said, "I don't know why." And I wouldn't be as worried about it as I am now when something happens. That has come with time, kind of get bits and pieces of information from other people about the reasons why this could happen. And store it up and frame it for the next time you have to use it, and then use it.

There is a qualitative change in the advanced beginners' anxiety. At first there is a pervasive anxiety about oneself and one's inabilities, accompanied by a pervasive fear the patient might die. This anxiety is experienced alongside a naive ease about aspects of the patient's situation that are not understood. New anxiety comes from understanding that small aspects of the patient's condition can herald important problems that must be attended to. Advanced beginners relate, for example how vaginal discharge in postoperative patients, eating problems, and elevated temperatures in post-GI patients suddenly take on new importance, because they mean something in relation to patients' status. Before, these changes were noted, but they weren't tied to specific implications for recovery and thus didn't raise considerable concern.

ADVANCED BEGINNER CLINICAL AGENCY

Clinical agency is set up by the advanced beginners' way of seeing and living within the clinical world. They dwell in a clinical world in which four things stand out: (1) the requirements for action, particularly in relation to particular tasks to be accomplished; (2) the need to define and explore the bounds of what patients present clinically, particularly in relation to past theoretical learning; (3) the need to define what guides to practice are appropriately applied in each situation; and (4) the challenge to the nurse's knowledge and abilities. Given this particular clinical grasp, which is distinct from that of nurses at all other levels of skill, advanced beginners' clinical agency is also somewhat unique. We have defined clinical agency as the experience and understanding of one's impact on what happens with the patient and the growing social integration as a member and contributor of the health care team. As clinical agents, advanced beginners attempt to manage patient care according to the specified plans and orders of care, maintain the patient at a stable level during the tenure of their care, handle patient care independently so long as it is reasonably safe, and delegate to others the overseeing and management of care that is beyond their capacities. As members of the health care team, advanced beginners experience complex agency in which they doubt their own contributions, see themselves as secondary participants, and at the same time experience incredible responsibility for breakdowns and failures in patient care. These aspects of advanced beginner agency are elaborated in the following section.

Procedural Practice

Advanced beginners organize their work and structure their days according to the demands and requirements that are external to the immediate patient care situation. In relatively stable situations, and with patient populations with which they are familiar, beginners attempt to manage care in a fairly independent yet methodical fashion. They feel secure with the structure of a specified routine and attempt to adhere to that routine, despite the unstructured and changing nature of the clinical problems and the continual fluctuations in the resource environment. Their care is guided by the medical orders, the nursing orders contained in the cardex, their understandings of "standard care" on the unit, and the unit and hospital rules and procedures.

Requirements for advanced beginners to record certain activities place these activities more firmly into their plan of action. Most units have standards for recording that require the nurse to note on a flow sheet hourly vital signs, medication flow rates, IV flow rates and so on. In addition, most units require the nurse to record her physical assessment once per shift and make notes each hour on the patient's status. Advanced beginners place high priority on aspects of their practice that require such recording. It seems that the system demands for monitoring standards sets the standard of care for many advanced beginners.

For example, one beginner was observed during the first few hours as he cared for a fairly complex neurological patient. When asked what he hoped would happen for the patient in the next few hours, he recited a list of treatments and medications, and admitted that he had to fully assess the patient sometime on his shift. His concern for completing this assessment arose from the fact that he had to record a full physical assessment on the flow sheet. It was striking that the advanced beginner didn't feel the need to complete this assessment in the first half hour with his patient, as did every advanced clinician we observed. Experienced clinicians use the physical evaluation of their patients to structure their care. With advanced beginners, the assessment is more a task which has been identified by others to be an important aspect of care, but the ability to structure clinical work based on that assessment has not yet been realized.

Records of prior nursing actions also guide advanced beginners' ongoing care of patients. Indications of care decisions that are reflected in the flow sheets and charting of nurses who have cared for the same patients in prior shifts are consulted for routine as well as more imminent care. This form of information provides advanced beginners with enormous practical guidance for filling in the gaps between the medical and nursing orders and the patients' actual moment by moment requirements. For example, advanced beginners who were managing diabetic patients who had orders to keep the blood sugar between certain parameters looked to past nursing records to see how to titrate the insulin drips. Similarly, when managing hypotensive patients, advanced beginners would consult the flow sheet to see how much and which vasopressor drug the past nurse had given when the patient's pressure had dropped to the same level. Invariably, the beginners then administered the exact amount that had been charted in the previous incident. While this action made sense in terms of managing patient care according to the particular patient's responses to particular drugs, it's clear by the adherence to past action that current patient conditions were not also factored into the plan of care.

Anxiety is generated when advanced beginners attend to immediate patient needs rather than getting their work done on schedule. At times patients' changing needs and concerns are experienced as an interruption in the flow of the nurse's care, rather than the focus of that care. For example, in the following exemplar, a nurse received a quick report on a very anxious postoperative patient, who was intubated and fairly stable. The prior nurse had restrained both of the patient's hands for fear he would dislodge his E-T tube or his arterial line. The advanced beginner explains in detail how she worked with the patient's anxiety.

> So I went in and we (the patient and I) spent the first hour and a half—I was lucky to get his blood pressure taken and the rest of his vital signs because he was writing me so many notes and I had to hold the piece of paper while he wrote. But it ended up, all of his question were totally legitimate. Like, "Why is my throat sore? I feel like I'm choking." And I said "No, the tube's new and your body naturally wants to cough it out. And it will get more numb, probably about the time they decide to take it out." (Laughs) And that helped. And I untied his hands and I had him explore all his tubes. He also had a chest tube and he couldn't understand why he had this low pain when he coughed; why it hurt down there. So I had him feel the chest tube and I showed him where it went. Then I had him feel his nose, because he had a scratch on his nose. It was the tape, so I had him feel his NG tube and then the E-T tube in his mouth and so he got to feel everything on his hand. . . . But he still was kind of panicky and asked "Aren't I really dehydrated?" So I showed him his IV line and took it down and said "Look, you get bag after bag of this so you're getting plenty of fluid." And he calmed down. . . .

And he wrote me a note that everything was ok and that it really helped, my telling him I would be back and look after everything. And he was really calm the rest of the night.

This intervention was skillful and time-consuming, particularly since all of the patient's communications had to be written. The nurse responded to the patient's anxiety and focused on his concerns until he trusted her and was calmed. She had seen another nurse intervene with a vent-dependent patient in this way and had noted how helpful it had been. Although this nurse was proud of her intervention, she had nagging concerns about getting out of synchrony with her personal schedule, as is evident in her follow-up statement: "Here he was my only patient, and his whole body assessment was not done until quarter to twelve. But he was much better through the night." Even when they provide impeccable care that is sensitive to the patient's immediate concerns, advanced beginners strain to meet prescribed routines and schedules. They cannot move out of their routines because they have difficulty differentiating an appropriate and an inappropriate change in priorities.

Advanced beginners seldom have sufficient practical experience to manage rapidly changing critical care situations smoothly. Consequently, in situations that call for rapidly changing perspectives on the problem and rapidly changing priorities for the patient's management, they miss cues and continue care in a relatively unchanging and rule-governed way. This is illustrated by the care that we observed an advanced beginner providing to a critically ill 38-year-old woman who had calculi in the common bile duct and who was possibly septic. The patient was extremely uncomfortable, thrashing about in the bed, moaning and crying. The beginner entered a chaotic situation at start of shift since the prior nurse had recently admitted the patient, had not transcribed the admitting orders, and had barely managed to get the patient's IV's hung. In the first half hour of care the new nurse demonstrated his concern to transcribe the orders, no matter what intruded. As he stood at the chart writing, alone in the room with the patient, the cardiac monitor alarm sounded. He did not look up to check the monitor or the patient when this happened, but maintained his focus on the orders. Each time the alarm sounded, 9 times during the next 20 minutes, the nurse ignored it, and frantically continued to transcribe orders. After the alarm had sounded 2-3 times, a resident entered, stood at the foot of the patient's bed and observed the patient as well as the monitor. The advanced beginner may have been aware then that someone was monitoring the patient. However, in the presence and absence of the resident, the nurse continued to ignore the alarm.

While this is an extreme example, it does illustrate how a plan or list of things to do orders action for the practitioner who does not yet have a well-formed sense of what is most salient or urgent in the patient's care. In this instance, the beginner understood that he must transcribe and note all medical orders before proceeding with care of the patient. He did so, despite clear indications that the patient's cardiac status was unstable and despite tangible signs that the woman was extremely distressed. Presumably, if asked in the abstract, this advanced beginner would correctly answer that checking alarms takes precedence over transcribing medical orders. The demands of the practical situation clouded the nurse's judgment about action.

Without an experientially learned sense of salience, the care of critically ill patients can become a flat landscape of anxiety-producing tasks to be accomplished. Advanced beginners speak of "prioritizing" their actions, but the basis for their judgments about what to do first seems most driven by what they know how to do (physical care procedures) and by what, in their limited experience, seems most important. Experienced nurses can and do highlight what is most important for the beginner to address, but this can happen only when the experienced nurse is monitoring the situation closely, or when the advanced beginner recognizes his or her limits and calls for help.

Reliance on the Experience and Judgment of Others: Delegating Up

Advanced beginners in this study demonstrate a range of acceptance and reliance upon their own clinical judgment. Particularly in the early phase of their practice, they rely almost completely upon the judgment of others whose advice is immediately and unquestioningly followed. They delegate complex clinical observations and decisions up the clinical ladder to nurses and physicians who have greater experience and authority. When situations arise where advanced beginners feel inept, they call in the expert to assess and advise. This strategy provides an effective means of providing for safe patient care in situations that outstrip beginners' capacities, provided they recognize they need help and provided there are adequate resource people on hand to help.

Delegating up the clinical ladder is evident in the language advanced beginners use in their clinical exemplars. They attribute clinical decisions to others and don't even include themselves in the reference. The team caring for the patient is referred to as "they" rather than "we."

> It breaks your heart to have to hold this child in like a headlock and have somebody else hold his legs and force him to take these meds that are absolutely disgusting. But you have to keep telling yourself that he really needs

them. *They* wouldn't make him take these. I have to keep telling myself that *they* wouldn't be forcing this child to do this if it wasn't really important. So that's kind of the way I get through it. (emphasis added)

The practice of delegating up is also evident in observations with advanced beginners where the moment-by-moment decision making comes into focus. Advanced beginners unquestioningly rely on those around them to decide when to give PRN medications, order extra laboratory tests, call the physician and in general, suggest what is clinically required in an evolving patient care situation.

A particularly vibrant example of delegating authority occurred in a pediatric ICU. The patient was a 6-month-old girl with multiple system problems including a kidney transplant and recurring seizure activity. The new graduate learned in report that there had been no seizure activity in the last 12 hours, and she had no description of what the seizures looked like. By chance, the baby had a seizure when a more experienced nurse was standing at the bedside. She called it to the advanced beginner's attention. The advanced beginner observed the baby for a second or two, and left the bedside to find the resident so that he could see the seizure in process. She was not concerned with observing the seizure herself, but with getting someone with authority to observe the seizure. In this instance the beginning nurse delegated both the assessment and the decision for action to the physician. A more experienced nurse might have stayed at the bedside to monitor the baby's airway and the oxygen saturations and to see how the seizure progressed. In this situation, the advanced practitioner who originally saw the seizure did just that.

A sobering aspect of this exemplar is how the delegation works only to a point. It can break down if those in authority misjudge the capacities of the advanced beginner, if they give unclear directions, or if they leave the scene before the situation is totally resolved. In this instance, a resident was located and came to the bedside to observe the baby seizing. The resident observed in silence and left the bedside without saying anything or giving the advanced beginner any new orders. After the physician left, the advanced beginner surmised aloud that "they don't want to do anything about the seizures." She understood the physician's minimal communication to mean that no further action was required. In fact, when seizures occurred in the next hour, she didn't call it to anyone's attention and merely observed that the baby was adequately oxygenated during each episode. A more experienced nurse might have closely monitored the nature and rate of these seizures and might well have called the resident again to re-evaluate the need for treatment.

This episode highlights some of the dangers in delegation. Beginners who are attuned to their own anxiety and lack of grasp search the actions of those around them for clues about what is significant and what requires action. This illustrates the way that practical knowledge is socially embedded (see Chapter 8). Unclear or nuanced communications and directions can be misread and patient care can suffer. In this instance, the beginner misread the resident's noncommunication as an implicit order to maintain the same care. Understanding this, the beginner perhaps feared correction for calling the resident to see the same clinical situation again, even though it was repeated several times in the next hour or two.

From the perspective of advanced beginners, unfamiliar developments in a patient's condition raise multiple concerns about what is happening with the patient, whether the more experienced staff know about the change, and whether that staff can guide the beginner's action. As their experience grows, advanced beginners note more and more situations they can handle on their own. They remain, however, emotionally and practically reliant on experienced nurses and physicians in their immediate environment. Beginners monitor carefully the availability of resource people in present and future shifts and considerable tension is expressed about shifts in which many inexperienced staff are scheduled to work together. During interviews, advanced beginners worried aloud about working night and evening shifts with few resource staff, even though these shifts would take place months in the future.

In some advanced beginners' practices there are beginning signs of capacity to take more responsibility for judgments and to disagree with the authorities. Nurses describe this as personal development and feel their relationships with experts in the situation are qualitatively different from before.

> Your thinking is different. You're not so task-oriented, you're not like: well if that's what they say, then it must be ok. . . . Now I'm kind of coming to the point where I see different attitudes, different options. You see it evolving. You can't say, yesterday I didn't question but today I do. But as the time goes on, you start questioning.

Advanced beginners remain on the brink of this developmental task. Unlike the competent nurses we studied, advanced beginners never rejected or seriously doubted the authority of more experienced clinicians. Rather, they began to wonder when and if they would rely on themselves rather than others to determine action. When disagreements about an assessment or a plan arose with more experienced staff, advanced beginners experienced considerable distress.

> I felt that I was, not battling, but coming up against more experience than I had and I didn't trust my reasoning. . . . And I really had to challenge them,

and I felt very uncomfortable doing that, because here I am just hot-shot, thinks she knows everything.

Advanced beginners consistently followed the advice of more experienced clinicians when there was a disagreement. However, strong emotions marked narratives where breakdown in patient care resulted from following others' advice. In this group we see the early glimpses of the disillusionment about other's knowledge that becomes a central crisis for competent nurses.

Learning the Skill of Involvement

One of the frustrations for me in doing this job is that in the beginning, because all the skills were new, my focus was (on the patient). Although I understood family process, I couldn't put the attention there because I was so caught up, and still am for the most part, caught up with learning how to do this and that, that my energy goes there. And until I'm confident about those things, I can't take in the bigger picture.

One area that seems particularly alive for advanced beginners is the caring practices of nursing. They admit that in the most troubled of circumstances, where they are overwhelmed by the biomedical needs of the patient and the complexities of the treatments, they feel unable to attend to the "psychosocial" needs of the patient and family. At the same time, they are challenged to use this aspect of their practice when the patient is familiar and relatively stable, or when the care of the patient has by consensus shifted to comfort and support.

Beginners observe that the more human side of practice becomes salient in unexpected ways and times. They have new revelations about caring for patients and families that far exceed what they were open to learning about in nursing school.

I think in nursing there's a little bit more emphasis and focus on kind of like holistic medicine. And when you're in nursing school, you're thinking, "Yeah, right. Let's just get to the meat and potatoes of this stuff." But when you get out into practice, its true [what they tried to teach you in school] . . . that you take a holistic approach to giving medical care or psychiatric care. . . . Not just focusing on just the patient and the physiological needs. There's a family with emotional needs and things will just come out of left field and knock you right down. Things that you just wouldn't even think of until it was too late.

The caring practices of the nursing role require demonstrations to the patient and family that they are not just another number, not "objects" to be processed. Benner (Benner & Wrubel, 1989) has shown in her previous work that nurses have an elaborate dialogue about getting the right kind and level of involvement with patients and families. It takes experience to learn involvement that is both authentic, or true to one's own sense of self and feelings, and yet not overinvolved, or inappropriately taking over for the patient. In the following statement an advanced beginner describes her initial steps at having a genuine discussion with a mother about the possible death of her son.

> The last couple of days that I've been taking care of him, she's (patient's mother) really been opening up, before I would even bring it up. "You know Ann, this is really hard. I'm having a really hard time with this." . . . She really was kind of talking about how hard it was.—And we really talked about it. At first it was a little uncomfortable for me just because it's one thing to talk to parents on one level. But it's different when you're talking about—she's worried about graft versus host and she knows it's fatal. And she knows there's nothing that can be done about it. She's telling me this and I'm thinking and telling her, "You're absolutely right," and inside I'm thinking this is the worst thing that anyone could go through.
>
> And I told her that, but I was finding it a little difficult the first day. By yesterday I was feeling a lot more comfortable about it. It was almost like an afternoon thing that we would start to talk about it and see how she was feeling.

This was a new turn for the advanced beginner which involved taking a risk and extending herself in a new way to the patient's mother. It felt risky, more intimate, and at the same time it felt right. The advanced beginner got over her initial discomfort and began to look forward to these "afternoon chats" with the child's mother. She recognized how important these talks became for the mother to express her honest feelings and concerns about what was happening in this situation.

Advanced beginners look to nurses and other professionals for examples of how to relate to patients and families properly. They actively notice the types of relationships that more experienced nurses establish with patients and families. They report both positive and negative role models and consciously try to structure their interactions like the former. Here an advanced beginner recalls a conversation he overheard between a patient's family and a physician.

> It was a cardiac surgeon who was explaining a cardiac cath to a mom. They had to get consent. He just sounded to me like he was being very condescending and patronizing on one hand, but at the same time, he was talking *way* over their heads, to me anyway, maybe I'm wrong. It's just from my perspective.—Because they just assume these people who look like suc-

cessful people, like they're well educated, and they're talking this high tech bit about the left ventricle and the right ventricle and the small bowel and the large bowel, and the electrolyte balance and the fluid balance, and da ta da ta da, nine hundred million things. And mom and dad just sit there and nod their heads. They're too scared to ask a question because they're so intimidated and they don't want to look stupid.

This advanced beginner quickly identifies the family's need for basic information and compassion and rejects as unhelpful the professional's technical and distancing form of explanation. Perhaps because beginners are so new to the clinical arena themselves, they more readily "hear" the foreignness of the ICU language and structure of explanation. As beginners struggle to take on the mantle of professional nursing, their understanding for patients and families that comes from not being entirely a part of the ICU culture might be explicitly valued and fostered by other staff. In this aspect of their practice, the promotion of the "naive view" may help beginners maintain their natural, helping and nurturing countenance which over time the ICU culture may impede. It is here that experienced nurses could learn from the openness of the beginner.

Agency Within the Health Care Team

Advanced beginners experience agency in which they express doubt about their own contributions to patient care, and yet, at times they experience incredible personal responsibility for patient outcomes. They often feel like marginal team members because they must ask "a thousand questions" of fellow nurses to complete a day's care. In addition, they recognize that their role is more peripheral than central in patient care decisions.

Int: Does it look like the picture's coming together at all yet?
Nurse 1: Slowly.
Nurse 2: It depends. If you get that experience, then yeah, it's there. But if you haven't had that experience, then you are just listening and you are just there for everybody else.

Despite advanced beginners' clear recognition of their limited skill in complex clinical situations, and despite their reliance on more experienced clinicians to complete care on their patients, personal agency is an *issue* for this group. They judge themselves and fear that they are being judged by others regarding their capacity to contribute and to make a difference.

Several instances were reported in which advanced beginners felt unable to manage the patient independently, sought the help and advice of experienced staff, and yet felt completely responsible for the patient outcome. This overarching responsibility for that which they cannot control may be one of the hazards of learning nursing agency in undetermined and uncontrollable clinical situations. Since they are always practicing at the border of their own skill and are continually dependent on others, they may have difficulty understanding where the borders of their responsibility lie. In particular, they may feel more responsible in situations where nothing can be done to change the clinical course. Lacking the practical experience to recognize inevitable trajectories, they may assume that they have more power to make a difference than is actually possible.

Advanced beginners' overarching sense of responsibility is demonstrated by a nurse who was caring for an 82-year-old woman who was admitted with a potassium of 7.1, was dialyzed, and who continued to be unstable despite extensive interventions. The nurse was busy and admitted that she did not manage to check the patient's monitor for about 1½ hours before the incident. This nurse felt very accountable for not catching the patient's widening QRS an hour earlier, suggesting that if she had, she may have averted the woman's death.

Once she alerted others to the situation, she wanted the team to act more quickly and with greater vigor to save this woman's life. She felt a moral obligation to "do everything" even though everyone else in the room felt satisfied with minimal resuscitation measures. Even after the fact, she never learned what actually led to this woman's death—hyperkalemia, digitalis toxicity, Lidocaine side effects, or other unmentioned possibilities. The nebulous outcome seems to add to her sense of personal responsibility and failure.

Nurse: So she did die.
Int: God bless her. [*Referring to this as a natural and reasonable outcome of events.*]
Nurse: Well, I didn't feel that way. I was really shook up. I felt really responsible. And I even asked the doctor, was there anything more I could have done? And he said, "No. Well, did you think there was?" And I said, "Well, if I had only caught that widening QRS sooner, like at 4:00 instead of 5:00." And he said, "She was going to die, There was nothing that could have been done." So now, I watch my monitors.

Although this situation is tailor-made to teach a new practitioner the limits of medical intervention in the face of old age and chronic illness, this advanced beginner does not learn that from her experience. Rather, she learns that she must be more vigilant in preventing this situation from arising again.

This nurse, like other advanced beginners, has a persistent belief in the power of medicine to prevent suffering and death. At this stage in their experience and skill development, trust in the power of medicine seems to serve them while situations that offer no possibility for healing or relief of suffering severely challenge their developing sense of nursing agency. When the patient's need for comfort or relief of suffering cannot be adequately met, advanced beginners often feel personally responsible and thus defeated.

Another advanced beginner expressed similar frustration regarding her capacities to meet patients' needs.

> Those kind of things are so frustrating for me when I can't meet somebody's needs. The hardest thing for me, is when I can't meet those needs, whether it be pain or not. And those are frustrating but even when they are not IV drug abusers, we have a real hard time getting someone's pain under control. Or people who are vomiting and you can't, you give them everything . . . I mean, we have this one woman, we gave her everything, I mean she had like eight anti-emetic drugs and nothing seemed to work. And it was just horrible, you know, to try and fix people when you can't.

These new nurses are facing head-on the limits of the medical treatment for curing patients. Their background understanding of medicine's capacity to heal is challenged when they witness "failures" and they become frustrated or distraught. They do not yet fully see what their role *is* in this situation. While they are clear about their role in the project of curing the patient, they don't seem to have as clear an image about their part in standing by patients during their suffering or in helping patients and families endure suffering and death.

Clinical agency of advanced beginners derives largely from directives that are external to the immediate patient care situation and is largely dependent on the resource environment. Beginners attempt to manage patient care according to physician and nursing orders and by following the example of more seasoned clinicians. They are acutely aware of the limits of their clinical competence and actively involve experienced clinicians in the oversight and management of care of patients assigned to them. Concern for patient well-being and safety is emphasized as is their concern for their own competence and knowledge. While they recognize their role in the health care team is secondary or facilitative, they are unclear about whether this secondary position is sanctioned in the institutions and profession in which they work.

EDUCATIONAL AND ENVIRONMENTAL IMPLICATIONS

In the nursing literature considerable attention has been focused on the aims and organizational structures of clinical programs designed to move advanced beginners into practice roles in hospitals (Shamian & Inhaber, 1985).

A recent survey of preceptor/orientation programs for new graduates entering critical care practice (Hartshorn, 1992) suggests a typical program includes at least 60 hours of didactic instruction along with 3–4 months of practical instruction, utilizing staff nurses as preceptors at the bedside. A third of the hospitals surveyed reported that their preceptor period lasted longer than 3 months and, of historical interest, most had instituted their programs in the year prior to the study, presumably in response to the nursing shortage. The content of these programs is quite varied and specific to the needs of each institution.

Research on the outcomes of preceptor programs for new graduates is fairly minimal but points to aspects that may increase success of the program. Supervised experience with preceptors bolsters new graduates' confidence in their leadership abilities, improves job satisfaction, and communication skills (Hamilton, Murray, Lindholm, & Meyers, 1989; McGrath & Princeton, 1987). Experience with preceptors has also been associated with the capacity to take on the full range of nursing responsibilities and lower rates of staff turnover. Aspects of a preceptorship program that predicted better outcomes on participants' self-ratings of nursing leadership, professional development, and capacity to plan for and evaluate patients were the quality of the preceptor's nursing skill, teaching ability, and emotional support given the learner. The best predictor of overall development in that study was the support of peers who were also new graduates at the institution (Brasler, 1993). Contact with more than one preceptor and support from the nurse's family also seemed to make a positive difference in aspects of new graduates' development.

Teaching/Coaching Strategies Tailored for Advanced Beginners

Preceptor Involvement

Advanced beginners' unique ways of being involved in their clinical world and their particular forms of clinical agency call for special preceptorship or teaching strategies. Since advanced beginners live in clinical worlds where the patient situation shows up as elemental, partial, and dominated by tasks and procedures, preceptors can help beginners fit the seemingly disjointed components of report, chart, and physical presentation of the patient into a meaningful whole. By working through this process with particular patients, beginners can begin to see patterns and glimpses of the whole patient's condition. Drawing on the experience of the preceptor, beginners can start to find order in the immense amount of information that they are given on each patient moment by moment.

Preceptors can also provide for beginners the historical context and possible future course of a patient situation. Beginners simply haven't had time to see patients with varied disease processes through complete illness trajectories. Lacking this experience, beginners can't place into perspective new symptoms or patient responses. When new symptoms arise, beginners may focus excessive attention or worry on them, rather than recognizing them as part of the expected pattern of recovery. Preceptors can readily contextualize a symptom for advanced beginners and let them know what is and is not to be expected with particular illnesses and patients. This teaching cannot replace first-hand experience, but allows beginners to have a broader focus and to recognize patterns of recovery when they actually come up.

In their efforts to match patient conditions with past theoretical learning, preceptors can validate the beginner's observations of new and unfamiliar conditions, encourage further exploration, and present some of the variations in the condition and its management that beginners should be watching for. At the same time, preceptors can help beginners appreciate the immense individual variation in patient responses and the tailoring of care required for addressing this variation.

Providing care in ways other than "by the book" requires practical reasoning in evolving situations. Beginners can ride the coattails of the competent through expert nurses' practical experience and break the rules with this careful oversight. Experiential knowledge is best shared ad hoc and in relation to particular patient dilemmas while the learner is deeply involved in the patient care situation. Beginners learn from preceptors how to weigh and balance competing concerns and attend to the most important concerns in concrete experience with many patients they encounter together.

Preceptors can additionally help advanced beginners improve their clinical grasp by offering opportunities to review and puzzle over situations that did not go particularly well. Advanced beginners often live with considerable ambiguity about past clinical episodes in which they felt they did poorly. A beginner's questions about why a particular patient died, why certain actions were or were not taken, and what the actual patient outcome was often go unanswered. Lacking resolution about such experiences leaves the beginner ill prepared to move into similar clinical situations in the future. Preceptors might review complex or ambiguous cases with advanced beginners. Calling up the patient record and reviewing the specific decisions that were made is one way to recreate the situation and provide for learning from experience that is grounded in a concrete case, yet is more distant from the beginner's emotions in the situation.

Specific training for preceptors and staff nurses on the learning needs of new graduates can reduce conflict and confusion. For example, it is sometimes confusing to staff nurses to discover that although new graduates have a good grasp of pathophysiology, they may not recognize when that knowledge is relevant for clinical work. Likewise, when advanced beginners are inundated with patient care demands in a rapidly changing clinical situation, they may not be able to request the most salient help. It is most helpful if the expert nurse can assess the situation and offer to do the most pressing tasks while at the same time offering any perspectives and judgments on what is occurring with the patient. Such well-placed assistance in high-demand situations can accelerate beginners' clinical learning.

Resource Identification

Many of the coping strategies used by advanced beginners depend upon the availability of a cadre of experienced and knowledgeable nurses, physicians, and ancillary personnel. Preceptors can help advanced beginners make their way more safely through dilemmas by pointing out those persons to whom the beginner should turn. In some hospitals, clinical excellence and resources are clearly identified by status and title. Clinical nurse specialists and other gradations of rank actually mark out those experienced and knowledgeable persons to whom the beginner can safely turn. Other hospitals have less developed systems for demarking the most experienced and knowledgeable nurses. It serves the beginner poorly to level clinicians to one rank, when their skills vary. Even in systems that have clear ladders for advancement which recognize advanced skills, nurses develop pockets of expertise and excellence. One nurse on a unit is particularly good at reading rhythm strips, another is a master at titrating sedation. These distinctive skills are usually known about and tapped by staff informally. Preceptors can help advanced beginners recognize the various skills of particular resource persons available to them in the unit.

Exploring the Nursing Role

In the beginners' interviews there was a substantial and continuing dialogue about what it meant to be a nurse in intensive care. Advanced beginners raised questions about what the nursing role encompassed, what were appropriate forms of relations, and closeness of relations with patients, families, and co-workers. They additionally were concerned with personal competence and how to present themselves to patients and staff in situations where they felt incompetent.

Advanced beginners can benefit by structured and unstructured opportunities to explore the nursing role with experienced as well as new nurses. Although there is some question about whether formal support groups contribute to role development, support from peers who share the new nurses' situation is strongly associated with new graduates' feelings of competence as nurses (Bellinger & McCloskey, 1992). In the small group interviews new graduates were visibly relieved to find that others had similar experiences and feelings. Discovering that their experiential learning is similar to their peers curbs self-blame and makes the demands of mastering practical clinical knowledge visible (Kramer, 1974).

Informal, ad hoc discussions of the nursing role at the bedside also allow advanced beginners to get validation for their behaviors or ideas about possible alternative responses from experienced nurses who are engaged in the immediate patient care situation. New nurses who have completed preceptor programs report that the emotional support of the preceptor, along with the preceptor's clinical skill and teaching ability, contributes to the developing nurses' sense of proficiency (Bellinger & McCloskey, 1992; McGrath & Princeton, 1987).

Coaching Beginners to Obtain Appropriate Physician Response

There is a substantial teaching role for preceptors in helping advanced beginners manage aspects of nursing that occur away from direct patient care. Included in this are: obtaining appropriate physician response, and managing interactions with ancillary services such as dietary, laboratories and pharmacy, as well as coping with nursing administration. Many of these skills simply cannot be the focus of advanced beginners, occupied as they are with patient care. Artful interactions with the larger system may be a learning edge for the competent clinician. However, the first of these skills, working with physicians, is essential to everyday beginning practice.

Advanced beginners benefit from experienced nurses who highlight clinical situations which require questioning, reinforce beginners' correct judgments about situations when they conflict with physicians' assessments or plans, and help beginners formulate a report or proposal to the physician so that it has a greater likelihood of being acted on. Experienced nurses support advanced beginners in maintaining the argument for the overall good of the patient as the beginner encounters inaction, resistance, or disagreement from a physician. Refinements about how and when to pursue disagreements "up the ladder" with physicians who have more experience are also essential aspects of teaching beginners how to get an appropriate physician response in settings where medical residents train.

Environmental Supports to Clinical Learning

It is imperative that advanced beginners work in environments where they feel safe asking questions. For the prudent care of patients, it is key that beginners' clinical inexperience not be judged as personal inadequacy, but recognized as an expected phase in the development of clinical judgment. Understanding the gap between theoretical and practical knowledge can help the discipline identify areas of experiential learning and qualitative distinctions that must be learned in practice. Certainly advanced beginners must know they are responsible for the judgments and actions they take. But the extent to which they operate on their own in making those judgments must be adjusted to their actual clinical experience and knowledge. Most hazardous to patients are environments which are interpersonally threatening, which punish early mistakes in judgment or set up barriers to the free flow of questions from advanced beginners. When advanced beginners feel they must hide their mistakes, cover their gaps in knowledge, and hide their inadequacies, their opportunities for learning are severely curtailed and the safety of patients is placed at risk.

Maintaining a preceptor to whom the advanced beginner can go for support and questions for the first 6 months of practice provides a safe way to encourage clinical inquiry and experiential learning. The nature of supervision with beginners' practice will vary during this time from extreme intensity at the beginning to a more distant and consultative tone at the end of the time. A variety of structural arrangements between preceptor and new nurses is possible. One option is to maintain a recognized relationship between each advanced beginner and one experienced nurse for the full time, which in one study was found to be most efficacious (Giles & Moran, 1989). Alternatively, after an initial period in which each nurse has a unique preceptor, a teaching/coaching nurse might be assigned to each shift on which advanced beginners work. In support of this option, Brasler (1993) found that nurses who spent more time with a secondary preceptor had higher ratings on their professional development and capacity to plan and organize. Despite the structure, the key to the success and safety of beginners' practice is the availability of a pool of experienced nurses who are explicitly assigned to teach and coach the new nurse about qualitative distinctions in practice, patterns of patient response, and perspectives on patients situations.

Providing adequate back-up support for the advanced beginner to safely practice delegation of decisions (delegating up) also requires that experienced clinicians be available each shift. Within the first six months of their practice and beyond, advanced beginners panic at the thought of working shifts which are predominantly staffed by inexperienced nurses like themselves. This unbalanced mix of staff leaves advanced beginners with inadequate resources for checking or delegating their clinical judgments. It also places enormous responsibility on the charge nurse on those shifts to monitor, support, and teach a cadre of nurses who are not clinically seasoned.

Given that practical clinical knowledge is socially embedded and dialogical, integrating newcomers into the community is key to both their clinical knowledge development and social support. Advanced beginners who are struggling with their own inadequacies do not immediately feel a part of the group of nurses with whom they work. Thus planned formal and informal support from colleagues can assist with social integration. There is an enormous amount of practical knowledge which is shared in informal, unstructured exchanges that go on in the coffee room, over lunch, while turning a patient, or in the locker room at change of shift. If advanced beginners are segregated from these discussions, and cannot feel comfortable participating, their learning and development will be stunted.

There is a way in which the advanced beginner can be accepted into the fold, albeit as the new kid on the block, that is inviting and accepting. This is in contrast to an initiation that tests their physical and emotional endurance and puts every aspect of their behavior up for evaluation. There are ways in which advanced beginners can be accepted without judgment and evaluation from the start. They can be invited to participate in the emotional life of the unit and often can instill refreshing enthusiasm and idealism to that life. Being cut off from this participation, even for an initial "hazing" period, creates undue stress on new nurses and is an unfortunate welcome to the profession. If there is hope that advanced beginners will become fully participating members of the nursing community, it's essential that they be engaged from the start as fully participating selves in the life of the nursing unit and the larger nursing community.

SUMMARY

Nursing practice as an advanced beginner is a time of extraordinary transition in terms of knowledge, situatedness in the practice environment, and self-understanding as a nurse. Clinical knowledge development is primarily about learning the concrete, practical exigencies of clinical situations that were earlier studied only in the abstract. Experiences with many patients suffering from varied conditions and at various stages in their illness trajectories helps beginners to build a foundation of practical understanding that bolsters prior theoretical training. During their first year in practice, advanced beginners continue to work with clinical dilemmas using disengaged reasoning, but they have a tremendously increased capacity to work within the realities and limits of clinical situations. Advanced beginners' anxieties remain a large part of their clinical narratives, but shift from unfocused overriding anxiety to anxiety that is more tied to specific concerns about the patient's condition. Finally, advanced beginners move from "acting like a nurse" to the early stages of coming into their own as nurses and developing their sense of what it is to embody the nursing role.

Chapter 4

THE COMPETENT STAGE: A TIME OF ANALYSIS, PLANNING, AND CONFRONTATION

BECOMING COMPETENT

Two years into practice, nurses typically perform at the competent level of performance, differing primarily from the advanced beginner by their increased clinical understanding, technical skill, organizational ability, and the ability to anticipate the likely course of events. The focus of these nurses' narratives is now more on clinical issues, i.e., the clinical condition and management of the patient, and less on getting tasks organized and completed. Through experience the nurse develops competence in handling familiar situations. Indeed, the ability to recognize a situation as a particular kind of clinical situation is experientially learned. At the competent stage the nurse has gained the ability to anticipate certain typical progressions in the patient's recovery and likewise begins to perceive discomfort when the patient's progression violates experientially gained expectations. The competent nurse is more discriminating about the performance of other members of the health care team, and the exposure to increasing divergence and complexity in patients' responses creates a search for broader and more extensive explanations. This is a time of heightened and broader clinical reading and study in order to better understand the newly perceived complexities of clinical presentations.

In the design of this study, we puzzled over the best sampling plan to capture practice at competent and proficient levels, as well as transitions in between the two stages. We expected to find a mixture of competent, proficient, and expert performance within the same person, because skilled performance depends on prior clinical learning and is always related to a particular situation. The sampling for this "intermediate" level was further complicated by hiring patterns in critical care units. Except during periods of acute nursing shortage, as was the case at the beginning of this study, new graduates are seldom hired directly into the critical care unit. Therefore we decided to sample nurses who had at least 1½ to 3 years of experience in critical care, but who may or may not have had other types of nursing experience, because the pool of critical care nurses with only critical care experience was small.

CLINICAL WORLD

Typically, nurses with more than 1½ years of experience and without experience in other units practiced at the competent level of the Dreyfus model of skill acquisition. The change from advanced beginner level to competent level is incremental, rather than discontinuous. The qualitative, discontinuous shift in performance seen in the transition from competent to proficient is absent. Rather, nurses practicing at this level differ from advanced beginners in their improved organizational ability and technical skills. This increase in skill opens up possibilities for noticing and developing new clinical knowledge so that in familiar clinical situations they have an increased understanding and ability to anticipate the likely course of events. While the focus of the advanced beginner narratives was on the challenge of task completion within the time demands of clinical practice, the competent level performer focuses more on managing the patient's condition. The temporal focus is broadened to include the experientially learned typical progression of illness and recovery. These narratives point to organizational skills as newly acquired triumphs, but the focus is increasingly shifting to the near future. The clinical world of this nurse is organized by planning for and anticipating likely events in the particular patient situation.

The progression of experiential learning sets the stage for disillusionment as the nurse is now more capable of recognizing the fallibility of other clinicians, at the same time as she begins to recognize the gaps in scientific knowledge and clinical understanding.

ORGANIZING THEIR WORK

On observation, the gain in organizational skill is apparent. The performance is more fluid and coordinated. Improved time management and organizational skills, while a source of gratification, are seldom the primary focus of concern and tension in the narratives. Many report their increased ability to handle busy complex situations:

> I think the more experienced you are, the better able you are to handle the stress and the different experiences that you're going through. And you're so much more organized and pulled together that you can divert and reduce the stress by sending the different problems different ways instead of taking, you know, not knowing what to do with them, which way to send them.

Increased understanding of the team and the nature of the work allow the nurse more reflective time and energy to more effectively seek help. Finesse in handling a situation that would have been overwhelming in the past, increased technical skills, and the ability to order multiple demands are described as triumphs. For example, the following nurse is describing a night in a neonatal intensive care unit "that went perfectly:"

> I have this little tiny baby and a ton of blood to draw and I've got this radial stick which was the best one I had ever seen, I have to say. It was perfect. And I went up to (another unit) and started an IV for them and it was just like "I'm really hot tonight." And last night I had three babies; one of them was intubated, two weren't but I just organized them fine and it was just wonderful.

The nurse is aware of the progress in organizational ability that includes difficult tasks (the radial arterial stick) and the organizational demands (three infants). She feels exhilarated with the progress in her skilled performance and her organizational ability. Skilled performance and organization enhance one another. The competent nurse has enough experience to anticipate what will occur and the definition of "organization" enlarges to incorporate planning ahead during a crisis. For example, a nurse describes caring for a 2-year-old who had accidentally taken aspirin and antihypertensive medications:

> There was a big hustle and bustle to get the charcoal and flush out the stomach with saline lavage and all this and that . . . The child had become hyperactive and screaming and carrying on in the emergency room and then would kind of lose it. And they weren't quite sure what to make of it . . . I got everything together and they did an electroencephalogram. And I had all the supplies and everything together to do saline lavage. And we got literature from the poison control center and Dr. M. said "I really like working with you. You stay so calm when it is so crazy." I felt very good because you do remember the times when you have not worked up to par . . . It wasn't

a code or anything. It was just a matter of getting stuff organized and having it there anticipating.

Being able to anticipate the demands and possible eventualities places the competent nurse in a new relationship to the situation. Organization now comes to mean not just completing tasks on time, but also anticipatory planning for rapidly changing, nonroutine events, preparing an environment, having the appropriate equipment and resources at hand, and performing calmly and efficiently.

Performance in a crisis requires mastery of one's emotional responses and the ability to imagine what will be required in what sequence for a range of clinical responses. This practical mastery is learned in a variety of ways beginning with "mock codes" in nursing school. In the following example, the nurse enters her first successful code with the experience of having closely observed and recorded several successful infant codes. She has mixed feelings about her "successful" performance because the infant is suffering and has a number of problems that are incompatible with life:

Nurse: . . . It would have been better if he hadn't survived and I think in a way I was hoping he wouldn't. So I was a little upset when we got a heart rate back, but at the same time, it was good. It was the first time I had been in a code [*she had discovered the respiratory arrest and initiated the resuscitation*] and for it to be successful . . .

Int: You haven't been in the situation where you . . .

Nurse: Right. Well I've seen a couple of baby ones that were successful . . . but this was one of those "baptisms by fire" where you are not absolutely sure that you can do it until you're confronted with the situation.

Int: What do you think helps you be ready for it?

Nurse: I think watching. I used to stand back and just watch and I really think before somebody participates, being a recorder is really good because you get to see everything that happens. You have to watch very closely, write it all down, and writing it down helps you remember later what order everything had been done. I had done that a couple of times before and I think that was probably the main thing and also knowing the baby, knowing what he's like, knowing every inch of the back of his neck. He didn't have an IV. Just things like that all added together. But I really think being a recorder was the biggest thing; much better than participating in a mock code in nursing school . . .

Practical mastery of the likely sequencing, the nature of the teamwork, and knowing a range of clinical eventualities, in addition to knowing this particular infant allows the nurse to anticipate and respond to the action needed. Experiential learning has been gained by actively participating in the recording role, sorting out the multiple instantaneous therapies and patient responses. She is troubled by the infant's suffering but has little sense of the social power or means to deal directly with this concern. She has not yet developed the experiential wisdom and ability to integrate ethical and clinical concerns. She was ethically and legally accountable to initiate the code since there was no familial and medical agreement to stop treatment. In this social context, her actions to prevent the code would have had to precede this particular crisis. However, she does not actively pursue this ethical concern after the code. This is in sharp contrast to the proficient and expert nurses in the study, who have a more developed sense of moral agency, foresee the ethical implications of clinical interventions, and typically seek an organizational response to their ethical concerns.

DEVELOPING CLINICAL UNDERSTANDING

Developing clinical understanding ultimately requires developing historical and clinical understanding in particular situations, reasoning in particular transitions. But advanced levels of clinical understanding require much experiential learning about (1) the nature of signs and symptoms in their various practical manifestations; (2) gaining a more holistic clinical grasp; (3) anticipating future possibilities; and (4) recognizing the distinctions between standardized and individualized care and reconciling them in particular situations.

Identifying Significant Clinical Signs and Symptoms

Textbooks make signs and symptoms seem far clearer and more explicit than the variations and subtleties confronted in practice. In addition, the recommended courses of actions seldom cover the range of actual clinical possibilities. Furthermore, it is impossible to convey the temporal nature of clinical understanding in written texts. Recognizing signs and symptoms and their significance continue to be a major part of experiential learning for the competent nurse as well as for the beginning nurse. Clinical and ethical reasoning require an engaged understanding of the historical unfolding of the clinical situation. Experience teaches that things are not always as they seem:

Nurse 1: . . . You explain to somebody "Well, just because they're resting more comfortably may mean that they're getting far worse; not far better." And you try to explain that to somebody. So you know that you've learned a lot, but the review part becomes actually kind of difficult because the book learning part is incorporated; and you can't spell it out . . .

Int: And a lot of it is from your experience probably too.

Nurse 2:   Like if somebody's resting quietly.

Nurse 1:   Yeah, and if that's a change, that may be something very bad and you have to watch that guy just to make sure that that's not—maybe they're septic or there is something going wrong in their heads. You've got to know how to handle it until you're comfortable. Go wake them up (laughs), whatever it takes to see if that really is a level of consciousness change, if that's good or bad. But telling that to somebody that's really new, they wouldn't know that. They say: "Oh, the patient was so restless before, and now they're quiet." And it could be real bad.

Nurse 2:   "Didn't offer complaints." [*Laughter. They are joking about how a new graduate might erroneously chart the above incident.*]

This example illustrates experiential learning about the historical context of patients' clinical presentations. The instructions to the new graduate about watching the patient are broad and necessarily vague because the clinical possibilities are too numerous to name without limiting them to a particular time-bound clinical situation.

Recognizing what constitutes a sign and symptom in real life, complete with variegations and subtleties, comprises a major form of clinical learning and clinical knowledge. Meshing of clinical (practical) knowledge with formal theoretical knowledge is evident in the beginner but becomes more nuanced and sophisticated in the competent nurse and, for the first time the competent nurse becomes a source of firsthand perceptual knowledge for others:

Nurse 1:   I have a tendency to go to more experienced nurses and say this is what I found, is there something I missed? Is there something that's not quite making sense? Or, "I haven't seen it quite this way before." It's really nice now to find people coming to you sometimes, not too often.

Int: How do you know when to go to a more experienced nurse when things don't fit together so well?

Nurse: I know I don't feel as comfortable with head traumas. I'm not familiar with some of the signs about herniation or head injury. We have a couple of nurses who are just excellent. You just say: "I just want to make sure I'm doing this okay. Could you just verify with me what I'm finding?" . . . Also, I don't feel comfortable with cardiac patients because we don't deal with that a lot. We have a lot of healthy hearts.

Textbook descriptions do not automatically lead to recognition of the actual signs, and recognition of contextual and relational responses requires time to assimilate. A nurse describes this transition in perceptual grasp in taking care of a heart transplant patient:

I was being a good nurse and turning him every two hours and he had really bad breath sounds on his left side. So I gave him P.T., elevated his left side so he could drain, had him cough. But it took me a couple of times to realize that when I turned him on his left side, with his bad lung down and his good lung up, his oxygen saturations showed great readings and his heart rate was wonderful, and then I would turn him on his back, or turn him up on his right side and within a few minutes, he would go into bursts of SVT [*supraventricular tachycardia*] and his [*oxygen*] saturations would drop. I had called the doctors and they didn't seem too concerned about it. They said: "Relax, he has a healthy heart." I said, if he has a healthy heart, why is he doing this? It spontaneously resolved after I turned him off his side. And I said okay, now I know what's going on. I'll keep him off that side. It was just a hypoxic reaction because he wasn't oxygenating well enough with his bad lung . . . It could be a bad situation if we left this so now we know that we just have to work on that lung and get it back aerating again, and he did fine. He's out walking around.

This demonstrates correlating the physiological responses with practical activity, the kind of "know-how" that must be learned in the firsthand way described above. As long as the nurse focused on standard procedures (turning the patient every 2 hours) and on the usual conceptual expectations for the situation (thinking, for example, "the heart is healthy and should not go into supraventricular cardiac arrhythmia,") she did not notice that the response to positioning was reasonable for this patient's lung capacity. The absent physician is less likely to imagine practical contingencies like patient position and agitation.

Gaining a web of clinical perspectives requires experience with a variety of patient situations that provide contrasts and corrections about the same clinical condition. For example, clinical expectations can become too esoteric or complex and the basics may be overlooked, as in the following situation:

I think I was looking for more complex things instead of just saying this is basic shock. It was pretty much the basic shock symptoms and I don't know, maybe she would not have coded if everybody would have acted more quickly.

The kind of reflection this nurse is practicing is crucial for clinical learning and illustrates the experiential distance between learning conceptual information on signs and symptoms as they are learned in the classroom and identifying them in the actual clinical situation. The clinical learning goal is to prevent formal codes by diagnosing clinical changes early in the cycle. Indeed, this clinical learning does occur, so that in a unit staffed with more experienced nurses, very few formal codes are called because interventions occur in increments in response to early patient changes.

Gaining a More Holistic Clinical Grasp

Nurses talk about getting the "big" picture—seeing and understanding the interrelationship between physiological states. This is illustrated by the following nurse's memory of learning the importance of seeing the big picture:

Nurse 1:   When I first started, after I had taken the heart class, one of my first hearts, I had learned a lot of theory about the hearts and the hemodynamics that are going on, the filling pressures et cetera. It takes a while to put all of the information together to get the big picture to see what's going on, and I hadn't really gotten that yet, and I had this patient and he was hypotensive. That's all I could see, the patient was hypotensive. I had to fix his hypotension, but I wasn't really looking at everything else. I wasn't putting together the big picture. I was very focused on this man's hypotension. He cycled downward and ended up coding. It was a bad code. It wasn't run well, and I felt really lousy. I felt like I hadn't put things together well and I should have seen this coming the second I walked in the door.

Int: Did you know that then, or do you know that now?

Nurse 1:   No, I learned it awfully quick after that. I said now I've really got to look at things and look at the whole thing and see what's going on. But, no, at that time, I just knew he was hypotensive and that I had to fix that. Not fix what was causing the hypotension or all the other things that could be involved with that. Since then I've learned.

Int: Have you taken care of a person with the same hypotension?

Nurse 1:   Oh, many.

Int: What kind of questions go through your mind now that didn't go through your mind then?

Nurse 1:   Are they volume depleted? Do they need blood? Are they dilated, do they need a little tone?

Int: Do you have a checklist that you go through?

Nurse 1:   Yes.

Int: You didn't have a checklist before?

Nurse 2:   You have little bits and pieces but it just doesn't all fit together.

Int: Didn't they present the checklist in the heart course?

Nurse 1:   They do present it in the heart course, but it's still, different things happen with different patients, so it's not exactly as the heart course presents it. Every patient is a little bit different. So, it's not always, as easy as going down the list and saying this and this and this, no, you have to sometimes consider other factors. But they did present a list. A sort of list, but it's not always that easy. Plus, understanding the concepts of preload and afterload, that doesn't come from—you don't understand that for awhile.

Nurse 2:   They give you a definition and you can spit it back.

Nurse 1:   Right, you can spit out a definition like that, but you can't picture what is going on in that heart until you've had a few of these hearts and realize what is really going on.

Int: What was the big picture?

Nurse 1: They wanted to put him on Levophed, but it wasn't really appropriate. His cardiac output was low and he wasn't vasodilated, it wasn't that he needed tone. That's one thing that stands out specifically, and I think we ended up putting him on Levophed. I think what had happened was that he had just had a massive MI, which you couldn't really see that coming. We did see some EKG changes and we picked up on that quick enough, but it's hard enough to see something like that right away. But now I'm much better at seeing things coming.

The nurse's developing sense of agency or responsibility is evident. Recognizing the needs of the particular patient in relation to general rules about caring for a class of patients and learning the concrete manifestations of theoretical categories of illness states—both major aspects of experiential learning in the advanced beginner stage—continue in this stage. The nurse no longer looks over her shoulder expecting others to augment her observation, although indeed it is their job to notice. She takes more responsibility than is realistic, given her experience. Even though these unrealistic expectations contain inevitable disappointments, they propel the nurse's clinical learning as the nurse learns to see relationships between therapeutic actions and patient responses.

The inadequacy of the "checklist" is apparent to the competent nurse. It is no longer enough to have an analytic template to guide a variegated and continually shifting patient situation. The nurse struggles to learn to read the situation because typically his/her understanding is post hoc. The competent nurse experiences a crisis in trust about two sources of knowledge and guidance for practice that were previously unquestioned. First, scientific knowledge and analytic approaches to managing clinical situations are now recognized as incapable of standing alone. Second, coworkers are now recognized as fallible both in their fund of knowledge and in the correctness of their clinical grasp and capacity to manage all situations. The breakdown in trust in this resource environment contributes to the competent nurse's hypertrophied sense of responsibility.

Anticipating Future Possibilities

As the above example illustrates, another major shift in perspective at the competent stage of experiential learning is temporal. The competent nurse has enough of a grasp of possible future scenarios in the patient's condition, and enough mastery of the present task demands to project into anticipated possibilities in future care. In contrast, the beginner's practice is focused on the present shift or even the present hour.

The competent-level nurse actively thinks about the future in order to plan present care. This is a conscious attempt to anticipate what is likely to occur in the future in order to provide guidelines for the present. This is not an integrated grasp of the present situation in terms of the most likely eventualities for this particular patient which is characteristic for the expert (see Chapter 6). Thinking about predictable and typical eventualities provides an analytical tool for the competent level nurse, whereas for the expert anticipated futures are more closely related to the particular patient and are incorporated in the understanding of the present situation. In the following exemplar, a competent nurse deliberately uses her past understanding of how new heart transplant patients usually respond:

> I had a patient who had his second heart transplant. He kept going into bursts of SVT [supraventricular tachycardia], which really frightened me with a new heart. New hearts shouldn't be doing this. He has a healthy heart. . . . It just made me really nervous.

The nurse knew that it was too soon for infection or rejection, both possible occurrences that she easily thought about in planning care for a heart transplant patient. She has enough experience to notice failed expectations, i.e., the absence of cardiac arrhythmias with normal fluid and electrolyte balance. "Failed expectations" are necessarily situated in one's understanding of particular clinical situations, since it would be impossible to have an explicit list of expectations for all clinical situations. In everyday practical understanding, knowledge and salience are located in concrete situations associated with perceptual expectations, so that the limits of formalizing the situation are not encountered by the situated, embodied skilled performer.

Reconciling Standardized and Individualized Care

Having mastered the more standardized task world, the competent nurse is now for the first time in a position to alter protocols and standardized care according to the patient's particular course of illness and individual and familial needs. The routines and rituals developed in nursing school and at the advanced beginner stage can now be individualized. The hospital has both professional and bureaucratic organizational structures and processes and these sometimes conflict. Consequently, learning how to put standardization and professional judgment together begins to loom large in the second year of practice:

> When you've been there for a while, you've picked up your own ways of doing things and you know that your way might be different, but it's just

the same outcome as someone else's. You might tell the newcomer, this is the standard way of doing it and this is my way, now you can try both and come to your own conclusions.

This is evidence of a loosening of the fixed rules and procedures that pre-occupy the beginner. The nurse now recognizes when there is room for flexibility and variability, but this recognition is part of the realization of the relative importance of other stances and perspectives that they might take. Because nurses at the competent level now recognize from experi-ence that they must *choose* a stance or perspective and that their choice makes a difference in patient outcome, the occasion of choice becomes in-creasingly apparent:

> Some nurses will say absolutely that the baby cannot come out every day to be held. But I might have a different feeling about that . . . and say I will wait to see when the mother comes in . . . It's just learning to be the primary and where to step in and say, would you mind? It is kind of hard to learn.

The difficult learning she refers to is the ability to trust her own judgment in particular situations. She is describing a judgment based upon the infant's responses to the mother's handling, and the mother's developing relation-ship with the infant. Postponing mother-infant interaction may imperil the mother-infant relationship, but this risk must be weighed against the infant's response to handling. Can the nurse be confident that she is reli-ably adjusting the rule of thumb of minimal handling? Empirical studies give guidelines but cannot provide clinical judgments about the compet-ing goods of infant stimulation and mother-infant bonding. When such clinical judgments about competing clinical goals and notions of the good are at issue, real-time judgments will vary daily based on the infant's con-dition. The combination of competing clinical and ethical goods, as well as the need to make judgments about these in relation to the patient's condi-tion, create a crisis in the analytic way of being in the situation.

THE ROLE OF EMOTIONS IN CLINICAL AND ETHICAL LEARNING

Although advanced beginners' practice can be impeded by their consider-able anxiety about knowledge or performance, competent nurses begin to talk about how they feel about a situation (comfortable, anxious, unsure, confident) in much more differentiated ways. Emotional responses are no longer characterized by diffuse or global anxiety. Instead, competent nurses' emotional responses to a situation now give them a better access to what is happening to the patient. Emotions in practice thus begin to be a screening or alerting process rather than a perceptual impediment or block. As competent practitioners settle more comfortably into their roles, their emotional responses become more informative and guiding. For example, not having a good grasp of the situation, or having the situation seem vaguely off what the nurse has learned to expect, provides guiding and alerting information. As competent practitioners settle more comfortably into their roles, they can more reliably trust their emotional responses to guide problem identification and they are more emotionally available to perceive the emotional needs and responses of patients and families.

Emotional Responses as a Source of Perceptual Awareness

Competent level nurses can now use their emotional responses more reliably as indicators of distinctions, significance, and threat. They "feel good" or pleased when their chosen action makes a positive difference for the patient and proves to be the best course of action. And they feel badly when they are slow to recognize a patient change or when things do not go well. It is here that the development of excellent practice demands that good patient responses are sought and recognized by the practitioner. For example, if a nurse is pleased to elicit ever-greater control over patients, and takes compliance and subdued responses by patients as evidence of excellent practice, then practice will become distorted and violate an ethic of care and responsiveness. This is similar to the disastrous consequences for a driver who feels pleasure over careening around corners on the outer edge of two wheels. The pediatric nurse must learn that a quiet, subdued child in a hospital setting is coping by withdrawal and depression, ominous signs for the child's well-being and not hallmarks of successful nursing management. Discussions about good, better, and poor outcomes and attendant emotional responses in the caregiver and the one cared for are crucial to both clinical and ethical learning.

Competent nurses have experienced and can talk about feeling comfortable when they have a good grasp of the situation. They talk about not feeling as overwhelmed as they did in the beginning of their practice because they now understand the situation better. In an earlier example, the nurse who entered her first successful infant code felt "wonderful" when she was able to marshal all the necessary equipment and stay calm. And even though the wisdom of resuscitating the infant was questionable, the nurse could feel sad for the infant but still feel a sense of success due to being able to perform well in a crisis. This grasp of the situation is global and embodied, registered by feeling tones. Competent level nurses also experience dread when things are too busy, too novel, or too complex for them to understand the situation. When nurses do not perform well they feel varying degrees of disappointment, when things go well, the success is laden with import, giving nurses hope that they can be good nurses. For example:

Nurse: I had a good week. I really did. The last [*interview session*] I could not think of anything good at all, it was like: "Oh, I hate nursing!" I want to get out of here so badly and then this last week I had two nights that went absolutely perfect where I could not have—I just feel good. I could not have done anything better than I did. I was so perfect (laugh). I needed those, didn't I?
Int: Save you from leaving nursing. What does perfect mean to you?
Nurse: Yeah, well but not just where you do all your tasks right, but where you get the art of nursing down to where it just feels like the night went absolutely perfect for you; not just good, not just the really nice night but it went great. And I was good . . . I don't know. Usually there are nights where you don't do anything wrong but there's a lot of things you could have done better. I could have positioned the baby a little bit better. I could have been brighter at the bedside, just little tiny things that you think, "Oh, it was good, but there were certain things I could have done better and these nights went perfectly" . . . It was a good feeling to feel like, I'd put the baby up on her side in a little fetal position and she stayed there. She didn't flail all over the bed (laugh). Just little things really made the night go well.

Feeling good when performance is good and poorly when things do not go well provides an emotional guide that sharpens the nurse's perceptual acuity and guides the development of skilled clinical know-how and ethical comportment. The nurse takes up the ethos of nursing through experiencing the appropriate emotional responses to good and poor performance, and good and poor health care practices. Embodied emotional responses allow the nurse to perceive discrepancies and poor fit with less than explicit clinical situations.

Developing the Skill of Involvement

Response-based learning and the role of emotions in developing perceptual acuity are related to involvement in the clinical situation (problem engagement) and in caregiving involvement with the patient as person (interpersonal involvement). At the competent stage the nurse demonstrates increased problem engagement, as a result of a greater understanding of the situation, and the suffering of the patient becomes more apparent, challenging the nurse to confront new demands for interpersonal involvement. The advanced beginner primarily talks about social exchange and negotiation of taking up the nursing role and identifying with patients and families in ways that resemble their lay experiences as families and friends. At the competent stage, the nurse typically begins to notice the patient/family suffering in new ways. It is a time of conscious repersonalization of patient and family. According to the participants' narratives, this rediscovery of patient/family as fellow human beings is qualitatively distinct from their initial confrontations as a new graduate. A major difference lies in the nurses' discussion of the skill of involvement in relation to the self. The nurse is now more reflective about his or her impact and reflectively discusses different qualitative distinctions related to the skill of involvement. They now have usually had the experience of becoming "overinvolved" or involved with patients and families in ways that were not helpful, and subsequently may err on the side of too much disengagement or detachment as a way of avoiding overinvolvement. Learning the skill of involvement is necessarily experiential, and existential. One learns the comfortable and effective zone of engagement by getting it better and worse in different circumstances. Nurses are pulled along in this skill by their observations of other highly skilled nurses as well as the patient/family expectations.

Developing the skill of involvement is set up by the culture of the unit, the styles of practice available on the unit, and the vision for the skill of involvement and for what is excellent practice. The subculture of the unit determines what kinds of expectations the advanced beginner and competent level nurse will have. They have mastered the task world, but unless they take up a new focus for their clinical learning, they may imagine that clinical learning is limited to learning new types of procedures, and learning to care for new patient populations. They will not easily shift their focus to knowing a patient and learning the particular in relation to the general. The role of the subculture of the unit in forming learning expectations and standards of excellence is so important that it is taken up in a separate chapter on the social embeddedness of learning. The unit level of expertise and standards of good and poor practice are highly influential in guiding experiential learning for the competent level nurse. For example, the work group may be focused on mastering technology and completing tasks rather than creating continuity in the care of the whole patient. While "mastering new technology and techniques" is essential in a rapidly changing field such as nursing, when expertise is viewed as the number of things one knows how to do, the more complex forms of clinical learning may be overlooked. The focus on mastering an array of technical skills may inhibit focusing on patient responses and gaining the "big picture" described earlier. The tension between mastering the technical demands and refining the art and skill of working with particular patients and families can show up as a deliberate choice for the competent level nurse.

AGENCY

Competent nurses' sense of agency is directly related to what they can plan, predict, and control in their delivery of nursing care. While one's sense of agency is never overtly visible, narrative accounts reveal the author's sense of self-efficacy, engagement, and sense of responsibility in the story. A narrative may be told as an outside-in account, with the narrator being an outside observer to events, or as an inside-out account, with the narrator being an engaged member-participant in the situation with a more or less well developed sense of the impact of their action in that situation. The challenges of newly gained experiential knowledge make the competent nurse's sense of agency a source of reflection and conflict, they may experience a sense of hyper-responsibility and they may experience discomfort as they come to recognize the extent to which they influence clinical decision making by the way they present the case for their clinical judgments to physicians and other health care workers.

A sense of agency and responsibility is not just a matter of assertiveness, social negotiation, or "choosing" to take responsibility, though all these interpersonal skills play a role. The nurse must be in a position to "see" that certain choices are possible and that these choices typically have certain consequences; she must be able to contrast the various perspectives and options available in particular situations. This was evident in the excerpt above about seeing the big picture. The ambiguous phrase, "the big picture," reflects this perspectival learning.

Coping with a Sense of Hyper-Responsibility

At this point in skill development, knowledge for safe practice is still primarily comprised of knowledge about discrete facts about specific situations, the amount of knowledge needed to make complex clinical decisions is daunting. Nurses expect to find scientific guidelines, principles, and rules to cover every action required by the practitioner, even though the evidence for this belief is beginning to crumble. This creates anxiety and a sense of hyper-responsibility. It is at this point that nurses begin to buy more textbooks and increase their reading.

Nurse 1:   Today we are required to know so much and it's like our role is kind of overshadowing the doctors' because we're there and we're taking on their responsibility. You have done so much and you've done beyond probably what you're even required to do because your knowledge base is so extensive. You've read at home or you've researched something that you are interested in so you're a little bit more knowledgeable about something. But then, this is just for me personally, I go home and I think, "Oh, God, what else could I have done?" Maybe if I knew a little bit better, I could have done that . . . And it's like today you're required to know so much. You get into situations where patients are so sick, if something happens where maybe that one little thing you didn't think about [occurs] it's like the guilt and the fear that you have during that time is just unreal. And you have to go home and you have to deal with that and you know that puts a lot on you.

Nurse 2:   You make a mistake, you can't erase it.

Nurse 1:   You can't just leave and go to lunch.

Nurse 2:   And you can't take it out of the computer. I mean, that's somebody's life. I mean you are dealing with life and you are dealing with death, and a lot of professions don't have that.

The work itself is life and death and calls for an appropriate level of responsibility. At this point the number of tasks can proliferate and the nurse curbs her anxiety by setting priorities. The situation presents itself to both the advanced beginner and competent nurse as a concrete need for setting priorities. However, as pointed out in Chapter 3, the advanced beginner seems to lack an adequate structure for doing so. These nurses are likely to do first what she or he knows how to do, whereas the competent nurses set priorities in relation to their goals and plans. Setting priorities must usually be a conscious and deliberative decision-making process, since the competent nurse does not have a sense of salience of the relative importance of aspects of the situation:

> But for me the hardest thing in codes is the priority, like the one that I wrote about was the first code of a patient that I had and that was my problem. People were shouting things all the time and yet you have to prioritize and figure out what is the most important.

The work is critical in every respect so that efficiency *and* reliability are fused. Finding procedures that will help the nurse get it right helps the nurse act in the situation, but it also helps her cope with her sense of responsibility for performing reliably in life-and-death situations. A major coping strategy encouraged both in school and in practice is to structure the work through setting goals and plans. As one expert nurse explains:

> I think one of the biggest assets of nursing is being organized. Competence, confidence, and conscientiousness are real important, but the biggest, biggest thing in nursing today because of time constraints, because of pressures, because there are so many things that you are doing . . . you really have to be organized. You have to know what's going on. You have to be able to set priorities, and I think that organizational skills are by far the most important.

This nurse refers to the additional time constraints placed on nursing care by cost controls and understaffing, but her perspective on organization is typical of the competent nurse. The understanding of work organization is radically different for the beginner who organizes through the structures and procedures designed to guide task performance, the competent nurse who organizes by setting goals and plans, and the proficient and expert nurse who organizes in response to understanding the changing demands of the situation (see Chapters 5 and 6). For the competent nurse, "making a difference" literally shows up in terms of what the nurse has achieved through setting goals and plans for the day. For example, the nurse in the following excerpt is frustrated because she had worked hard with few results, to get a suspension of what she thought was futile treatment for a dying man:

Nurse: I think you get into a kind of thing where you are deluding yourself and you are working so hard, you want to think you are making a difference. And you have to examine whether you are deluding yourself when you are working so hard, and you want to make a difference. And you have to look at the fact that maybe I can make a difference by preparing this family. I tried to do that; I arranged for the patient to have last rites while his son was here. It didn't help him much but it helped him a little bit. And the way I maintained [myself in the situation without getting too frustrated] was by being able to say, I can give you sedation. I will fight for his sedation. I will fight for his comfort issues, and I will fight for the right to be heard because I know him. And the fact was that I was being pretty vocal. I mean, being able to know what I could do from when his hair needed to be cut, when he needed a shampoo, the little things that I knew were making him comfortable, or making his family comfortable helped me maintain even though . . . they weren't going the way I wanted (them) to go.

This nurse's practice is constituted by goals that determine the action even when the nurse cannot achieve her preferred goal of allowing the patient to die with dignity. She keeps her goal of advocating for less aggressive therapies, but since that is not being heard, she sets up accomplishable goals that sustain her in the situation.

Preferred actions are those that fit goals and plans. Consistency, predictability, and successful time management show up as important, and gaining a sense of mastery through planning and predictability provides a sense of accomplishment. However, this organizational ability is nurse-structured rather than in response to patients' needs. From the nurse's perspective, it can seem like the goal is to organize the work despite "patient interruptions." This is a distinct conflict for skillful caregiving, because it is inadequately guided by the responses of the patients:

Nurse 1: I'd rather have a difficult patient two days in a row than two different easy patients.

Nurse 2: Yeah.

Nurse 1: Just because you can't anticipate—even if they're demanding patients—Or say, for instance, you have a demanding patient and everybody says, "Oh, they're such a grouch." But if you have them two days in a row, you can figure out the first day and anticipate what they need. And I've got patients like that and so, they say, "Oh, nobody ever brings me blankets." So fine, you offer them a blanket. Or people say, "Oh, she always wants to go to the bathroom right when I'm busy doing something else." So think about it and offer to take her to the bathroom when you've got time, not when she's asking but when you've got time. "Oh, do you need to go to the bathroom?" Here, let me unplug your IV."

Nurse 3: It just improves your body care if you can have consistency in your practice.

The focus is on gaining a sense of mastery through prediction, planning, and achieving specific goals. This causes the competent nurse to try to limit the "unexpected," to achieve a "status quo" as illustrated in the following nurse's account of an unexpected event:

Int: What kinds of things did you use to get through that?

Nurse: It kind of humbles you. At one point, I'm feeling like I have things straight now, and I can handle the situations, and when something like this happens, I think, well, I still have a lot of learning to do. I can handle the situations that are status quo; it's the unexpected that I have to learn to deal with now. But then I think back to situations when I was brand new. Things that are status quo now weren't back then. Things I can troubleshoot and solve now were much different back then. I usually needed help.

Not needing help, ordering the task world, and planning based on goals and predictions structure what the nurse notices and what are considered issues. It is not accidental that this vision of performance and agency is institutionally rewarded and encouraged as "standard."

Structuring the day by goals and plans, however, interferes with perceiving the demands of the situation and with timing interventions in response to the patient's responses and readiness. The competent nurse seldom sees changing relevance in a clinical situation. Their skill of seeing is hampered by the need to organize data collection and to achieve goals. Inevitably the clinical situation intrudes by not matching the goals and plans and the nurse must adapt. As noted above, conceptual descriptions do not automatically lead to recognition of actual signs, and varied responses require time to assimilate and interpret. Slavishly following one's plans and holding on to preset expectations can limit perceptual grasp. This was illustrated in the nurse's discovery of the cause of the heart transplant patient's supraventricular tachycardia. Holding on to this form of agency (sense of personal influence in the situation) prevents the nurse from having expert clinical and ethical comportment because response-based organization is not yet achieved.

Negotiating Clinical Knowledge, Learning to Make a Case

Negotiating clinical knowledge and learning to make a clinical case for action to physicians show up as major learning issues in narratives of the competent nurse. Indeed, the analytical structure of diagnostic reasoning fits well with the competent nurse's approach to practice. However, these nurses are now acutely aware that identifying a clinical problem is not sufficient for obtaining appropriate medical action. They must make a convincing case for their clinical judgment. Indeed, they are becoming more aware that clinical judgment is involved and not just a presentation of clinical information or facts. Therefore, after many difficult negotiations of clinical knowledge, the competent nurse begins to focus on learning to make a case for her/his assessments and preferred clinical interventions. A nurse talks about building a case to physicians:

Nurse: You've looked at all the facts, and you present them in a certain way that they know that you know what you're talking about.
Int: So you sort of build your case?
Nurse: Yes, I have everything prepared and anticipate any kind of questions that they might have.

Another nurse states:

Nurse: Many of us are new on nights, so we all try to figure everything out before we start calling and get yelled out by physicians. We get real aggressive, too. We do try to call before they go to bed and say: "You don't have morning labs ordered, you don't have this ordered, or that ordered. You know this patient has a history of getting fluid overloaded in her lungs and has renal problems and decreased urine output. Do you want a standing order of Lasix? Do you want any standing orders for titrating meds? You know we can do those without any problem." If the physician says: "No, no, no." We respond, "Okay, the minute the urine drops one cc below 30, I'm calling you." And we do. Usually I do it the same way, but we eventually get our way if its the right way.

Note that the competent clinician has a clear sense of what is clinically right for the patient. The argument can never be satisfactorily reduced to a mere power play because clinical knowledge, knowledge of the particular patient, science, and clinical evidence spell out the parameters for what can be "right" or good. Earlier in the discussion, these same nurses had stated:

Nurse: Before we call the doctor, we'll say: "What's going on? Why are these numbers this way? His wedge [*pressure*] is 5, his RA [*right atrial pressure*] is 20. What do you think we had better be doing here?"

This interview illustrates the extent of the problem-solving and selectivity prior to calling the physician. This is required for the system to work, since physicians are simply not available for every possible question. This kind of reflection on practice is essential to learn when it is necessary to go up the chain of command if the physician response is not appropriate:

Nurse: If you can't get through to the intern, and nothing is being done about it, you go up this ladder and it's okay to talk to attending physicians. Get hold of them even if they are out of town. It's perfectly okay to ask any kind of question, because they are the ones who are ultimately responsible for this patient. It is their patient and they would like to know. It is good to know the attending physicians and build a rapport and be very professional in dealing with them.

This excerpt illustrates the increased sense of agency of the competent nurse and the sense of responsibility she bears for her knowledge of the patient. Nurses note a shift in their seeking assistance from physicians:

Nurse 1:   That's a point you get to do trouble shooting [about] possible physical causes before calling the physician, whereas when you are fairly new and before you develop this sense or whatever, you might not have thought about the tube, or you wouldn't have suctioned, you would have just gone right to the physician.
Nurse 2:   Right.
Nurse 1:   And then you get to the point where you do a lot of things first before you go looking for the physician because you know, you learn . . .
Int: How do you learn those things?
Nurse 3:   From the senior staff. A lot of stuff I learned on the night shift where you had time to kind of observe. When I first started, you just never sit down, you're just watching people. You just go around and just being in the room helping someone boost the patient up in the bed. You just kind of watch the senior staff, what they do and how they do it.

This excerpt illustrates the nature of clinical knowledge and the typical distance between formal education and informal learning about actual practical situations. Gaining this knowledge requires critically evaluating reliable sources of clinical knowledge and contrasting the performance of various nurses and physicians in many clinical situations.

EXPERIENTIAL LEARNING AND COPING
WITH FAILURE

The narratives and discussions of nurses at the competent level reveal the tensions and conflicts experienced at this juncture. Competence is also a time of questioning, of confronting extreme societal and personal break-down, and of losing illusions about the certainty of scientific knowledge in particularized clinical realms and about the limits of one's own and other's clinical and ethical competence. The learning and coping issues focused on:

1. limits of elemental and scientific knowledge and need for experiential learning;
2. confronting new levels of distress over patient suffering;
3. moral conflict over prolonging dying;
4. confronting the cultural crisis in caring; and
5. institutional breakdown and its impact on practice and career.

Each of these areas are discussed below.

This is clearly a time of evaluation and questioning for nurses about whether nursing measures up to their expectations and whether they feel that they measure up to the demands placed on them by nursing. Competent level nurses are better able to recognize their own shortcomings as well as the lack of clinical competency of others. In contrast, beginners could naively feel that others had more experiential wisdom, and that their own shortcomings were to be expected as a newcomer.

The Limits of Elemental and Scientific Knowledge
and the Need for Experiential Learning

In nursing education the nurse is confronted with elaborate discourses on explanation, prediction, and control and offered limited practice with the engaged practical reasoning of clinical and ethical practice. Now she needs to learn to deal with the situated possibilities and constraints in the real world (Benner & Wrubel, 1989).

It is not surprising that nurses engage in critical questioning about whether nursing or intensive care is the right career choice. Confronting the need for experiential learning in a practice becomes a more acute transition in a society that recognizes traits and talents rather than skill, and knowledge as the possession of theories, concepts, and science rather than knowledge experientially gained. Practitioners may feel that they simply do not have the correct talents and traits, or that their education has been defective. Openness to experiential learning, i.e., openness to having one's preconceptions and assumptions turned around, is essential for the nurse to move beyond competency to proficiency and expertise.

The advanced beginner moves to competency in part as a result of a crisis in confidence, but also as a result of being taught by actual clinical situations and the actions by other health care workers. Experiential learning requires a change in one's assumptions and expectations in a situation. Change, not passage of time, is the defining characteristic of experience. Therefore, experience is laden with false starts, challenges, and failure. How nurses cope with their emotional responses to experience is crucial to clinical learning. That they even sense surprise, disappointment, or failure grows out of their increasing involvement and agency. Failure means something distinctly different for the competent level nurse than for the new graduate, for whom failure typically means not meeting external standards or experiencing self-mastery that may or may not be attuned to the situation. Failure for the competent nurse is closely linked to failed expectations, unmet goals, and disrupted planning in specific situations. Also the competent level nurse is beginning to have a perspective on breakdown and failure, whereas failure is less differentiated for the beginner. For example, in an interview excerpt presented earlier, a breakdown in expectations was described where a critically ill patient on a balloon pump cardiac assist device got out of bed while in a state of confusion, endangering his life. Reflection on that situation by the nurse demonstrates an ongoing internal dialogue about self-improvement related to specific caregiving situations:

> I still have a lot of learning to do. I can handle the situations that are status quo and it's the unexpected that I have to learn to deal with now. But then I think back to situations, when I was brand new, things that are status quo now weren't back then. Things I can troubleshoot and solve now, were much different back then. I usually needed help.

This nurse exemplifies good clinical learning. She acknowledges her need for continued learning and reminds herself how far she has come. For her, learning is gained over time. She has gone beyond the common cultural barriers of viewing performance as merely a display of formal knowledge or talent. Clinical know-how requires attentiveness and openness to learning from new situations.

Competent nurses confront the limits of disengaged reasoning taught by scientific and technological training. Clinical knowledge is covered over and relatively underemphasized in comparison to technical and scientific knowledge in nursing and medical education. Competent practitioners discover the nature of clinical and ethical knowledge as different from the application of science and technology. For competent nurses, the limits of elemental analysis and the importance of understanding the particular situation becomes evident. In the earlier example (see p. 85, this chapter) of learning about postoperative hypotension in an open heart patient, the nurse recognizes the limits of the checklist offered in the course on caring for postoperative open heart patients. Her narrative demonstrates her corrective dialogue about the usefulness of the checklist:

Int: Didn't they present the checklist in the heart course?
Nurse: They do present it in the heart course, but it's still, different things happen with different patients, so it's not exactly as the heart course presents it. Every patient is a little bit different. So, it's not always, as easy as going down the list and saying this and this and this, no, you have to sometimes consider other factors. But they did present a list. A sort of list, but it's not always that easy. Plus, understanding the concepts of preload and afterload, that doesn't come from—you don't understand that for a while.

Fortunately, this nurse recognized that her need for experiential learning did not reflect a lack in the content of the "open heart" course, but rather the necessity of experiential learning in specific clinical situations. Learning to administer response-based therapies requires experiential learning and engaged practical reasoning. This is a critical juncture for recognizing the limits of formal knowledge and an increasing sense of responsibility.

Nurses at this stage are reflective about their own sense of achievement. For example, the following nurse describes a faltering in her confidence that she will progress further and achieve the level of expertise that she had expected:

Nurse: I'm in my third year in critical care and that's one reason why I'm thinking of getting out of it, because I'm not sure. I have backed away from taking the difficult patients whereas once I liked to do that. And I'm not really sure why this is happening. There are other things in my life where I feel like I want to devote more energy, but it's partly because I don't know if I ever will become that nurse that I'd like to be, so it's a little uncomfortable.
Int: Are you saying that you don't think you will ever become the kind of critical care nurse that you would like to be?—What about the community health nurse you would like to be? [*This nurse had described an interest in community health nursing earlier.*]
Nurse: Yeah, that seems possible [to be a community health nurse].

She went on to describe a problem with short-term memory, which she found improved once she was no longer working night shift. She is clearly suffering a crisis in her confidence and self-esteem:

I am somewhat ashamed of myself that I'm not going out there like I did to take the difficult patients and some people have noticed that. I'm intimidated by them when I didn't used to be. I am just not that interested. Maybe it'll change, I don't know.

She thinks that her grasp is not what it should be and in commenting on her role models she states:

I met some nurses when I first started that I would have picked as role models and that pretty much stayed the same. I esteem them more highly now than I did originally, if anything.

A Crisis in Confidence in Others' Competency

The experiential learning gained in the first year and a half to 2 years creates a crisis in confidence in health care team members. Nurses at this level describe incidents where experienced nurses and physicians make faulty assessments or prescriptions that undermine their confidence about the authority of these coworker. In reality, these nurses are confronting both incompetency in some coworker and a necessary correction of their own inflated expectations of experienced staff from their earlier lack of ability to accurately judge clinical knowledge. At this point in their competence, nurses are experienced enough to recognize that not all health care workers are reliable, but they may not accurately discern the complexity and novelty of the situation. In the following example, the nurse is weaning an infant from a ventilator and phoned a resident unfamiliar with infants and received an unreasonable oxygen order. The nurse refused to follow the order and the physician became very angry and yelled at her. The conversation ended without resolution about taking the next blood gas and using a pulse oximeter, so the nurse phoned the physician again:

Nurse: I decided I was going to get yelled at either way and I went ahead and called him to get another order, I had taken a few minutes and I had calmed down a little bit, took a few deep breaths. And I thought I just hate to call this man back, and he had probably been doing the same thing I was, taking some deep breaths and going over what had happened over the phone. When he answered he said: "Look I'm really sorry I was yelling at you. Why on earth do you accept that kind of a gas in babies?" And I said: "It's a different hemoglobin than adults have. It doesn't hang on to oxygen in the same way." [*A lengthy discussion and question and answer period ensued about acceptable blood gasses and oxygen saturations for infants being weaned from respirators*]. That was what I was trying to tell him: that if we don't wean this baby down, we're never going to be able to. We won't get her off if we don't do it now. So he finally agreed to let me dial the oxygen [down] but refused to decrease the rate which is why I got another blood gas in the middle of the night and called him back. And he responds: "Well what do you think? Do you think we should cut down on the rate?" I said, "Everything is fine." So things did work out in the end. . . . [*she talked to another doctor on the unit who counselled her:*] "You've got to realize one thing; you guys are excellent nurses in here. You know your job very well and that's wonderful, but to people who don't know babies it can be very intimidating, especially when they're going through a service where they are expected to know everything and to be on top of everything and to know much more than the nurses do. That will create a lot of friction." She said: "Really he is a nice person once you give him a chance." But if I had it to do all over again, the one thing that I would do exactly the same is question that order to make sure that I understood what he was saying, because I've never had anyone say: "Leave the kid at l00% oxygen and don't try to wean him to 80 and leave him there all night." So I would have continued to question that and to trust my clinical observations and hopefully I would do that a little sooner.

Int: Where did you learn all that about babies' blood gasses?

Nurse: Experience. I didn't learn it in nursing school. I was shocked when I came into that unit. I had learned typical adult blood gasses. I learned very little about babies. So I was really surprised when you'd have a kid with a PO_2 under 60 and we were weaning him. So I can understand his point of view better now, and I think it's more just being maybe a little bit more assertive in getting my point across and realizing that with some people you are going to have to go the extra mile.

The competent nurses' gains in clinical knowledge expose the resident's lack of experiential knowledge. The loss of the nurses' confidence level in others may not necessarily be replaced by knowing who is reliable. Narratives frequently focus on incidents where experienced nurses and physicians make mistakes. The loss of confidence in the knowledge of others makes these nurses feel a new level of obligation to know about and manage clinical problems themselves. In the following excerpt, the nurse is confronted with a patient's imminent demise after coronary artery bypass and is unable to marshal the resources she needs to handle the crisis. She is confronted with the limits of her own knowledge, the limits of medical interventions, and a breakdown in support:

Nurse: My patient had an angioplasty, and ended up crashing and going to surgery really late for a five-way coronary artery bypass surgery . . . About 3:00 AM he needed suctioning. So, I had another nurse come in and help me, and he started flinging himself all over the bed. We didn't know if he was just really agitated or if he was hypoxic or what, so we just bagged him [*hand ventilation*] and tried to calm him down. I phoned his surgeon and was going to ask him for some sedation, it was pretty soon after surgery, but he is a pretty big man and sometimes they wake up very fast after surgery. As I went to the narcotic cabinet, I went to look first, he was on an intra-aortic balloon pump and he was on a lot of drips. Only myself and the charge nurse were familiar with the machine, so I went to look at it to see how he was doing and his heart rate dropped down to like 20 and his pressure dropped to like 50 on the pump. So, I ran in and connected his pacemaker wires to a temporary pacemaker and flipped it on and turned it to 70 [beats per minute]. His pressure came up, but not a lot. So I turned it to 90 and cranked up the drips. I called the surgeon back and explained what had happened and said, "This man is not doing very well. He is going to have to be paced. His heart rate is 90 and his blood pressure is only 80 augmented on the balloon pump. We have these drips increased. What do you want me to do?" So, I'm reading him the numbers off the Swan and telling him everything that's happening. Before this episode happened, we don't know if he went hypoxic, or he had an infarct, or if he threw a clot to his head, because he went purple from his neck up. Right after we suctioned him, we drew a gas. Now he is diaphoretic. He is unresponsive, he is obtunded. I told him all of this and he gave me an order for some drugs and put him on another drug to try to maintain him.

Int: Do you remember what the drips were?

Nurse: Yeah, Epical, bolused him with calcium, and put him on an epicalcium drip to keep his pressure between 90 to 110. [*The story of rapid changes and crisis continues. The pacemaker stops capturing the patient's heartbeats. The nurse had asked another more experienced nurse to come in from home, and had again requested that the doctor come in.*] I am trying to do stuff with the pacemaker and calling the surgeon in and telling him: "Something is going on. He's—I'm scared, I don't know what else to do. I've done everything that I can think of. I think you better come in. The nurse asked the doctor to call the family and he responded: "Well, I'll deal with the family later. I'll call them in the morning. We don't know what's happening right now." And he says: "What do you think is happening?" He's asking me these questions on the phone, and I'm saying, "Get in here!" The charge nurse was now talking to the physician. [*The situation deteriorates further and the nurse calls a code getting people from the other ICU and from the doctor from the emergency room. The patient's physician comes in a half-hour into the resuscitation. The patient dies and afterwards the nurse talks to the physician.*] I went to the surgeon after and said, "Can you please give me some input into what happened to this man?" And he said, "Well I think he had a massive infarct and he lost his conduction system. And that's why you saw him brady out and drop his pressure and he was pacemaker-dependent only for a short time." I cried all the way home. And I cried when I got home. . . .

Int: So you were at the end of your resources?

Nurse: Right, one other nurse who's trained in open heart surgery care, besides the other nurses who were just there. And it's just like, basically I and she and the other nurses doing everything in our power, not to so-call save this man, but just try to do something to correct the situation, but we really didn't know what the situation was. But we were trying to think of everything that we could to know what was wrong and why this was happening. This might sound kind of funny, in a sense, I can see the physician's viewpoint of it, but he should have come in. But once he was there, there wasn't anything that he could do because we pretty much did everything. But, I think in that kind of case, they should come in regardless whether they do can do anything or not.

The nurse is in a situation that exceeds both her theoretical and experiential knowledge. Her patient is dying before her eyes and she is unable to marshal the resources to alter the course. In retrospect the course sounds unalterable, but she is left without adequate medical backup and the physician is slow to respond and slow to believe her reports. Early in the incident he asks if she had checked cuff pressures to validate the changes in blood pressures. Indeed she had, but this validation was hardly needed in light of the other parameters reported.

The expectation is that the physician will manage rapidly changing and dangerous medical situations. In actuality physicians seldom arrive in time to manage rapidly changing situations, especially in private nonteaching hospitals. The nurse has the illusion that the physician has resources that he and the nurse have not tried, that there is magic to offer in this situation. Only in retrospect does she realize that there were no other options—no magic. Every heroic effort had been tried. She experiences first-hand the responsibility placed on the one who is there, and a sense of abandonment when she must continue all the heroic efforts with no physician present evaluating the patient's response.

Confronting the Moral Conflict of Prolonging Dying

The moral context of nursing practice is more than "ethical decision making" since the nurse must continually act in the situation. The nurse's action forces her to intensely confront the moral predicament of administering futile treatments that prolong dying, rather than fostering cures. Concrete action in the face of strong evidence of suffering is a different moral situation than disengaged ethical reasoning about suffering that can only dimly be imagined. Because of an intermediate level of experiential knowledge, the competent nurse is often assigned to patients who are chronically critically ill, who, while relatively stable, require complex extensive therapies. This assignment pattern and an astute new awareness of the patient's suffering create moral conflict and tension for the nurse:

Nurse: Well, I'm kind of at a crossroads right now. I'm trying to decide if I want to go on with being at the bedside, even, or if I want to leave the bedside. . . . I sometimes enjoy the work, but I just don't want to take care of these entities anymore, and it's just getting depressing, and I'm just ready to leave that aspect behind me. I feel like I'm not really giving nursing a fair chance when I don't like going to another area, and if I just leave with a kind of a bad taste in my mouth. So I'm kind of wondering if I should stay and do something else, do differently, and see if I like it better. I'm even thinking of doing some kind of consulting or something for a company that makes medical products that are used in cardiac diagnosis and treatment. . . .

I've always been interested in cardiology, and I will be interested in it for a long time. I'm kind of deciding if I should pursue taking the peds [*pediatric course*] also and getting more experience there with cardiac kids . . . I think what I'll probably end up doing is staying where I am a little longer and taking the peds course and go through that, and probably try to pursue my current position a little bit, and give it a time frame and see if it changes or if I change or whatever.

When I got out of nursing school, I just loved being at the bedside and part of me still does, but part of me doesn't like dealing with these people that don't respond and don't even talk or open their eyes. So I think that's really kind of burning me out, and [I] can't really feel like I'm doing any good for anybody anymore.

This nurse is experiencing a breakdown in the meanings that constitute and sustain her practice. She, in the same interview, wonders whether she has made the right career choice. She has been given a prolonged assignment of taking care of chronically critically ill nonresponsive patients. She cannot feel worthwhile in suspending someone in a prolonged dying process through technical interventions. Her work no longer makes sense and she is considering other options. As an intermediate level nurse, she is frequently assigned to complex chronically ill patients because the experts are assigned the most unstable patients, and the new graduates are assigned with preceptors to care for more typical acutely ill patients. This assignment pattern contributes to this nurse's discouragement with the nature of the work, and the moral weight of prolonging death rather than fostering cures or respectful deaths.

Nurses practicing at the competent level also confront the inequity of "enlightened" reasoning that delegates caretaking to lower-status groups, and devalues care of the body. Since there is little public language for caregiving work, they encounter a cultural silence around the care of the sentient, social body. The limits of medical interventions and the realities of misguided futile care become apparent. Competent nurses confront daily the relational ethics of their practice. The formal ethical principles typically taught in school do not cover the gamut of ethical issues they confront in practice, and once again the issue of matching the practical manifestations and variations with the formal teaching are present. Because the nurse is the one who is there and operates in between patient, family, and physician (see Bishop & Scudder, 1990) she can be left standing in the breach both clinically and ethically:

An elderly woman, living alone, had been in to see her doctor because she was complaining of shortness of breath. He [*the physician*] prescribed a diuretic and a tranquilizer. The woman's son, a nurse, called the physician because his mother wasn't any better. The next day the son found his mother unconscious at home, called the paramedics and started CPR. She was rushed to our unit, where she coded again . . . and was again resuscitated.

She was on the ventilator, her pupils fixed and dilated. She was on Lidocaine, Dopamine, Nitroglycerin, and Levophed. And the family was very upset with the physician, because the son kept telling the physician that he thought his mother was in pulmonary edema. She wasn't doing very well, but the family didn't feel like they wanted to make her a no code blue at that point. The family left around midnight, and around two in the morning, she started dropping her pressure. First, I would turn up the Dopamine, then the Levophed . . . dicker with this drip, dicker with that drip . . . and nothing was really working, so I call the doctor and he's says, "Oh, all right, just make her a no code blue." And I said, "She's going to die imminently . . . will you call the family?" And he flat out refused, because he was afraid he was going to get sued. I was really angry. You are left holding the bag. I'm left with all that responsibility, but no real decision-making [*power*].

The nurse is left to solve problems related to impending death and the human issues of coming to terms with death. The stark realities of practice do not match promises or expectations. The nurse experiences anger and moral outrage. Persistent remnants of this developmental crisis can be found in the experienced nurse who does not move to the level of proficiency or expertise (see Chapter 7).

Confronting Crises in Societal Caring

Confronting extreme deviancy and social disintegration shatters cultural illusions. For example, caring for addicted babies and their mothers confronts the nurse with issues that are centrally at odds with the goals of nursing care, and nurses must come to terms with this cultural conflict on a personal level:

Nurse: I really like what I do. What's interesting is how my attitude's changed since I left school. When I was doing my preceptorship in the nursery I couldn't even take care of druggy moms and their babies because I was so angry. And I had no sympathy for them. I thought they were the worst people in the world. I couldn't empathize with them at all. In my community health part of the education, they had a person come for the methadone program and tried to show the mom's side of the methadone program, why it was so good. And I had taken care of methadone babies. I knew how terrible they were. I just left because I just couldn't even listen to it. And now I think I went through a period of desensitization where every other kid I was taking care of was a crack baby or a cocaine baby or something like that. And now I just accept it; it happens and I have my crack moms.
Int: What changed that for you? You mentioned desensitization, but how?
Nurse: The more I took care of these kids, and maybe getting involved with a few of the parents' lives and really understanding probably why they abused

drugs, because they were abused and their parents used them. They had horrible childhoods. There are all kinds of reasons. I don't condone it, and I don't think that it is right, but I think I can relate to it better. I can deal with it, and I can be nonjudgmental. And I think that just took a little growing up on my part, because I was so young right out of nursing school . . . Drugs weren't a part of my life ever. And then seeing the real world and the cruel realities of it probably helped a lot.

Nurses must come to terms with the pain and with the differing values of those for whom they care. This same nurse went on to say that she was glad to have confronted these issues:

Nurse: But I think there is something worth confronting. I guess I wanted to confront that because otherwise it sort of was nebulous fear out there.

She has faced what she considers to be the worst and feels stronger for now being able to stay in the situation and be helpful. Like policemen, nurses in critical care must confront extreme deviancy. In response to the above excerpt, another nurse told a story of being confronted with a murderer sneaking in to finish the murder, though the victim was "brain dead." The man had weapons and was a physical threat to the nurses. This level of violence and threat is not in most nurses' consciousness during school or in their thoughts as they make their career choice. Therefore, the confrontation challenges their idealized version of nursing. In the same group, another nurse told about her responses to caring for a murderer:

I took care of a man who had shot one of the guys he was dealing drugs with and he was handcuffed to his bed because he was being held for murder. It was weird. The guy was very nice and very pleasant and courteous. Of course, I don't know that he had much option since he was handcuffed to the bed. But it was weird knowing that this guy killed someone else and we're supposed to take care of him.

Confronting deviance, and violence that may even be life-threatening, is an issue for all health care workers at all levels of experience. To come to terms with being a nurse, the recent entrant must now incorporate this understanding of their work and how they will respond as nurses.

Institutional Breakdown and its Impact on Practice and Career

Not all disillusionment and sense of failure can or should be attributed to the nurse's lack of experiential learning. Systems do fail and staffing is often inadequate to meet the caregiving requirements. Learning to recognize when working conditions are beyond safe practice is also experientially learned and tested. The nurse may feel failed by unreasonable demands and limited resources:

> I was scheduled to take over charge at 11:00 PM which was fine. Unfortunately, I was the only person on the schedule with any kind of experience . . . the patient census was very high acuity . . . and no one else was trained to go to codes even. We told staffing and the charge nurse of the intensive care unit, and the charge nurse of ICU was upset with us for being overstaffed . . . So there was no support for me whatsoever. While I was giving report, I noticed this one particular patient kept coming off the monitor. I went in the room to put him back on the monitor, and noticed that he was in extreme respiratory distress. He was becoming diaphoretic, his pressure was dropping . . . he went into acute pulmonary edema. I'm charge [nurse]. I walk into this situation where this patient is crashing. The nurse [taking care of the patient] didn't have a clue. . . .
>
> When I was new, I had expectations. This is how it should be. And two years down the line, I'm seeing very, very obviously that this is not how it is . . . There's a breakdown in your ideals . . . that you learned in nursing school . . . [You have this idea that] this is the kind of nurse I'm going to be and this is how it's going to be . . . and then finding out that that's not the case at all.

This nurse describes a common experience for nurses 2 to 3 years into their practice. She is placed in an untenable situation and she feels disillusioned. This situation should have been declared unsafe and additional help should have been marshalled. The union contract with this hospital allows for such action, and the nurse thought about it, in retrospect, but received very little support from the nurse manager for such an action. Nurses with 2 to 3 years of experience know their own limits better, and the limits of the resources available. But even in the worst conditions, their effective performance is still linked closely with their identity as nurses.

Because of the frequently unacceptable working conditions and increased sense of vulnerability and responsibility at this point, more nurses at the competent level than nurses in any other group talked about looking for another job or even leaving nursing altogether, indicating that this is a critical point of adapting to or rejecting work life demands. Advanced beginners who have worked less are protected by a secondary ignorance. They do not know what they do not know, and they do not yet bear the weight of expectations for complete role performance. But with time, performance expectations increase, as do the worker's expectations of the organization. Failed expectations at this point of disillusionment and a sense of hyper-responsibility make the entrant feel vulnerable and question whether the work demands are worth the personal cost.

EDUCATIONAL IMPLICATIONS

Studying the disillusionment and crisis of the competent nurse presents an ethical, professional, societal, and institutional challenge because the crisis of the entrant reflects the crises inherent in the health care system and in nursing education and practice. Their concerns and learning demands present an agenda for institutional and societal reform. Attending only to the nurse's "adjustment" problems makes us overlook the societal and institutional problems that create the problems for nurses, and reduces the social issues to psychological ones. Giving language and taking political action to correct the sources of the nurse entrant's crisis of "adjustment" avoids blaming the victim and placing the burden on the entrant to correct all the ills of a faulty system.

Breaking the silence is a first step. Giving these nurses a political platform within the organization and listening carefully to their struggles rather than insisting that they "cope" or manage are essential steps for creating institutional renewal that can alter this cycle of extreme disillusionment. We will discuss broader revisions in Chapter 13 on organizational impediments to patient care.

The competent stage is a critical developmental step in becoming an expert nurse. It is a point where nurses may change positions or careers in order to solve the crises they experience relating to the limits of their ability to cope with increased organizational demands through setting goals, planning to meet those goals, and struggling to keep things stable or in a status quo. They are beginning to understand that the nature of critical care nursing limits this coping strategy. Critically ill patients, by their very nature, change rapidly and sometimes unpredictably. Overreliance on structuring one's actions through goals and planning limits the nurse's ability to notice changes in the situation when goals and planning must also change. Too much emphasis on controlling the clinical situation decreases the ability of the nurse to notice alterations in the situation that call for new goals or altered plans.

A staff development intervention at this stage of skill acquisition is highly warranted to clarify common experiences such as hyper-responsibility and disillusionment, and to learn an appropriate level of involvement in patient and interpersonal problems.

Confronting Suffering, Coping, and Learning the Skill of Involvement

It was common to find nurses 2 to 3 years into their practice confronting suffering in new ways. Small group sessions with other nurses at the competent stage, key leaders in the unit, ethicists, and psychiatric liaison nurses may be highly beneficial at this point. Participating in more open collaborative discussions with physicians and other health care workers about prolonging dying and the excessive use of medical heroics could help improve the clinical judgment about the limits of medical intervention and also help these nurses articulate their ethical concerns. At the very least, it would demonstrate to these nurses that they are not alone in their perception of the patient's suffering and the limits of medicine.

Open discussions about learning skills of involvement with patients could also be highly beneficial to all nurses on the unit. The danger is that nurses may conclude that disengagement is the only viable coping strategy. If they reason in this way and disengage from patients too completely, they will lack sufficient involvement for engaged reasoning, perceptual acuity, and for connecting with patients/families in healing and therapeutic ways. Choosing small group discussions with highly effective nurses who manage to be skillfully engaged with patients and families, and who have found ways to cope with the suffering and ethical dilemmas around caring for the dying, can be extremely helpful. Staff development sessions with first-person narratives about confronting suffering, excessive medical intervention, and clarification about appropriate levels of care for those who are not to be resuscitated would be extremely helpful. Here we recommend joint meetings between nurses and physicians to establish clear guidelines for care of the dying, for setting limits on allowable medical interventions, and for defining the care of patients who are not to be resuscitated (see Pike, 1991; Wros, 1994). Making public these sources of ethical concern and conflict can improve the care and alleviate the isolation nurses feel, especially 2 to 3 years into the practice.

Coaching for Improved Perceptual Acuity

Precepting of competent nurses by proficient-to-expert nurses could be highly beneficial for showing the competent nurse how to read the situation and develop the skill of seeing changing relevance in patient care situations. Proficient nurses could be encouraged to develop and present narratives around changing their understanding of a clinical situation as it evolves. Narrative accounts that contain emotional responses provide better guides to enhancing problem identification and a vision for tailoring one's care and goals to patient/family changes.

Developing a more response-based approach (i.e., altering one's plans according to the situation and to the patient's responses) may appear to the competent nurse to be a loss of newly developed organizational skills. Stories of changing relevance, seeing changes in the relative importance of different aspects of the situation (see Chapter 5) can be an effective way of capturing the possibility and vision for a different approach to practice (Dreyfus & Dreyfus with Athanasiou, 1986). Because competent nurses rely heavily on analytical strategies, goal setting, and planning, they can benefit from practice in problem identification. Exercises in determining which among competing problems is the most salient can increase their powers of discernment. Similarly, practice in seeing the big picture, through detailed case analysis and following the patterns of response captured on the ICU patient flow sheets, can teach relationships between patient responses and related therapies (e.g., the titration of vasoactive drugs, or pain medication). This strategy was used by a competent nurse who had begun precepting new nurses:

Nurse: Now I am looking at the whole picture. Does the person need it? Does this cardiac index need it? You know the whole thing. So now I am not such a narrow-visioned person where I'm just looking at this one order.

Oftentimes when I orient nurses, I see that they are narrowly focused. They are just looking at one spectrum of the whole picture just like I was doing [*she refers to an error she made using Isuprel*], and I am never going to do that again. And my horror stories really emphasize this to the people I orient.

Int: You use horror stories to help someone?

Nurse: You bet. And I always tell them they can never make more errors than I did (laugh) because I can win [such a contest] no matter what they say. . . .

I take our 24-hour flow sheets, specifically with the heart patients and those with Swan Ganz and I say, "See how this affected urine output and this affected that and the heart rate affected this and going down on the dobutamine affected this." So I'm always including the whole spectrum so they can see it on the paper. And then I also give little scenarios: "O.K. so you see this and this and this, what do you think is going on?" Because they don't always cue in that cardiac output increased. They may be thinking of drugs or more concrete things rather than, "Oh, the heart rate went up just a little bit, so I use the whole spectrum."

The use of flow sheets to trace the effect of regulating fluid volume, administering vasopressors, antiarrhythmic drugs, and diuretics on the patient's cardiac perfusion, respiration, and vital signs allows the learner to see clinical patterns in the real situation. The goal is to teach the kind of modus operandi reasoning that is essential for administering response-based therapies. All of the nurses in this group agreed that precepting a beginner stretched their own abilities.

Many nurses, but particularly, the new graduates and competent level nurses talked about the value of "mistake stories" and "horror stories." These stories, when told with all their drama and immediacy, can be far more effective than procedural accounts because they are remembered complete with the sense of threat, danger, or relief. What was salient in the story becomes salient for the listener, and the perceptual world is changed so that the nurse's powers to notice without deliberation are enhanced.

As pointed out earlier, active involvement in actual codes in the role of recorder is an effective learning strategy that could be enhanced by debriefing and comparison of different resuscitation efforts. This would also be an excellent learning experience for undergraduates.

Addressing Organizational Impediments to Practice

Entrants to an organization with 2 to 3 years of experience offer a rich potential for organizational development. Creating an opportunity for them to meet with nurse managers, physicians, and key committees, after helping them identify their frustrations and concerns, can help the organization address the central function of patient care. These organizational development strategies diminish the invisibility of nursing practice and empower the nurse to become a part of improving the organization rather than becoming alienated or exiting the organization. Employers would be wise to spend time evaluating the adjustment demands of their organization for the person 2 to 3 years into the organization. Organizational design and development that fosters the satisfaction, success, and retention of the practitioner at this point could improve the practice of nurses at all levels of skill acquisition.

Telling and listening to narratives from practice that capture the best of practice helps identify and extend innovations in practice. Narratives of breakdowns, conflict, and ethical dilemmas can be a source for correcting barriers to good practice. Many of the frustrations of patients and nurses alike are related to real organizational impediments to good patient care, and work on these impediments can be a source of organizational renewal. Shared problem-solving with expert clinicians, physicians, and managerial staff can offer vital new suggestions for organizational renewal.

SUMMARY

The competent nurse experiences a critical juncture of increasing sense of agency and responsibility with the growing awareness of the limits of scientific knowledge for particular situations. This is coupled with firsthand experience with the varying levels of competence of coworker and the system. S/he is still experimenting with learning the skill of involvement. Indifference and detachment do not work, but many forms of involvement also do not work, and are sometimes painful. Furthermore, this stage of skill acquisition calls for new strategies for performance that are not so analytical and elemental. These new experiential demands create a difficult stage of transition. Unless the nurse can come to grips with these issues in ways that create new possibilities without too much personal distress and confusion, he or she will feel compelled to leave critical care nursing and perhaps leave nursing altogether.

Understanding, finally, that choosing a perspective alters what they do, and experiencing the ambiguity of open, evolving clinical situations, the nurse must come to terms with these newly perceived realities while gaining fresh personal and organizational skills and resources. This appears to be a critical developmental juncture. How nurses solve the crises and disillusion at this level of skill acquisition will determine whether they will make the qualitative leap to proficiency and expertise, and for many, whether or not they will stay in nursing.

Chapter 5

PROFICIENCY: A TRANSITION TO EXPERTISE

T he proficient stage is qualitatively different from the advanced beginner and competent stages and once entered will most usually lead to expertise with additional experience. Proficiency is a transition stage because once the nurse begins to see changing relevance, it seems that seeing a clinical situation in terms of a past clinical situation, complete with all its sense of salience, is a next step in the skill of seeing. The crucial shift is the perceptual ability to read the situation and respond appropriately. At this juncture, the nurses' organization may appear to deteriorate as they gain a qualitatively different approach to organizing their task world. Practice is transformed in six major ways:

1. the development of engaged reasoning in transitions;
2. emotional attunement to the situation—doing what needs to be done;
3. the ability to recognize changing relevance of aspects in the situation;
4. a socially skilled sense of agency; and
5. improved and more differentiated skills of involvement with patients and families.

Increased perceptual acuity and responsiveness to the particular situation are hallmarks of this stage. We expected that the movement into proficiency would be uneven and variable depending on the nurse's familiarity with particular areas of clinical caring practice. Proficient and expert performance require an experiential base with particular patient populations because these skill levels depend on a perceptual grasp of qualitative distinctions, which can only be acquired by seeing and contrasting many similar and distinct clinical situations as they evolve over time. Clinical reasoning in transitions, a sense of salience (i.e., having some things stand out as more or less important), and the recognition of changing relevance are perceptual skills that assist in identifying significant clinical problems. These skills of seeing require shifts in skilled know-how that are *qualitatively* distinct from the earlier stages of skill acquisition.

Experience, as defined here, is not the mere passage of time, but rather an active transformation and refinement of expectations and perceptions in evolving situations (Gadamer, 1975). The nurse shifts from exclusive use of objective characteristics and quantitative measures as guides to understanding and action with particular patients. Clinical reasoning is based on understanding patient changes through time, that is, reasoning through transitions.

As noted in the last two chapters, the move from advanced beginner to competent stages of skill acquisition is incremental in nature. Though the advance in actual performance is remarkable, it is occasioned by increased planning, familiarity with the environment, and increased skill in managing the environment and technology. Performance of tasks becomes smoother and quicker, so that organizational ability is further enhanced. Thus increments in skill development are continuous between the advanced beginner and competent stage. However, with proficiency, a qualitatively different way of being in the clinical situation emerges that is based on experiential learning. New perceptual and relational skills radically reshape performance capacity. Actions are now much more structured by the perceptual grasp of similarities and differences of the current and past clinical situations, and with perceived trends and meanings in the patient's situation.

As noted in Chapter 4, we sampled for nurses who had at least 2 to 3 years of experience in the critical care unit, but who may or may not have had other types of nursing experience. This sampling strategy yielded more proficient narratives than competent narratives, with nurses who had nursing experience prior to critical care being more likely to have proficient level narratives. Since our research goal was to describe the characteristics of the level of skill in particular clinical situations, and since we did not study nurses longitudinally, we did not address the question of typical time frames for developing a level of skill, nor the actual progression of skill levels within particular nurses.

ENGAGED REASONING IN TRANSITIONS

The knowledge of the particular patient contains many embodied, environmental, cultural, and therapeutic commonalities. A Cartesian view of the subject as a private separate subject representing and interpreting an objective world seeks to establish similarities and differences based upon objective disengaged criterial reasoning (Benner & Wrubel, 1989; Dreyfus, 1979, 1991). But the clinician must understand the distinctions and commonalities within the clinical situation as it evolves. This form of reasoning in transitions is engaged in historical or modus operandi reasoning (Bourdieu, 1990; Taylor, 1993). The nurse proficient in caring practices connects with a particular patient and his or her concerns. It is this connection that enables the nurse to understand and respond to what is salient in the situation. This greater facility at engaged reasoning in transition is characterized by a global understanding based on the integration of past experience:

> You're with the patient, you take care of them and you see them hour to hour exactly. They [*the physicians*] don't see every little drop in the blood pressure or every little change in the rhythm. They just kind of get an overview, where you are in there constantly ... They can go read the chart, you're in there. You're turning this patient, you're doing this, you're seeing every little aspect.

This excerpt illustrates a new level of skill of seeing and interpreting patient responses. The interviewer asks the nurse quoted above:

Int: Can you give a specific example of when you saw something very differently?

Nurse: They come in and look at the flow sheet and we don't, you can't write every, every change you know. Everyone always says, you may take hourly signs that you put on the chart, but if we had a little computer in our head that really wrote down every little blood pressure or heart rate we looked at for the day, it might be just fine. So they might come in and say, "He looks stable, why don't we take him off the dopamine." And we say, well, wait a minute, I didn't write everything down. I turned him and his blood pressure dropped—you don't know that. "Let's give him some Lasix." "No, he's not ready for that." . . . I notice that they're good about talking to you before making decisions.

The nurse is now synthesizing the meaning of patients' responses through time. She imagines that a computer could capture all her readings, but she fails to recognize that her understanding of the patient is now situated and based upon a practical understanding of the patient's response over time, rather on than a collection of data points. The clinician struggles with articulating this practical grasp:

Nurse: I had drawn a [*blood*] gas on a person and the gas was pretty poor and I took another gas to the house officer and he looked at it and said: "I don't believe this gas, the patient hasn't changed." And at that point—it takes a while to get to this point, but I felt comfortable in saying to him: "What do you mean, this patient hasn't changed? This patient's blood pressure has gone up to 200," and I presented him with a picture of this patient that he had obviously overlooked. It takes a while to get to the point where you can feel comfortable saying this to the doctor and feeling comfortable, feeling that you can go with your instincts.

Int: What happened in that situation?

Nurse: I was right.

Int: But what led you to believe that gas was correct?

Nurse: Well, there were a lot of objective things. This patient had been in a Pentobarb coma for a few days and they had just discontinued it that day. The nurse who gave report said: "Oh, he won't wake up tonight." But of course he did. And his respiratory rate was 36. He was breathing 24 over his vented breaths. His blood pressure had gone from 120 to 200 over a period of 3 hours. There was just a look about him that wasn't the same. You could look at him and tell that things had changed drastically in the last 5 or 6 hours.

Int: How did you learn that the objective signs that you were seeing were correlated with blood gas?

Nurse: Just experience and seeing different patients and different breathing patterns and knowing by looking at the patient that this breathing pattern is effective and this one isn't, knowing whether there is air exchange there or not. These breaths aren't effective and he's wearing himself out and that could be the cause of his deterioration in his gas, and just experience and seeing different cases and how people adjust to physical things that are going on.

Though difficult to articulate, this practical grasp is not mystical. It reflects the skill of seeing practical manifestations of changed physiological states and patient responses, and engaging in practical reasoning about these transitions. The nurse actively interprets the direction of the change and keeps track of what can be ruled in and ruled out. Practical grasp is perceptually grounded and response-based and requires being open to correction and disconfirmation as the situation unfolds. The clinician is always in the situation with some practical understanding, and it is that practical understanding that is revised or confirmed. In situations where patterns and trends are clear and have definitive interventions associated with the clinical trend, the practitioner can make quick decisive responses. When the practitioner's grasp of the patient's clinical situation is jarred by changes or unexpected patient responses, the practitioner searches for a new grasp and if all goes well, experiential clinical learning occurs. Engaged reasoning through transitions requires being open to correction and dis-confirmation. The ethos of openness, rather than prediction and control, and fidelity to what one sees and hears, rather than excessive suggestibility and confusion, are embodied and linked to emotional responses to the situation. Thus, one's skilled emotional responsiveness guides perceptual acuity *and* responsiveness to changes in the situation.

The proficient nurse's possibilities of engagement in the situation are radically different than those of the new graduate nurse because the technical mastery of skills and task performance no longer demands so much of their attention. Also, they have experientially learned to recognize clinical changes and diverse ways patients respond to suffering and comfort. They can now trust that their loss of practical grasp or discomfort in a situation is meaningful, i.e., connected to what is occurring in the situation. Therefore, these emotional responses can reliably guide them in a search for a more definitive understanding of the changes in the situation. This is in stark contrast to the advanced beginner, who may have a much more generalized anxiety.

At the proficient stage the nurse can develop an ethic of responsiveness to the particular situation. The ability to read the particular situation based on the sense or practical grasp and the emotional response to the situation increases the powers of understanding. An ethic and skill of responsiveness will prevent the practitioner from reading his or her own responses into the situation or be indifferent or blind to the patient's situation and concerns.

EMOTIONAL ATTUNEMENT TO THE SITUATION, DOING WHAT NEEDS TO BE DONE

Proficient practitioners are better situated, meaning that they can see aspects of the situation rather than understanding the situation in terms of rules and context-free attributes. They can see relationships among aspects of a situation. They have a growing sense of nursing concerns and contrast them with medical concerns. They are becoming at home in familiar situations. Whereas the new graduate suffers from the inability to recognize situations, and the competent nurse overdefines the situation, the proficient nurse's practical grasp of the situation is increasingly accurate, and thus when a practical grasp is missing, the nurse feels uncomfortable or a vague uneasiness. It is no accident that emotional response language increases during this stage of skill acquisition. Increasingly, nurses say: "I felt uneasy" or "I felt comfortable." Emotional responses, mood, and the climate of the situation become important in their narratives. These feelings are not just a self-reference to internal emotional states. They point to what nurses notice in the situation. To have a perceptual grasp of the situation is to have an emotional tone related to the situation. Emotional responsiveness and tone are central to having an embodied skilled know-how and signal an understanding of the situation as well as a way of being in it.

All of the examples depicting gaining a sense of salience, increased emotional attunement, and recognizing changing relevance demonstrate the role of emotion in experiential learning. They illustrate the process of gaining embodied know-how and illustrate the role of emotion in recognition of significance and in problem identification. Because emotion has traditionally been treated as primarily an interruption or distortion of "rational problem solving," delineating the role of emotional responses in acquiring clinical expertise is particularly relevant for the nurse at the proficient level. Emotional language is distrusted in our Cartesian legacy of separating emotion from thinking and knowing (Benner & Wrubel, 1989; Vetlesen, 1994). The Cartesian perspective is not so inaccurate for the novice or advanced beginner, whose emotional responses are likely to reflect a pervasive mood of fear and anxiety about the unknown or their awkward performance capacity. Novice and advanced beginner performance usually will improve by dampening anxiety and fear. But it is a mistake to overgeneralize detachment from emotional responses to subsequent levels of skill acquisition (see Chapter 1). While practitioners must be able to discern when emotional states carried over from other situations are falsely coloring current perceptions, eliminating or ignoring *all* emotional responses will prevent proficient and expert performance. Emotional responses enable fuzzy recognition powers that allow the practitioner to respond to dimly perceived changes in the clinical situation (Dreyfus, 1979, 1991; Wrubel, Benner, & Lazarus, 1981). Of course, the clinician must not proceed to interventions before the clinical situation is understood sufficiently to guide action, but emotional responses to early changes or nuances in the situation allow for lifesaving lead time in clinical detection.

The whole picture, as the nurse has now come to understand it, guides the way care is given. The nurse now has an ability to read the situation so that actions are guided by that reading. Emotional responses guide attentiveness and consultation with others. Based upon their emotional responses to the situation, nurses perceive whether or not they have a good grasp of the situation without calculation.

Giving patient information is a good example of changes brought about by developing better emotional attunement to the situation. Giving information can no longer be a matter of blindly following a principle of telling the truth. The practitioner now feels the demand for timing, and being oriented to what the patient and family can understand and are ready to confront. For example, a nurse talks about learning how to fit the giving of information to the patient/family's response to the information. The nurse's discussion can no longer be a simple matter of giving all the "objective information" based upon the ethical principle of the patient's right to know. The ethical tension encountered is to be truthful, but now the nurse recognizes that "medical truth" is not static. It changes over time and has unintended ramifications; therefore the nurse begins to be sensitive to the patient's response to the "current truth." This is an unsettling change from the initial simplistic understanding of what it means to be truthful and open with patients and families. The intent is not to deceive or cover over information, rather there is an increased awareness of the need to respond to what the patient/family is asking and wants to know:

Nurse: Transplant patients and families are very knowledgeable about their disease and about their medication because they need that control. They have spent so much time in liver failure or renal failure that they know what creatinine means, what bilirubin means, and their lab values everyday make a big difference to them for that day. If the bilirubin is up, they're really depressed for the day and that's really hard for them. I learned how much to tell them, what to tell them, how to tell them and when to start teaching. You don't want to tell them too much, because then they fixate and get stressed about everything. So you tell them little bits and pieces and try to tell them good things, but not blow the good things out of proportion because if the bad thing happens, they're just knocked down and they don't know how to deal with it . . . So I definitely learned to judge, to have a clue about how much families can take, how much they know, how much they need to know . . . I think it comes from knowing, having a good sense of people, and giving them as much as they can take in that day.

So nurses learn the perspective of the family and gradually tailor information to the clues about how much families want to know on a given day. Attunement to patient/family needs and desires for information is in the context of a strong nursing ethos for full truth-telling and openness about diagnoses and patient condition. In fact, it is this background ethical concern that shapes the narratives of adjustment and attunement. The nurse must learn when not to tell and how much to tell in response to the patient/family clues and guidance without slipping into deception or keeping secrets. This is the qualitative distinction between deception and humane sharing of information that fits the request and understanding of the information by the patient/family. The principle of truth-telling is an important background and safeguard that can provide correction to errors in judgment. From the principle of autonomy, this may appear paternalistic, but the nurse is clear in the narrative that she is learning to follow the patient's family's cues and guidance.

Without concrete first-person experience, emotional attunement to the situation is impossible. For example, the proficient nurse now has enough direct observation and experience to recognize trends and have strong convictions about whether a patient is deteriorating, improving, or on the road to recovery. These understandings and expectations are experience-

based and depart from clinically predicted timetables. The following neonatal ICU nurse illustrates this new confidence:

> Oh, of course he's going to make it. He's getting better every day. He's gain-
> ing weight. His heart and lungs do not sound as good as they should. He
> has to have the facial CPAP every 4 hours to open up the alveoli because
> they clamp down because he doesn't have any surfactants to keep them open,
> but he's strong. He'll probably be okay.

This level of confidence is possible because the nurse has seen other
babies with this degree of illness recover. It is interesting to note that most
experts perhaps would leave more room for doubt, based upon having been
surprised by unexpected turns in clinical courses (many experts made dis-
claimers about "never" being certain, having been surprised a number of
times, and even this nurse concludes that he'll "probably" be okay). What
is notable is the budding capacity to recognize a trend and probable outcomes. The nurse now has the experiential basis to recognize familiar trajectories and have confidence about the combined signs of progress which
signal recovery. Recognizing trends is the harbinger of the expert level of
performance where current actions are guided by the perspective about
the patient's future trajectory.

Predictions about a patient's future trajectory are based on engaged
reasoning in transitions and first-hand recognition, rather than matching
theoretical and objective criteria to features and attributes of the situation.
Attunement is now possible because the nurse's attentiveness is guided
by salient aspects of the situation. This allows for a smoother response-
based approach to the situation. Planning and deliberate reflectiveness
decrease.

The proficient performer perceives and responds to patients/families
with a qualitatively different kind of attunement. With repeated performance and increased confidence in her or his attunement to the situation,
the nurse is increasingly confident that she or he will be able to do what is
required. This is illustrated in the following excerpt, where a critical care
transport nurse describes the experientially learned ability to resuscitate
an infant:

Nurse 1:   The residents don't do transports very often. They are not used to doing
as much as the nurse is doing, and the nurses work better together and get the
baby "spiffed up" faster [resuscitated and stable] because we are just used to
doing it, and you just do whatever needs to be done. I was working on one new
baby by myself and I got a line in, and then he was working on the other baby
and put the line in. And he decided to let the referring physician intubate the
other baby, and I was going to intubate my kid and take my time to intubate

because my kid was a little more stable, so I had a little extra time to get things ready. And the referring physician was just watching like a hawk. He was amazed, like "Whoa, the pressure's on." He probably hadn't done it in ages himself. And so it was kind of fun. We would say, "My pressure's this, what's yours?" They go, "Oh well, we haven't done any of those." It's like: "We haven't got the blood pressure." It's fun, laughing back and forth about: "Oh, you do it."
Nurse 2:   Everybody has a specialized role, and you just kind of go back and forth and there's camaraderie. It's kind of a nice thing.

"Just doing whatever needs to be done" is a skilled response based on knowing how and when. As Dreyfus pointed out when comparing human expertise to computerized capacities, the human expert can respond in a way that is as orderly as the situation demands (Dreyfus, 1979, 1991). In the high time demand of the clinical emergency, increased perceptual acuity and skilled know-how help the nurse to respond to the situation in a fluid, nonreflective way. The skilled actions are themselves now a way of "thinking" because the actor is responding to experientially learned distinctions and timing. When the nurse talks about taking her time, she is probably talking about a process lasting less than a minute—which during a resuscitation can seem like a very long time.

CHANGING RELEVANCE AND SITUATED RESPONSES

Recognition of changing relevance is a major theme of the proficient nurses' narratives. Overturned expectations often constitute the themes and plot of the story. They now see contextual and situational changes that require actions other than those planned or anticipated. Discoveries of changes in the clinical situation now loom large in the narratives. These practitioners have an increased ability to recognize and respond to changing relevance in the patient's condition, as illustrated in the next excerpt:

We admitted a man who became very sick very quickly. He had a huge infarct. About two hours after he was admitted, he had vomited and obviously had aspirated his vomitus. He was hypoxic. He was blue and crawling off the stretcher. He was a huge man. I said to the intern. "You need to draw a blood gas." And he said: "I drew one when he came in." I looked at the resident and I threw the blood gas syringe and I said, "Could you please draw a blood gas." His P0$_2$ was 30 or something like that. He had to be intubated. I said: "You know, the situation changes often, and you can't say, 'I drew one.'" I said, "Look at him. Take a gander. Does this look like the same patient you drew the blood gas on?" He just didn't know what to do.

Here the proficient nurse recognizes a change in the situation, and the intern isn't responding to the change. While hypoxia seems obvious from the description, the intern probably had little practical experience with such rapid changes and in the urgency of the situation probably had little sense of the passage of time. Learning about the actualities of clinical change is a good example of experiential clinical knowledge. Any one of these clinicians would have been able to answer a formal test question about the possibility of blood gas changes within an hour, and correctly identify conditions under which oxygenation changes rapidly, so it is not "factual" knowledge that is at stake here. Rather, skilled recognition of salient facts and orchestration of skilled responses within the time demands of the situation constitute the relevant knowledge and skills.

Anticipation of likely changes and following guidelines for changes are different perceptual skills than recognizing a contextually determined shift in priorities. What is new at the proficient level is the nurse's ability to read the situation and notice when the patient's condition has changed sufficiently to warrant a redefinition of the situation and thus a change in perspective or actions. The skill of seeing has become a direct perceptual grasp through association; however, the proficient nurse may not immediately comprehend what action to take in response to the pattern recognition. This is illustrated in one nurse's description of learning to recognize needed shifts in therapies for post-operative heart patients:

> I feel pretty comfortable, and you learn when they're warming to start giving the volume and when to stop because now maybe they need a little bit of Levophed to keep their blood pressure up, when to shut off the Levophed because they're waking up and you know their catecholamines have kicked in and that kind of thing. It's almost routine, whereas before it took a lot of trial and asking questions.

This change is based on procedural knowledge and protocols, but the transition being described is the flexible recognition of patient changes in particular situations. These decisions cannot be based on quantitative physiological measures alone, but must be based on understanding the relationship between the numbers and the way the patient looks and responds. This form of response based action is crucial for performing well in a rapidly changing emergency, as illustrated in the following example of preparing a critically ill infant for transport:

> It was good that there were two of us [nurses] who were both senior. The kid's right lung was down and the doctor was able to get a chest tube in, but he wasn't getting any air back. We listened and there were no breath sounds and so it's like go through the process as fast as you can and try to think of what's wrong. We had a tube in one side and there were just mini-

mal breath sounds, and then it went to nothing, so one person started suctioning and got a mucous plug out. And I tried inserting a needle in one
side of the chest, but couldn't get any air out. Then while I was doing that,
the pediatrician pulled out the one chest tube that he had put in. And then
the kid had no breath sounds on that side again, so we were bagging him.
We started to have better breath sounds on one side, so I put a chest tube in
on the other side. [*The story continues with much troubleshooting and response
before and after the transport and concludes with a report that the child is now a
healthy 2-year-old with no brain damage.*]

The skill of resuscitating an infant requires rapid response to what is actually occurring. The practitioners must take into account the skill of the team
working with the infant, but the infant's actual responses must guide the
action. For such an action-oriented skill, the analogy of learning to play in
a sport is strikingly similar. As Bourdieu (1990) points out:

> The term academicism is inherent in every attempt to make explicit and
> codify a practice that is not based on knowledge of the real principles of
> practice. For example, research by some educationalists . . . who have en-
> deavored to rationalize the teaching of sporting or artistic activities by try-
> ing to favour conscious awareness of the mechanisms really at work in the
> practices, shows that, if it fails to be based on a formal model making ex-
> plicit the principles which practical sense (or more precisely, the "feel for
> the game" or tactical intelligence) masters in the practical state and which
> are acquired practically through mimeticism, the teaching of sport has to
> fall back on rules and even formulae, and focus its attention on typical phases
> ("moves"). It thus runs the risk of often producing dysfunctional disposi-
> tions because it cannot provide an adequate view of the practice as a whole
> (for example, in rugby, training draws attention to the links between team-
> mates instead of giving priority to the relationship with the opposing side,
> from which successful teamwork derives). (p. 103)

The clinician must not only learn the scientific and technological rules of
the game, but must also learn how to see and attend to the patient's responses and anticipate probable future courses of events in the clinical
situation. The clinical learner needs to focus on identifying and rapidly responding to chains of events. The patient's changing condition and concerns, like Bourdieu's opposing team, provide puzzles, risks, challenges,
and possibilities for the clinician's responses.

An experientially gained sense of perspective and timing allows them to
notice when past concerns are no longer the issue. This recognition may be
vague at first but become clearer with reflection. Nurses talk about noticing
new versus obsolete concerns in their narratives, and this ability to notice when
a change in direction is needed often shapes their stories. From experience,
they now have the capacity to notice when things do not go as they expect;

consequently, missed timetables in a patient's recovery, and an absence of expected patient responses, show up in their narratives. General patterns and expectations create emotionally toned perceptions in the situation. What is absent can now guide nurses' perceptions of the situation, because they now have enough experience to recognize when things are awry.

The changing relevance noticed need not be an emergency. Often it relates to recognition of slowly accrued changes and progress in patients' capacities for eating, sleeping, moving, et cetera. Responding to changed capacities can hasten recovery. For example, in the following excerpt, the nurse recognizes that the patient no longer needs the Kin Air bed (a specialized bed that prevents pressure sores):

> A bed doesn't seem like a big deal with all the clinical expertise that we have, but it is a big deal. That's something I have learned. . . . In terms of manpower it's a major decision to put somebody on a Kin Air bed, because if somebody is on bed rest and immobilized, it takes about five or six people to do the switch from a regular bed to the Kin Air bed. . . . I think that's one factor that causes a lot of nurses to forget about taking a patient off the Kin Air bed. To take them off, again, you have to mobilize all these resources.

This nurse notices the improvement of the patient; that she now has more mobility; that she needs some outward sign of her progress; and that the noise of the bed is now disrupting sleep since she is now capable of longer periods of sleep. All of these are indicators of changed relevance for different aspects of care.

The nurse herself recognizes that she can now make a difference in the patient's care and sees herself as an initiator of change, and this is a different form of agency than following the plans and expected guidelines typical of the competent stage. Recognizing changing relevance is not just a matter of timing, it also requires making qualitative distinctions, the hallmark of clinical and ethical judgment (see Chapter 7; Taylor, 1989, pp. 21–30). For example, the following nurse talks about learning to give control back to a transplant patient and makes the qualitative distinction between necessary dependency and lack of control:

> Transplant patients become so dependent on you for everything—Can I brush my teeth now? Do you think I should do this? And you have to really encourage them to take control back. It's a hard concept for a lot of them because they need to be dependent because it's safe for them to be dependent . . . I've learned how to give them control back slowly and how to encourage them to take that control back over their own life.

Qualitative distinctions are laden with tone and emotional and attitudinal qualities, as well as action and contextual qualities. In the context of extreme fatigue or the beginning of rejection or infection, the transplant patient may have to relinquish most independence, but with astute coaching the patient can often retain control over information and participation in decision making may be retained even in extreme periods of dependency.

Proficient nurses talk about their newfound ability to recognize changes in the meaning of signs and symptoms. The following nurse describes such a change in a woman who had been resuscitated successfully:

Nurse: She was so much better. She was out of bed and she had her makeup on and her perfume on and her pocketbook right next to her. It was a nice change from how I had seen her over the past 2 weeks.

Int: Did your priorities change in terms of taking care of her last night?

Nurse: Definitely . . . A lot of things didn't matter anymore. It didn't matter to me really if she was straight in the bed, as long as she was comfortable . . . It didn't matter if her A line read 80, because [her arm] was up over her head . . . That was really important last week, but it didn't matter because her blood pressure wasn't 80, and if she wanted to put her arms over her head, let her. I cared more about was she comfortable, was she able to get up when she wanted to . . . My priorities changed from the physiologic more to the comfort.

Though it sounds obvious, this ability to be confident in the changing physical state requires experiential learning. Initially, objective signs and symptoms are just that, objective, but with experience, the nurse can evaluate them more readily in terms of context and significance. The narrative typically depicts increased flexibility and fluency. The nurse's knowledge of the context has become more sophisticated and nuanced.

Identifying changing relevance improves response time. This is evident in the example of an early warning:

Nurse: I was taking care of a baby with a complex heart disease who had a shunt placed, and had been extubated earlier that day. Around midnight he started to get a little more pale and a little bit more [*inaudible*] and his lung sounds were okay. They had a few crackles, but nothing really significant. And by about 2:00 AM he was looking quite a bit worse and very wet which is like he was dumping fluid into his lungs. So I went ahead without—I just decided to try to get as much information as I could about the baby before I went and got the doctor up because this doctor tended to be less likely to take action. So I got a blood gas and the pH was 7.2. The blood gas was very low, but the CO_2 was 55. The baby's neck veins were distended. So I went and got the doctor up and told her what the baby looked like. She came over and listened to the baby and said there's no fluid in that kid's lungs. It's just the stethoscope rubbing against the chest wall. And I said "It doesn't sound like that to me." I said "I didn't hear this at midnight and I'm hearing it now." And she said: "That is not fluid. That baby is dry." The baby had a spell earlier in the day and she kept saying: "Well he looks so much better than he did earlier today. He'll come out of this by himself." And I requested that we could give some bicarbonate and Lasix, and she agreed to the bicarbonate and refused the Lasix saying that the baby's lungs were dry and then she said: "Well, let's go ahead and get a chest film so you can see for yourself." So she ordered a film and X-ray. Usually X-ray will just call and tell us that the film is ready but this time they called and said: "Your film looks awful." They usually never tell us what it looks like, so I said: "Does it look awful like the baby's doing bad? Or does it look awful because you need to take the film again?"

So the nurse who had answered the phone came down in the front and said: "They said it's awful, the baby's lungs are terrible." And the doctor said: "Oh, let me go down and look at it." She still didn't believe it was bad, so when she left the unit, I had five other people come over and assess the baby to see what they all felt. The baby had a lot of fluid in his lungs, and the doctor came back, and the film was completely whited out. You could not tell the heart from the lungs. There was just no evidence at all. And I asked about Lasix and she said. "But the baby's not wet." I said "I'm sorry, I had five other people listen while you were gone and they all think the baby's wet." And she stomped off the unit to call an attending physician on her own. She's absolutely furious at this point, and I was getting really nervous and I finished giving the bicarb about a half hour previously and I looked at the baby and he looked much worse, than he had before.

Int: How did he look much worse to you?

Nurse: His mouth was just open slightly. He was gasping to try to breathe. He just looked awful, looked absolutely terrible and so I asked the doctor if I could go ahead and get another blood gas. And she came out from talking to the other doctor and said: "Have you given Lasix yet?" and I said: "You haven't ordered it." And so she said: "Go ahead and give Lasix." So the doctor did tell me that she called at home and the doctor said that he wanted some Lasix, so I gave the Lasix, but at that point the baby was looking so bad that I didn't even wait for the Lasix to take effect before I went ahead and did another blood gas without the resident's order and the pH by this time was 6.74 and his CO_2 was 155. And so we had started bagging the baby before I got the results of the gas back just because the CO_2 was so high and the baby's saturations were dropping by this point so that we intubated the baby, and then by this point I think the doctor realized that she had made a mistake in being a little less willing to take charge and to go ahead and to do things for the baby instead of waiting for the baby to pull himself out of it, which he was obviously not going to do. So she went ahead and ordered the [*ventilator*] pressures to be given pretty high and the rate turned up to 80 and within minutes, the baby had started to pick up. His eyes were open. He was looking around and just got better and I guess three days ago, he got to go home. . . . When it came to a very, very critical point we [*the physician and I*] were able to work together and get the kid taken care of.

The ability to recognize that the infant "looks awful," and to hear the wetness of the lungs, are both qualitative distinctions that compels the nurse to respond. In the narrative we are placed into the field of tensions and appraisals. When the nurse's own certainty waivers in the face of the dis-agreement about how wet the lungs were, she asks her colleagues to listen and they agree that the lungs are indeed wet. Once the physician sees the patient as the nurse does, she too sees the same responses as appropriate. The nurse's early warning declares itself to be the correct appraisal, but the clinician cannot afford to wait until the situation is unequivocal, be-cause with infants there is little time between the recognition of impend-ing danger and catastrophic outcomes.

AGENCY

Because the clinical world is increasingly differentiated so that some things automatically claim attention (a sense of salience), the nurse is freed from the hyper-responsibility experienced at the competent stage. Deliberate anticipation of changes is no longer required. Numbers gain meaning, or salience so that the focus is no longer so much on the patients' charts as it was for the new graduate:

> It is the difference between staying in your room and writing down all those little numbers and making sure they're on a sheet, and getting to the point where you know what the numbers mean, you have done the typical things that you can do [standing orders and protocols for blood gasses, and medications] and then you call the doctor in the middle of the night instead of waiting until 6:00 AM so that when they do rounds they won't ask you why you didn't call them.

Knowing what things can and cannot wait has been experientally learned and now shapes the nurse's agency. Meaningful trends and patterns emerge. With an increased ability to make distinctions and understand the particular situation, flexibility increases. The performer no longer has to wait to be told what is relevant. These new perceptual skills and ways of being in the situation alter the nurse's agency, that is, the way she or he influences and acts in the situation. An increased ability to read the situa-tion and respond with as much order as the situation demands is less self-focused, in that the constraints and possibilities inherent in the situation are acknowledged. This is illustrated in the following comparison of the first 6 months on the unit with the second year:

> My organization skills have improved. . . . You know that if you have 12 things going on, some things have to be prioritized and left out. . . . The first 6 months you might dwell on it more and be harder on yourself . . . you feel

terrible, that you didn't get this done . . . [*You worry*] that something bad is going to happen to the baby later because you missed something. But you just learn what is important, I guess, as you have more experience.

With experience the nurse notices a shift in his or her ability to notice what is important. The nurse no longer has the level of anxiety about the consequences of what she might leave out because she has more confidence in her ability to notice the important things.

The emerging sense of salience is not infallible, but still is a real advance over the earlier undifferentiated dread or worry that a nebulous "something important" will be missed. The heightened skills of perception and judgment, coupled with the experiential learning that allows for missed signs and symptoms, make this a time when the nurse confronts the full level of responsibility inherent in the work. In the following interview excerpt, the nurse has a sense that more seasoned nurses do not feel responsibility in the same way as in the past. The discussion moves to how she is increasingly better able to manage her responsibility:

You are able to use more resources besides yourself and maybe at first you start to realize that there's a problem and you're not really sure which way to turn or even if you should turn, or whether you should even take action or not. But I think after a while you start to realize you can take action and you know where to go and where to get the help to take that action that you need. And where, if you can't handle a problem, where to turn or where to focus it. And that you do not bear the full responsibility. The doctor is in on this too, and the charge nurse is responsible too. So it's not shirking the responsibility, but it's sharing it instead of keeping it to yourself. Because I think you really take the weight of the world on your shoulders when you've got this whole person, and you feel: "Oh, my God, if anything happens to them, it's all my fault."

The above excerpt illustrates the increased sense of social integration and shared responsibility that can only come from learning experientially what the team members have to offer and the recognition of the limits of any one person's contributions (see Chapter 8). It is easier to ask for help when one can be articulate about what help is needed or even what the problem is. Proficient nurses talk about feeling comfortable when they have a good understanding of the patient situation (Tanner et al., 1993).

The task demands of the ICU are dense, and time is frequently parsed in 5-minute segments or less. Thus it is not surprising that gaining a perspective is a major aspect of experiential learning that creates new forms of agency. Competent nurses continue the dialogue begun at the competent stage of relating and synthesizing the interrelationships between all the medical realities. Nurses talk about seeing the "whole" picture and the "big" picture. The whole picture typically refers to the human side of the patient's needs, and the bodily care aspects, such as the need for skin care, nutritional needs, and monitoring comfortable levels of stimulation, as illustrated below:

Nurse: On [physician] rounds the doctors address the major issues and what steps they're going to take that day to improve the situation. There comes a time when you've been there for so long that you have to jump in with the other issues that are important to that patient. "What about feeding this patient? What about this decubitus, doesn't it need debriding?" Sometimes they overlook these things. You're thinking more about all the systems, where the doctors are more focused on what's the patient's main problem.
Int: When did that start happening?
Nurse: It took a while. It seems like once I overcame, getting used to the tasks and getting comfortable with the environment, and was able to focus more on the patient. I don't know, I really can't put a time on it.

Increasingly, practice is guided by good outcomes. It is no longer enough to have performed efficiently, or to know the right answers. The nurse feels satisfied when the outcomes are good and dissatisfied when things do not turn out well. These appropriate emotional responses are at the heart of developing expert clinical and ethical comportment. The community standards evident in dialogue and discussion among practitioners and from physicians, patients, and families set the conditions, for what the nurse feels good about may be sources of disappointment and embarrassment. For example, a nurse responds to the interviewer's question about what makes a good code in the following way:

The guy wakes up and talks to you. That's the only qualification. A code can be messy and horrid, but if he wakes up later and talks to you, it's worth it.

Nurses talk about their way of being in the situation as being comfortable or confused. They less often feel overwhelmed or lost. As noted earlier, since their anxiety is now generally lower, they can begin to trust their emotional responses to guide their attentiveness and calls for help. Having an increased perspective about the situation and past experience at feeling a better grasp of the situation than they do currently enables competent nurses to sense impending doom and experience dread. This is illustrated in the next narrative. Here, the nurse has been unsuccessful in getting the interns and residents to share her assessment that a child's condition is deteriorating. She calls the attending physician because a sedative has been ordered, instead of the resident coming to examine the child:

I called D. at home and I explained the situation of both kids to him and he at that point told me that my feeling of impending doom with J. was probably accurate because he's critically ill, and "if his heart stops, if he codes, we're not going to get him back." . . . The attending said, "Okay, I know what's going on. I understand what you're saying and the dose [of the sedative] is small and if he really needs sleep, then maybe we should go ahead and give it to him, but at least you've notified somebody else before you've done it." So we did end up giving it to him, which I didn't feel comfortable in doing. But when everybody else says: "Give it" what are you going to do? And he did need sleep, but that wasn't what his problem was. . . . He did end up coding and of course, they didn't get him back.

It is telling that the nurse breaks her identification with the resuscitation team calling the team a "they" even though she herself is a member of the team. This no doubt reflects her sense of alienation in the face of her helplessness to alter this situation. The child's death is a tragedy, and one that is recognized as impending, but one for which the nurse is not able to marshal adequate preventive resources. Indeed, probably few options were available, and no one had an adequate grasp of the situation because "one thing after another occurred" with no one understanding what was causing the child's distress. It is, however, a turning point for this nurse's sense of agency and responsibility. Her assessment is accurate, but she is not able to marshal effective help for the child. Instead she confronts avoidance on the part of the resident and acknowledgment of the grimness of the situation on the part of the attending physician. She is left with the instruction to give the sedative, which does not address the sources of the child's distress. She confronts the ethical demand of being the one to get help, to marshal support, and procure effective interventions, and in this situation confronts the limits of her ability to convey the gravity of the situation and the limits of medical interventions to alter the situation.

LEARNING THE SKILL OF INVOLVEMENT

Learning how to confront one's own anxiety in the face of suffering and loss is a major experiential learning never learned once and for all. We have much evidence that learning experientially how to be engaged in the clinical situation and be connected with patients/families in ways that are helpful is central to clinical expertise and skillful ethical comportment. Nurses must learn how close to stand in relation to the patient and families. They must guide their involvement so that they do not over- or underidentify with the

patient/family plight. Learning the skill of involvement is necessarily existential, involving personal knowledge. Nurses learn by being overinvolved
or too detached. The skill of involvement requires attunement, because what
is an appropriate level of involvement during a critically ill phase is usually excessive during the recovery phase. Learning the skill of involvement
is further complicated by different comfort zones and expectations of patients and families. Recognizing signs of trust and comfort versus threat can
only be learned by taking care of many patients over time.

In the following example, a nurse reflects on her relationship to the family in a situation where the medical treatment, after the fact, was considered to be inappropriate, prolonging the suffering and dying of a young
child. She demonstrates a strong sense of agency and responsibility in the
situation and indicates that it was the first time she ever knew a patient so
well that she was effective in predicting impending crises. Her reflection
has to do with how her intense involvement with the little boy influenced
the medical and nursing care:

Nurse: My emotions in the end did get involved because I wasn't sure if I was the
best person to take care of him because I wasn't sure if I could see over what
was really happening, if I was making the best judgment. Medically my care
was fine. Towards the end I really tried to push the mother [to recognize the
futility of the heroic measures], but it was hard for me because I really cared
about them. It was almost like I was too involved that I couldn't push her to the
point and say, "Okay, stop." But I don't know if that was the best point, though,
they were such a strong family. I don't think they would have. I really don't.

Int: It's very hard to go back and sort of second-guess it . . .

Nurse: At the time, I didn't really think about it. It wasn't until everything was
over when I went back and said: "Did I do what was right for that family?" Or
should I have pushed them way before, and said ["You are being selfish."] because they really trusted me. Or did I not push them enough because I was
selfish in myself? They were such a strong family. If I had tried to direct them
differently [to decrease the heroic measures] they may have turned against me,
because they did turn against some physicians who didn't think they were
doing the right thing for the little boy anymore and tried to get them to stop
heroics. And I certainly didn't want them to do that after 18 months.

This is a tragic case because the nurse's exquisite knowledge of the little
boy allowed her to provide many lifesaving early warnings of septic shock,
that later felt like contributing to the child's torture rather than helping.
The level of connection between the child and nurse is evident in the following excerpt:

I was real close to the mom, but the child—it was not as if he could talk to
me, or something like that, but there was just something—he really knew
me, and his eyes would light up when I came in on a daily basis. So of course

that would get to me. And people would say, "He just doesn't act like that with anyone else."

This was the first time this nurse had become a significant engaged caregiver for an infant. Her sense of responsibility and responsiveness was heightened by the infant's response to her over a period of a year and a half. In the course of the two interviews, this nurse explained that this situation was still emotionally laden and still guides her level of involvement with other infants. She felt that she "had given beyond her means" and she was afraid that her involvement had contributed to the child's prolonged painful dying. Since this incident, she has taken shorter assignments or staff resource nurse assignments that do not require close sustained relationships with infants. She did not indicate that the child's trust and relationship to her was a "good" for the child or for her because she was so acutely aware of the "bad" outcome (a prolonged painful, disfiguring treatment leading to death). She lives out the cultural fear that involvement is dangerous and leads to poor decisions. She confronts the pain of emotional labor and does not notice the other extreme negative possibility of an infant being cared for by strangers for a year and a half with no attachment and trust, though she is aware that the child would not have survived without the attentive care that she gave. She focuses on the poor outcomes and overlooks the moral worth of creating a human bond of comfort and safety for this child during the ordeal. She now recognizes that her attentiveness and responsiveness to the child are as potent as the medical arsenal of multiple surgeries and massive antibiotics and thereby confronts the agency and responsibility of caring. Clinical and ethical judgments are forged.

Overinvolvement, or misguided involvement, that takes on unrealistic rescue goals or usurps the patient/family concerns and control is dangerous, but its polar opposite, disengagement, is not the solution. Lack of involvement or detachment and disengagement interfere with attentiveness, noticing, and knowing the patient/family (Benner, Wrubel, Phillips, Chesla, & Tanner, in progress; Tanner et al., 1993). The disengaged nurse is ineffectively protected from the pain and effectively shielded from the possibilities in the situation. In fact, it is the nurse's connection and concern for the child that enables her to judge that the treatment has become both excessive and futile.

This nurse is currently avoiding involvement by taking assignments that do not require a sustained relationship with patients. She has not yet worked out the skillful possibility of being involved while remaining clinically astute about the qualitative distinctions between reasonable heroic efforts and unreasonable futile care that prolongs dying. One cannot learn the skill of involvement without experientially learning when it serves the ones cared for and when it harms or fails to help. An ethic of care and responsiveness depends on developing this skill for the sake of the ones cared for. The skill of involvement is different for parents, teachers, nurses, doctors, social workers, et cetera, because the cultural possibilities and expectations for each are different (Phillips & Benner, 1994). But each must learn the appropriate skill of involvement in order to be the parent of a particular child or the nurse of a particular patient, or the teacher of a particular student. Still, without learning the skill of involvement, standing in the right relationship of attachment and respect for the other, one cannot develop excellence in these complex relationships and practices. It would have been tragic had not the child been able to relate to a reliable known nurse in the hospital. The nurse does not reflect on this positive contribution of her involvement, only on the complicity of her care for prolonging suffering rather than preventing it.

With intimate knowledge of the other comes responsibility, in this case, the responsibility that comes with the ability to recognize early signs of sepsis. The nurse is confronted with the extent of the life and death power of her caregiving practice and she takes time out to reflect on her skill of involvement. There was little evidence that this nurse received any institutional support, guidance or counselling for dealing with her grief and for examining her practical moral reasoning. This represents a dangerous lack of care for the caregiver. The danger is that overinvolvement may be experienced only as personal failure and not as an occasion for learning. Rather than altering the quality of involvement, nurses may seek to avoid it altogether leading to excessive disengagement. Engagement and disengagement may be experienced as two stark alternatives, instead of experientially learned and situated skills embedded in concrete interpersonal relationships. Here expert coaching in actual situations is needed to assist nurses in sorting out the difficult skills of involvement in such tragic and demanding situations. This coaching should be offered at a similar level as that of debriefing and examination of transference and countertransference by a psychotherapist.

Expert nurses demonstrated keen abilities to engage with patients, and allow their involvement to guide their clinical and ethical comportment. Experienced nurses who did not become expert demonstrated difficulty learning workable levels and quality of involvement (see discussion, Chapter 7).

These nurses demonstrate a new level of experiential wisdom about the limits of medical heroics and now have confronted many patients whose dying and suffering were being prolonged by futile treatments. As new graduates they were often naive about the limits of heroic care, and were sustained by the goal of "saving lives." As illustrated above, nurses may find their increasing skill only adds to the patient's suffering. Finitude and vulnerability are inescapable facts of human expertise.

EDUCATIONAL IMPLICATIONS

Moving from competency to proficiency is discontinuous, calling for a different way of being in the situation and a different form of agency. The competent level of performance is reinforced with most educational theories and organizational rewards (Benner, 1984). In nursing school students learn that moving from a lay to a professional perspective with scientific and technical knowledge entails developing skills in planning, analysis, prediction, and control. To be an "expert" typically means possessing "expert knowledge" that is applied in the situation. Formal explanations are highly valued for their ability to predict and control outcomes. This model of theoretical knowledge covers over the reasoning in transitions, skilled know-how, and emotional attunement central to *any* practice, and crucial to clinical and ethical expertise (see Dreyfus, Dreyfus with Athanasiou, 1986).

Relationships Between Theory and Practice

The widely held institutional and cultural valuing of abstract professional knowledge may make nurses entering into proficiency feel that they are losing rather than gaining ground, because the transition to reading the situation and becoming more responsive can feel like a loss of organizational skills and a loss of clarity. We recommend a new level and kind of staff development for the nurse who may be becoming proficient. Narratives of learning told in small groups, that focus on changing one's perspectives and expectations in a clinical situation, can be very instructive and support this crucial shift in the skills of problem identification and responsiveness. The public storytelling of changed perspectives, and of recognizing changing relevance in clinical situations, can provide a new vision to competent practitioners who have not yet made this shift. Equally important, recognizing changing relevance can be publicly sanctioned and legitimized as astute and flexible, instead of being mis-attributed to having held the "wrong" perception or plan from the outset. Perfectionism can hamper learning from experience and from turning around preconceptions because the person is trying so hard to be beyond experience, i.e., perfect. The powers of understanding *in* the situation and the nature of experiential learning can be articulated and valued in the narratives.

Particularly in areas where there is a high time demand for performance, as is the case for patients with highly unstable conditions, the shift to response-based practice is potentially lifesaving. But this shift is also crucial to the nurses' comfort and ease in the situation. Developing ever more elaborate planning and organizational schemes can block recognition of changing relevance and thus prevent effective timely interventions. Successful clinical forethought and prediction seem to be essential for learning to recognize changing relevance. However, if plans and predictions are held too tightly, they block the recognition of changing relevance. The one who is prepared to "see" certain anticipated changes in patients is best prepared to notice when these changes do not occur. The paradoxical and difficult perceptual skill is to anticipate and plan with openness rather than rigidity. This is why skilled emotional responses and the ability to attend to them are crucial to the development of proficiency and expertise. Being emotionally attuned to the situation and to patients and families allows for feelings of uneasiness, when broad, vague experientially based expectations are not encountered. Knowing the patient (Tanner et al., 1993) allows the nurse to recognize subtle changes in the patient's condition. Knowing a particular patient population gives the practitioner a fund of clinical expectations and qualitative distinctions that enhance perceptual acuity and the ability to understand patient transitions. Since proficiency develops unevenly and in relation to knowing particular patient populations, comparisons between well known and less familiar populations can make the skills of reading the situation more apparent to the nurse making the transition into proficiency. The educational strategy at the competent level is to enhance the practitioner's awareness of the skills of reading the situation. Increased awareness of the shift to moving with the situation, rather than laying a plan upon it, can increase the nurse's active learning to respond to the situation and turn around preconceptions.

At the undergraduate level, clinical knowledge development could be taught more interactively with more focus on problem identification and reasoning in transitions. This requires that the nursing instructor engage in dialogue with the student's clinical reasoning. The value of openness to responding to the situation can be taught, balancing the quest for planning, prediction, and control in the current approaches to teaching problem solving that focus on assessing, planning, intervening, and evaluating. Teaching the student to make practical comparisons between two similar and dissimilar clinical situations can enhance the ability to make qualitative distinctions and improve problem identification and recognition of meanings in the situation.

Response-Based Skills and Overadaptation

Developing response-based skills runs the risk of overadapting to unreasonable situational demands. For example, heroic performance against all odds and persistent institutional impediments is too risky, costly, and, ultimately, unsustainable. Planned reflection on both excellence and breakdowns in practice can provide guidance for redesigning environments and resource allocation. In clinical situations where the nurse is fully engaged and responding to the demands of the moment, including the limitations of the way in which the system is designed, there may be little or no time for reflection on improving the system. Narratives from all skill levels are instructive for redesign, but the proficient and expert narratives provide a vision for redesigning the system for the best practice. There are troubling silences in proficient narratives about correcting the unsafe clinical situations in the immediate telling of the story, but upon reflection, these narratives provide examples of innovation in practice and also ideas for ways of better facilitating diffusion of these innovations into practice. Overadapting to unreasonable organizational demands threatens the development and the ability to sustain proficient and expert practice.

In the press for cutting costs and improving efficiency, reliability can deteriorate, and these narratives typically provide accounts of delivering reliable care in the context of real time. Aggregate patient outcome data are critical evaluative information, but they cannot provide information on the means for achieving these outcomes and the ways that means and outcomes are linked (Borgmann, 1984). Excessive focus on outcomes detached from practice overlooks or even devalues the means for achieving the outcomes. Clinicians must find ways to communicate and hold the organization and the economic policies accountable for adequate resources for safe and human clinical practice. System design must facilitate and improve the means–ends relationships. How to analyze and create strategies for correcting problems at the system level can be effectively taught to the nurse at the proficiency level. Narratives of system breakdown and innovation can provide the basis for exploring ways to translate experiential learning into better system design.

Enhancing Moral Agency at the Proficient Level

In the western tradition we have two major visions of moral agency. The first is an individualistic oppositional one, in which the individual stands over against the group in opposition to the status quo—notable examples being Socrates drinking the hemlock, Martin Luther nailing the theses on the door in opposition to the Catholic church, and Martin Luther King, Jr. engaging in civil disobedience. A second major view of moral agency is one in which the individual, in leadership, service, and solidarity with other practitioners, constitutes a community that facilitates coordinated and concerted action. Both kinds of moral agency are needed within the same person and in all communities. The extreme view of the individual in opposition prophetically judging the community without building the solidarity necessary for community life and coordinated action is an unreasonably restricted view of moral agency. Caregiving, by its nature, is intensive and extensive work (Benner & Gordon, in press). No one person can replace the community of caregivers. This is especially true in the intensive care unit, but can be generalized to all spheres of caregiving as they allow other human beings to be seen, to be who they are, and to be nurtured, challenged, and protected. Moral agency must encompass building and supporting coordinated community life and effort.

Similar to a community of caregivers, an improvisational jazz ensemble offers a concrete example of the combining of both the individual voice and responsiveness to others. Improvisation artists must improvise in relation to and response to their fellow musicians. Even so, each member creates and improvises. Each member contributes in response to the other, synergy occurs, and beautiful music is created. The proficient nurse is a budding improvisational artist. Experience has taught the limits of formal scientific knowledge for reasoning in transitions, and the nurse can now better recognize clinical knowledge in others. Individual agency can extend in synergistic ways to team members.

In proficient practice, more than at any prior skill level, negotiating with physicians becomes essential. Because here nurses' understanding is situated in time and in the context of the patient's situation, and because nurses have increasing skill in noting changing relevance in the patient condition, their capacity to communicate this situated understanding to those who are often operating outside of the situation (out of the room, on the telephone, or simply from a distance because they aren't at the bedside, as is the nurse) becomes ever more essential.

Negotiating clinical knowledge requires more than the skill of seeing; it requires interpersonal skill, trust in one's own grasp, and a capacity to anticipate and respond to an outside vantage point of the situation. With interpersonal skill, the nurse making the clinical case can further illuminate and substantiate the clinical situation.

Use of multiple perspectives to improve clinical understanding can improve clinical reasoning and visions for responding. Multiple clinical perspectives, as illustrated in the nurse who asked her colleagues to listen to the baby with fluid in the lungs (see p. 227), can improve clinical judgment. The planned use of multiple perspectives can improve the clinicians' ability to recognize qualitative distinctions and interpret trends in the patient's condition.

Planned staff development courses in concert with physicians can assist in better negotiation of clinical knowledge for the sake of improved patient care. Again, narratives of excellence, as well as breakdown cases, can improve the communication of clinical understanding and facilitate the development of clinical knowledge. Physician and nurse narratives are both needed. Struggling to understand the clinical situation can improve clinical judgment and patient care. Divisive power struggles can cloud the communication channels and impede clinical judgment. In life-and-death decisions, shared and individual responsibility to do well by the patient are essential.

Planned educational programs around criterial reasoning and reasoning in transitions can clarify communication patterns and the diverse warrants for legitimate clinical and ethical reasoning. At the proficient stage, organizational strategies for negotiating and adjudicating clinical judgment must be reinforced and clarified, so that when misunderstanding and breakdown in communications occur, the nurse will have routinized avenues for making a clinical case. In the end, a climate of open communication and trust focused on the goal of excellent patient care is the most reliable organizational resource. In-service strategies that foster open communication and trust between the health care team members should be designed especially for the proficient and expert levels of clinical practice.

Teaching for Response-Based Actions

Many response-based maxims taught early in nursing education can be introduced anew now that the nurse can recognize the situated cues involved. For example, nurses are taught to observe when the patient is ready to learn. Educators admonish students to wait for a "teachable moment." At the proficient level, nurses can compare their experiences with recognizing and responding to teachable moments. These concrete examples can enhance perceptual acuity and generate ideas for responding. At the proficient stage, nurses develop response-based skills, such as giving information, and here the experiential learning around giving too much or too little information or poor pacing or timing of information giving can be learned because the nurse is experientially ready to perceive these response-based demands. In-service education classes around response-based skills of managing fluid shifts, titrating vasopressor drugs, and managing pain can now be more effectively taught.

Emotional Attunement and the Skill of Involvement

Emotional attunement is required for understanding the situation and for developing the requisite interpersonal skills for helping relationships. Anxiety, foreboding, and uneasiness in situations where the practitioner does not have a good grasp of the situation provide signals that can prompt seeking clarification. Practitioners may mistakenly feel that they must dampen emotional responses even after these emotional responses become more attuned to real threats and significance in the situation. Therefore, reflection and follow-up on emotional cues to changes in the patient situation can improve perceptual acuity and the recognition of changing relevance. Emotional attunement to the situation and to the patient/family are related. Concern and emotional connection to the patient/family allow the nurse to perceive both patient distress and enable the nurse to respond in attuned ways. To be a skillful helper, one must be attuned to the patient's suffering, concerns, resourcefulness, and possibilities. This requires knowing and connecting with the patient (Tanner et al., 1993).

Interpersonal anxiety can interfere with developing the experientially learned skills of involvement. The western bias of considering emotions as "irrational" or distorting noise to be coped with in order to improve performance can block the development of emotional attunement to the person and the situation. At the proficient level, nurses would benefit from planned opportunities to talk about their developing skill in relating to and caring for patients and families. Currently, outside of basic nursing education, professional structures for fostering the skill of involvement are almost nonexistent. In contrast with, for example, psychotherapists, psychologists, family therapists, and psychiatric nurses, who have normative expectations for ongoing supervision and advice for developing the skills of interpersonal involvement, nurses in acute care settings have few of these structures, even in caring for dying patients. It is evident in our study that there is enormous variation in nurses' capacity to relate to and help the other in these highly charged critical situations. The development of emotional attunement to the situation and the skill of interpersonal involvement are critical to moving to the proficient and expert stages. Indeed, failure in this area of skill development seems to play a key role in blocking the development of clinical expertise (see Chapter 7). It was evident in the small group interview sessions that nurses were surprised at the degree of commonality in their experiences of emotional involvement and grief work, yet these experiences had seldom been shared with others. Planned consultation and support groups for dealing with developing the skills of involvement and for dealing with suffering and grief could be helpful at all experiential levels. Such support could reduce the stress of nursing work and increase the nurses' ability to stay open and flexible. One cannot dictate or prescribe perceptual acuity, openness, and emotional attunement. However, these are gifts and commitments that can be supported and which are enormously rewarding in their own terms. Expert helping requires being with and not just the performance of skills. Skills are necessary, but must receive their direction and guidance from the relationship itself. It is at the proficiency stage that the nurse develops new experiential capacities for reading the situation and being emotionally attuned to patient/family concerns. Focusing on these existential and interpersonal skills at this point can be very rewarding.

SUMMARY

Proficiency marks the transition between competency and expertise. Educational support at this stage can enhance the development of expertise. At the proficient and expert stages, the organization has much to learn from the practitioner. The practice of the proficient and expert nurses should guide the design of the system in order to enhance their practice and improve its quality.

Chapter **6**

EXPERT PRACTICE

s noted in the preceding chapter, the shift from competent to proficient performance is dramatic, marked by a qualitative change
in what the practitioner is able to see. Proficient performance is
characterized by an increased capacity for recognizing whole patterns and
a budding sense of salience where relevant aspects of the situation simply
stand out without recourse to calculative reasoning. Proficient practitioners can read a situation, recognize changing relevance, and, accordingly,
shift their perspective on the whole situation. It is this ability to read the
situation instead of laying on a preconceived set of expectations that makes
expert practice possible. However, for the proficient nurse, ways of responding are not yet linked to ways of seeing the situation, so the nurse at
the proficient level still has to think about what to do.

Expert practice is characterized by increased intuitive *links* between
seeing the salient issues in the situation and ways of responding to them.
This is evident upon observing the nurse in the situation, and is partially
captured in the following account of a situation where a patient who was
hemorrhaging stopped breathing. The links between patient condition and
action are sufficiently strong that the focus shifts to actions taken rather
than the problems recognized. This a "natural" shift, since in extreme circumstances the possible responses are fewer, but experience is required to
make this shift in performance:

> So we didn't even call the code. We just called the doc[tor] stat [emergency]
> and got him up there. [They had sufficient people available to resuscitate
> the patient, so no formal page for additional help was needed.] I looked at
> his heart rate and I said: "O.K. he is brading down. Someone want to give
> me some atropine?" I just started calling out the drugs that I needed to get
> for this guy, so we started to push these drugs in. In the meantime, I said,
> "can we have some more blood?" I was just barking out this stuff [the things

142

that were needed and had to be done]. I can't even tell you the sequence. I was saying, "We need this." I needed to anticipate what was going to happen and I could do this because I had been through this a week before with this guy and knew what we had done [and what had worked]. The anesthesiologist came in and did a good intubation. He asks: "What kind of [IV] lines do we have?" I said, "We have a triple lumen and we have blood. All [IV] ports are taken. We need another kind of line. He's got no veins left." He goes, "O.K., fine, give me a cut-down tray . . ."

The recognition and assessment language are minimal, in part, because the number of actions per problem are limited, but also because recognition and assessment language become so linked with actions and outcomes that they become self-evident or "obvious" for the expert practitioner. In this situation, the response was even more fluid and knowing because this nurse had taken care of this patient during a previous successful resuscitation where she had learned, first-hand, what worked and what did not. This is not just a rote repetition of the previous resuscitation; rather, her responses are based on the understanding gained in the previous situation.

The practice of the expert, like that of the proficient nurse, is characterized by engaged practical reasoning, which relies on mature and practiced understanding, and a perceptual grasp of distinctions and commonalities in particular situations. While nurses at this level know what to anticipate and how to prepare for possible issues and problems, expert practice requires remaining open to what the situation presents. When deeply involved in the situation, nurses practicing at this level do not see problems in a detached way, needing to work out how to solve them. Rather, their actions reflect an attunement to the situation that allows responses to be shaped by a watchful reading of the patient's responses without recourse to conscious deliberation. With expertise comes fluid, almost seamless performance. Organization, priority setting, and task completion do not show up as focal points in their narrative accounts.

Nurses at this level of practice have reached an increased facility and comfort in their level of emotional involvement with patients and their families. Rather than becoming uniform or standardized, emotional involvement varies considerably depending on the needs and openness of patient and family. Unattuned emotional attentiveness is a sentimental focus on one's own feelings instead of the other's (Logstrup, 1956/1971). Focusing on one's virtuosity and virtuousness in caring rather than meeting and responding to the other likewise is a form of sentimentalizing. In the narratives of connection and attunement, the focus is on the worthiness, needs, resourcefulness, and concerns of the other. When listening to and reading expert narratives, by virtue of the expert's engaged access to and way of being in the situation, the listener/observer is placed *in* the situation and is helped to see what the expert sees, rather than a self-conscious focusing on the storyteller/agent.

Expert nurses readily describe those patients and families with whom they've had a special connection, where they felt that the connection was in some way either sustaining for the patient or brought new understanding to the nurse about the patient's world and what was important to him. The "unusual" connections are described without illusions that such connections are possible and sustainable for *all* patients. Nurses at the expert level know that they are not, and that they are not always wanted or available from the patient and family. Dreyfus' (1979) observation about human expertise being capable of being as "orderly as the situation demands" is relevant here. A vision of "treating everyone the same" is a distorted vision of "justice," since in situations of different levels of risk and vulnerability, responding to the vulnerability, needs, and possibilities at hand is the relational ethical demand. These connections are seen as necessary for survival in the case of extremely vulnerable patients, as illustrated in the following excerpt about a physician who was critically ill and on a mechanical ventilator. This story was a paradigm case for this nurse about an unusually close and lifesaving connection to a patient; the story will be re-visited throughout the chapter:

Nurse: He developed ARDS [*Acute Respiratory Distress Syndrome*] like I've never seen anybody develop ARDS. Within hours he was on a 100% O_2 and 15 of pressure, and then he had pneumos and bradycardia if they took him off the ventilator. This was all very sudden and unexpected for an elderly man who was healthy . . . He was a retired physician. So he really wanted to be interactive and you really couldn't let him be, because his airway pressure was so high that he would try to write or try to communicate and I was afraid that he would blow another pneumo. So with this type of balance going on . . .

Int: What made you want to pick him as a patient—what attracted you?

Nurse: He just was really vital. He wanted to know what was going on and he was writing and he had really bad spelling, and I remember thinking, he's so great, and yet his spelling is atrocious. He's really trying to communicate with me and I'm trying to sedate him and there was just a lot of me trying to allay his anxiety and his family's and to try to keep him going, and it was a frightening situation not to have that much more to offer in such a quick period of time . . . it wasn't like he was bleeding and you could give him blood. It was a pulmonary process which was going on and on for whatever unknown [reason]. No one ever knew, what happened to him. On this day in ICU, it was really stormy. He arrested a couple of times. Jean [another nurse] was taking care of him one time and he was very unstable, if you didn't watch his color, his eyes, if he tremored, you really had to pick up on it, much more than his numbers, much more than his monitoring. . . . Sometimes I just had to gauge what I was doing with him, and how quickly he would become hypoxic, . . . there weren't any numbers because I would have to get a blood gas, take it to the lab and do whate you had to do. You had to base a lot of what you were doing on what was ha pening right then, rather than get a test to say: "I've documented it," you had to more or less look at him, and just know. And to know his fatigue, know just how much he could do . . . You ask somebody if you want to get out of bed, you want to eat? There are so many things he didn't want to do after this withdrawal period or he would only be selective with people that he was involved with that he cared about. Was he tired? It was just a matter of *why* he resisted to it. Does it mean coax him or that you have pushed him too far?

Knowing the patient (Jenks, 1993; Jenny & Logan, 1992; MacLeod, 1993; Tanner et al., 1993) is essential to clinical judgment and ethical comportment in this situation. Knowing the patient's warning signs for having a cardiac arrest such as "his color, his eyes, if he tremored" came before overt changes in vital signs from the monitors, and this lead time was essential for adjusting his intravenous medications and ventilator settings to prevent cardiac arrest. As the nurse notes, it was necessary to know when he was just resisting movement or when he was indeed too tired and weak for planned activities and treatments. Expert care in this situation required this level of patient attunement along with linking the patient's condition to instant therapeutic responses.

The moral agency of the nurse practicing at the expert level is also a strong recurring theme. Central to expert practice is a concern for revealing and responding to patients as persons, respecting their dignity, caring for them in ways that preserve their personhood, protecting them in their vulnerability, helping them to feel safe in a somewhat alien environment, and comforting their family, striving to preserve the integrity of close relationships (see Benner, Wrubel, Phillips, Chesla, & Tanner, 1995).

In the following discussion, key aspects of the clinical world of expert practice are presented first: (1) clinical grasp and response-based practice; (2) embodied know-how; (3) seeing the big picture; and (4) seeing the unexpected. Each of these aspects must be thought about in relation to the other, since they are not separable in practice. Then we will take up the nature of agency for the expert practitioner. At the expert level of practice, moral agency becomes much more situated and socially embedded and is enabled by experientially learned clinical and perceptual capacities. Three key aspects of moral agency made possible by expert clinical and perceptual acuity will be described: (1) developing the skill of involvement; (2) managing technology and preventing unnecessary technological intrusions; and (3) working with and through others. Neither discussion can spell out completely the clinical and moral world of the expert nurse, but the examples provide a vision of expert practice that can be recognized and emulated by others.

CLINICAL WORLD

The nurse practicing at this level is always in the situation with some practical understanding. Indeed, this is what it means to live and move in a human world (Dreyfus, 1991). Even before they know the patient, nurses have expectations about the clinical situation that are open to revision or confirmation when they meet the patient. Mature practical knowledge of particular patient populations shapes nurses' expectations and sets. Expert nursing is also characterized by expert caring practices, that is, attending to human concerns such as concern for easing suffering, protecting from vulnerability, and preserving dignity.

Clinical Grasp and Response-Based Practice

When assuming the care of the patient for the first time, nurses talk about needing time to "get settled," meaning to get a sense of who the patient is, the patient's patterns of responses, and the immediate demands and concerns in the situation. This is evident in the following account of meeting with the family of a patient while he was in surgery:

> We had a patient that was in the OR [*operating room*] and I'd gotten word that he had been, I think he'd been in the CCU beforehand, had a really poor heart, had a lot of M.I.'s [*heart attacks*], poor ejection fraction . . . I was coming on to work that evening and had received word that his family was sitting and waiting in our waiting room . . . So I thought I'll go out and meet them which I try to do when it works out that way . . . They were like stressed to the max because the minute I walked out they jumped off the chair and— they knew I was coming to talk to them—"How are things going?" So I just introduced myself and explained that we really don't hear much until they [the patient] actually get up to the unit and just talked about what to expect and that they could come in after an hour or so. Anyway, they proceeded to tell me this whole story about what this poor man had gone through and how it was so rough on him, and how he'd been in CCU and was so sick . . . I went back into the unit, the patient came up and sure enough was sick as anything on every drip known to man, ballooned, [*heart assist device*] had a real hard time coming off bypass. And as I listened to report and I went into the room and looked at him, I'm thinking "it's going to be a miracle if this man leaves this hospital alive." That was the sense I had. So anyway, after I got settled, I went out and had the family come and just tried to give them a sense of what to expect, explained that it sounded like he'd been really sick before surgery and that his recovery was probably going to be very slow, might have difficulty weaning [*from the ventilator*], not to expect things to

go too quickly, and know that there was a possibility for complications and that kind of thing. And we just sort of clicked . . . we just hit it off or something. It was like they needed—when I went out to talk to them in the lobby before, it was like they were just looking for this release valve and I gave it to them and they seemed to appreciate that, and I think at that point we kind of clicked.

Here the nurse's clinical grasp includes her understanding of the family's situation. Through experience, she knows what to expect in this patient's recovery and gives this projection to the family so they can have a sense of what the patient will look like and what the likely events will be. As she says, she takes time to get the patient settled in, which in the case of receiving a patient back directly from open heart surgery requires much activity and assessment. The term "settled in" covers a wide range of activity but also refers to gaining a clinical grasp of the situation. And that grasp takes into consideration the immediate past, the present, and the likely future course of events.

Where patterns and trends are clear and there are definite actions associated with the clinical trend, the nurse can respond quickly and fluidly, giving little conscious thought. On observation, these nurses typically manage multiple tasks simultaneously, for example, adjusting intravenous drips, talking with the patient or family, observing the patient, and noting any changes in the clinical picture. This is illustrated in the concentrated and meaningful accounts of clinical actions taken by another nurse's account of receiving a very ill patient back from surgery:

He moved into a ventricular bigeminy rhythm and he was also in renal failure and knowing that his acidosis is all the way out of whack, I don't want any PVC's [premature ventricular contractions] that aren't going to respond to treatment. Because if he goes into the attack, being acidotic, he really won't respond to anything so I empirically just hit him up with some potassium [gave the potassium before the laboratory results could be obtained] because he'd been third spacing [fluid moving from the vascular system into the tissues], he had a large GI [gastrointestinal] output and the potassium that I drew came back at 2.8 and he was really down there. And after 60 total meq. [of potassium] over 3 hours, even though he was in renal failure, it was up to 4.4 and he had no more ectopy and we weaned him off the lidocaine without incident. I gave him a very concentrated dose [of potassium] because he couldn't tolerate having a whole lot of fluid extra, at that point, they'd cut his fluids back and they were resuscitating him with dopamine for his blood pressure rather than fluids and not wanting to give him a lot of fluid that was going to sit in his lungs or something, I put a high concentration 20 meq in 50 cc's over an hour for about three times and that's about as concentrated as we can get . . . and I thought that was the safest for this guy. And it worked out fine for him.

The abbreviated, somewhat cryptic account is an insider's story, told from a good clinical grasp of the situation that includes a prescient sense of the immediate future given the current clinical situation. Given the patient's clinical condition, the expert anticipates low potassium, and responds to the premature ventricular contractions as an early sign of low potassium. There are standard orders for potassium replacement, but any physician or nurse will uphold the practice standard of *not* giving potassium without knowing the lab results; yet any expert clinician, given this strong circumstance, would at least consider starting the potassium replacement as soon as cardiac dysrhythmias began if the lab values were not readily available. Of course it is best to have definitive laboratory findings prior to action, but this rule of thumb is bent when the urgency of the situation seems to require it. This brief excerpt demonstrates the multiple levels of action required in these high time-demand critical situations.

Response-based practice is based upon having a good clinical grasp and recognizing both familiar and individual patterns of responses. In the following discussion, neonatal intensive care unit nurses describe the distinctions that they make in practice, based on the particular infant's response patterns:

Nurse 1: Because the baby is telling you what he wants.
Nurse 2: And there are specific preemie patterns. But there's also individual baby patterns that may or may not jive with what your typical preemie patterns are.
Nurse 1: Or what they told you in orientation.
Nurse 2: Or what the primary nurse was enamored of 3 days before which may or may not still be appropriate anymore. And you have to make all these judgments fairly quickly if the kid decides to do it on your first 10 minutes into the shift. Which they so often do. [*laughter*]
Int: That's amazing to me. So there is this whole thing of learning this baby?
Nurse 2: Oh, absolutely. Especially for this kind of stuff, oh absolutely. [*Prior discussion had been about adjusting respirator settings*]
Nurse 3: You can put on the Kardex that this baby likes to be two-person suctioned and hand-ventilated, there's several different suctioning methods you can do. Or minimizing handling, that sort of thing, but you really have to evaluate that you can pass along what you did and what worked for you. But the fact is, the next person may evaluate the kid and find something that works better. You can't really argue with that . . .
Nurse 1: And, the other thing is that sometimes doing nothing is best and that's real hard to get your head around . . . So you better have that baggage in your brain too where sometimes you intervene and it's worse. So, if they said I shouldn't intervene, maybe I better wait this one out. That's hard to do. When you're trained to react, it's hard to wait it out and see if it really does . . .
Nurse 2: And also if the kid really does get worse then you have to explain why you didn't do anything.
Nurse 1: You have to decide how far you're going to let it go [respiratory distress]—when you're going to just say "That's enough and I'm going to at least

try to do something about it." This is going on so fast you don't always have time to look around in the other rooms and see where the resident is . . .
Nurse 2:   You're just gut-reacting here.
Int: Give me a sense of the time frame.
Nurse 1:   A minute. [laughter]

Certainty is not possible; practical reasoning in the particular transition (modus operandi reasoning) is the best that can be done in the situation with such a high time demand. Cumulative learning and courageous open learning from past situations where optimal and suboptimal responses were made is the best the practitioner can do.

In the following exemplar, these multiple aspects of clinical grasp, that is, responsiveness, understanding the immediate past, the present, and the immediate future, responding to both the clinical and human dimensions, and close linkages between understanding, action, and outcomes are illustrated. The nurse is describing the care of a man in his mid-60's who had been admitted to a general medical unit in liver failure. He was transferred to ICU.

He came up looking about as orange as that orange juice, but not in any real acute distress. I got him about 3 o'clock in the afternoon so I had him for about 4 hours that day. Then the next morning when I came in to report, they had just intubated him. By the time I got out of report they were setting up to put invasive lines in and by 10:30 in the morning he was being dialyzed. So all of this in a space of about 5 hours really kind of overpowered this guy who was still quite with it [*alert*]. He knew everything that was going on even though his liver enzymes were just sky high. I really thought that he should have been encephalopathic by then but he wasn't. And his family was all here. But none of this [*intervention*] made any difference in his lab work. None of it made any difference in his clinical picture. He continued to deteriorate and after being on dialysis for 4 hours and not having that make any difference at all.

The physicians were very involved and kept the family informed about the patient's lack of progress, being both "candid and compassionate." After several hours of dialysis, when it became clear that there would be no improvement, the physicians recommended to the family that the dialysis be stopped, and that they "let him go." After the decision was made to stop dialysis, the nurse talked with the patient:

At this point, this was the first time I had ever, ever, ever said this to a patient. And I knew that he could hear me. He responded to me. I said, "You're going to be taken off dialysis and you're probably going to die in the next couple of hours." His eyes just popped open, and then just this peaceful look came over his face. It was an amazing transition. He finally died about 6:30 that evening. And to have been with him through that really very critical period and make sure that he knew everything that was going on and make sure that his family knew what was going on. And to help him into the most peaceful death that could happen under those circumstances. . . . It seemed like he really did let go very soon after his family had come into the room. He became unresponsive probably within about an hour of that and I think having the permission . . . his family came in and said "we love you, we'll miss you, but we know you're going to die." I think having that realization from the family and having it spoken to him [*gave him permission to let go*].

The nurse later described what had solicited her actions and this response:

Our only interaction had been the night before. And it seemed like we had connected in some way. It felt like there was a, I don't want to say relationship, that sounds much too deep, but a rapport, a connection. Something between him and me and the family and me. There just seemed to be people that you connect with pretty easily and he seemed to be one of them. And it was also clear that he was going to die [soon]—medically, it was not intuition. It was total body failure.

The nurse described how she supported the family throughout the day:

Nurse: I tried very hard to have them be in the room as much as possible so they could see what was going on. See what I was doing. See what all the other technical people were doing.
Int: Because?
Nurse: I think so it wouldn't be a shock to them when the decision had to come that he was going to be allowed to die.
Int: Did you have the sense that was the case in the morning?
Nurse: Yeah, it was real vague. A real vague sense of doom at the beginning of the day, but when everything happened in that short time, it finally knocked me over the head. Gee, this man is really sick. I think my first clue was having gone home the evening before, having taken care of this fellow and things having gone fairly well. I knew he was sick but that's the kind of patients that we see in the ICU. Kind of the feeling that OK, we'll get him over this little crisis period and then he can go home and be with his family for awhile before he dies. And then coming in the next morning and just 2 hours before I got to the unit, he had been intubated, very, very suddenly. It was a very sudden deterioration of his pulmonary status. I think just the quickness of everything happening seemingly at once. His lines were in by 9 AM, he was on dialysis by 10:30. You know, I think probably not seeing his eyes nearly as much as I had the day before.
Int: Talk a little more about that.
Nurse: He kept them [*his eyes*] closed most of the time. He was exhausted, I'm sure. But not seeing his eyes. He would open his eyes once in a while when I

would talk to him. But most of the time he would just nod or squeeze my hand or help me turn him or whatever.

Int: Did you have any interchanges with the family, did you talk with the family?

Nurse: Oh yeah, as much as possible. In the morning it was real hard. I was really caught up in the technical stuff that was going on and it had to be. I tried to get them into the room as much as possible, but they would stay just for a couple of minutes and leave. Finally, after about the first 3 hours of dialysis, we knew things weren't going real well and I tried to get them in. I went out to the lounge and talked with them for a bit. That was pretty low-keyed because there wasn't anything that I could tell them yet. Just kind of getting a feeling of what was going on and how scared they were. Dealing with them in the afternoon was much different. Of course, I could see them more and pay a lot more attention to them and kind of interpret what had gone on during the day. I felt a great urgency to get all the peripheral junk out of the room, as many machines as possible. Get some chairs in there. Just a different accoutrement in the room. Instead of having all the technical equipment in there, to just get rid of all of that as much as possible, leaving just one IV pole, the pump, and the ventilator, and kind of hiding the arterial and PA [*pulmonary artery*] lines. And then setting up the room with some chairs and making sure there were several strategically placed boxes of kleenex and his water pitcher and several glasses. And then being able to leave the family for, say, half-hour periods and just kind of keep an ear out for what was going on and keep an eye on the monitor, then go back in occasionally and see how everybody was doing.

Set in the death-defying culture of the intensive care unit, the practices described in this narrative are quite extraordinary. It is remarkable and unusual that the physician, nurse, and family nearly simultaneously reached the awareness that the patient was unlikely to survive and that impending death was so openly acknowledged to the patient. The nurse's central concern was preparing the patient and his family for death, creating a caring space in which the family could be together. Through her connection with the patient, and understanding of the clinical situation, she was able to somewhat domesticate the alien environment of the ICU, and pave the way for the family to be fully with the patient, to say what they needed to say, and to begin to "let go."

The nurse had a strong clinical sense of a downward clinical trajectory. Correlating laboratory findings with clinical signs, the nurse was surprised at how alert the patient was ("His enzymes were sky high; I expected him to be more encephalopathic, but he was really quite with it.") But by the next day, the rapid change from the evening before, and subtle clinical signs ("I didn't see his eyes as much today as yesterday") signaled the patient's decline. The nurse responded to this change. During the morning hours, although she was occupied with managing the rapidly changing clinical situation, she still attended to the family. Throughout the day, she set up the possibility for the family to be with the patient, and to begin to understand how seriously ill he was.

Clinical grasp and clinical response are inextricably linked (Benner, Hooper, & Stannard, 1995). For the expert nurse, having a good clinical grasp also means knowing what actions are appropriate. Nurses practicing at the expert level read the patient and respond instantaneously. By being fully involved in the situation, knowing the patient and his usual pattern of responses, nurses can follow patients' responses and modify their own approaches. The following refers to the physician with ARDS described earlier [see pp. 144–145]:

> Sometimes I just had to gauge what I was doing with him and how quickly he would become hypoxic, so it wasn't a matter of there weren't any numbers there because I would have to get a blood gas, take it to the lab, do whatever you had to do. You had to base a lot of what you were doing on what was happening right then. Rather than get a test to say "I've documented it," you had to more or less look at him. And just know. And to know his fatigue, know just how much he could do. You really had to listen to him.

This ability to read the patient's responses allows the nurse to gauge what activity the patient will tolerate and what intravenous fluids and respiratory support to offer.

Embodied Know-How

Observation of expert practice demonstrates remarkably fluid skilled performance. The skilled performance of difficult technical tasks requires a good clinical grasp, however, having a good grasp of the situation calls for swift adept action. Thinking in action is lodged in the body, the hands, eyes, and practiced habitual responses to situations (Dreyfus, Dreyfus with Athanasiou, 1986; Benner, 1984; Benner, 1993). Typically, if the nurse mentions skilled performance, it is linked with anticipating likely future events:

> I was out on a transport for a 7-year-old kid with a lot of congenital anomalies. We heard that the kid was not doing well . . . Anyway, this little kid was way too pale, way too tachycardic and yet the referral physician and the parents were saying, "It's not too bad—why don't you just take the kid in the helicopter?" . . . And actually within 10 minutes of being there, we had to intubate the child . . . Heart rates are normally 120–130; this kid's were 160–170. They were wondering if she'd blown something out in her gut or she was septic or something like that because her respiratory rate was 60— just too fast. She wasn't responsive, and even though she was developmentally disabled, she would have still normally pulled away or whatever. So,

I asked the parents, "Does she usually do something if she doesn't like what you're doing?" "Yeah, she pulls away," they said. And I said, "I think we need to get her intubated right now" and I took her blood pressure and it was only like 38 and children typically keep their blood pressures until the bitter end . . . And this child had no IV and I was just told that it took them 7 hours to get the last one in . . . Anyway, I found a vein and I got an IV in!

Being able to perform skillfully under time pressure takes well-honed embodied skills, the kind of skilled performance that comes only with practice. Response-based practice, as described above, implies the skilled know-how to respond to the concrete demands of the situation. Both expert problem identification and expert skilled performance are required for expert practice. Taken in isolation, inserting IVs is not that notable, but in the context of understanding when an IV might be urgently needed, the skillful insertion in a timely manner becomes lifesaving:

Actually [this 4-month-old infant had an episode of bradycardia] and we did this little tiny code where we did chest compressions for a few minutes, and then right after he did that, this is where my expert clinical judgment came into practice—I said I need to get an IV in him just in case he does this again. And two people said "No, you don't need to do that, he's O.K." So I slipped an IV in, which is no mean feat on a kid that's 4 months old, in our unit, their veins are trashed anyway, I got an IV into him and within 20 minutes I needed that because then he really went into a full code and needed drugs.

Skilled performance is linked with judgment and is a form of knowing. The interaction of skilled performance, timing, and anticipation is evident in the following description of resuscitation of newborn infants who are in heart failure and have pleural effusions:

Unless you resuscitate immediately, these infants are just not going to survive. I find it really exciting. You have to be ready and you have to do everything just like that [snaps her fingers four times]. Otherwise, that baby is just not going to make it. We have it set up so that we have everything in the delivery room that we need. We draw up the meds. We don't put chest tubes in the delivery room, but we do use angiocaths to withdraw the fluid. And sometimes we'll withdraw the fluid from the abdomen at the same time. We'll go ahead and intubate and most of the time we need to give ephedrine . . . Then we take the baby to the nursery . . . We have everything set up in the nursery . . .

The skilled performance includes teamwork, orchestrating one's own skilled responses with others, having the environment prepared, and sequencing the tasks as needed by the infant's clinical condition. Indeed, recognizing the current response capacities of other health care team members present in an emergency is a skill that expert nurses develop. We observed a flexible shifting of roles and functions depending on the level and nature of the expertise of those present in a resuscitation effort. This is illustrated in the continued discussion from the above interview:

> The last time we had one of these kids, we had only one physician because they didn't know it was coming, and everything just went beautifully. He [*the physician*] intubated, no problem at all. He started bagging, and then he did a once over the chest [*listened to the chest*]. One of the nurses took over drawing fluid back. He did the other side of the chest and I took over drawing the fluid out of there. Then he took over the ventilation and we went over to the nursery. Everything went right in. Never had any problems. It was just great. . . . Sometimes having one physician instead of three helps.

The nurse is satisfied by the orchestrated teamwork that she and the physician have accomplished. Because of the infant's fragile condition and a high time demand for action, skilled embodied know-how is crucial. Knowing what to do and when to act are linked with knowing how to do what is needed. It is here that the typical analytical strategy of separating the means and ends and devaluing the means as a delegated skill that anyone could do makes no sense because thinking, knowing, and doing are all fused (Borgmann, 1984).

Big Picture

Experts often characterize their clinical understanding by phrases such as "seeing the big picture." The big picture for the expert nurse goes beyond the immediate clinical situation typical of the competent and proficient level of practice. Seeing the "big picture" takes on new meaning for nurses practicing at this level. The big picture includes a sense of the future, recognizing anticipated trajectories, and grasping a sense of future possibilities for the patient and family. These nurses also have an expanded "peripheral vision," sensing the needs of other patients in the unit and the capabilities of nurses assigned to care for them, and recognizing when greater expertise may be required. The preeminence of the patient's world, and the role of the family in preserving that world, is prevalent in the narratives (see Chesla, 1990). Thus, the expert nurse has a strong sense of future possibilities, through following the course of many similar patients and this understanding shapes his or her understanding of and response to the present situation.

In addition to this greater temporal grasp of relating the past, present and future, seeing the big picture also means seeing what else is going on in the clinical situation or on the clinical unit. Expert nurses have expanded peripheral vision. They have a sense of the timing and pace of the unit. They are attuned to the skill level of other nurses during the shift, and notice when the demands of the patient situation may exceed the capabilities of the nurses involved:

> We had a young man, who was hit by a motorcycle and had multiple injuries. His primary nurse was experienced in trauma care; but then she had an extended period of time off, and very much of a novice nurse took over caring for him. And you could just kind of see things coming to a head over the weekend. I had nothing to do with this patient other than her coming to me from time to time as a resource and me kind of overhearing things and me always feeling compelled to intervene in situations like this. There were a lot of communication problems going on with the family, the physician and this young novice nurse. I think the family wanted a lot of questions answered and this young nurse really couldn't answer them, and she really wasn't making any attempt to get the questions answered. Now I can't always answer a patient's family either, but one of the things that I have learned is that there is always somebody that generally can . . . Now I had a very busy assignment of my own that weekend, but it was kind of where you see out of the peripheral vision. I knew that the primary nurse was going to be gone for several more days. We ended up being on opposite shifts over the weekend and I signed up to take care of the patient on the novice nurses' off-shifts. There were injuries on the patient that hadn't been picked up because of lack of experience [with trauma patients].

Identifying injuries in trauma patients takes good detective work and is aided by being familiar with patterns and signs and symptoms associated with different kinds of trauma. This is an area where experienced-based pattern recognition is irreplaceable.

> I had an incident a couple of weeks ago where there was a traveler nurse taking care of a patient who was having some respiratory problems. I had worked with this nurse a few days before, so I knew that her experience level was not as good as somebody else. I had also taken care of her patient. I knew enough about the patient's history to know that he had respiratory problems, and I knew that this was a shift, that he needed more suctioning. It went from every half an hour to every 15 minutes, and then it was interrupting the report to suction him, then it was every 10 minutes after report. This man desaturated very rapidly when we suctioned him, so they really wanted two people, and there wasn't anything happening. I thought something needs to be done here. I went over to help suction and sort of eyeball the situation to see if I could help or make a suggestion about what needed to be done. He was definitely getting into more trouble. But you see something going on, you have to decide, is it important enough to jump in and get involved.

The expert nurse knew the patient and knew the skill level of the nurse caring for him. She was attuned to the situation. When the clinical trends became clear, that he was deteriorating and nothing was being done, she decided that it was important enough to intervene. This heightened attunement to needs of other patients in the unit and the sense of responsibility in supporting less experienced nurses is characteristic of expert practice.

Seeing the Unexpected

In the previous exemplar the nurse recognized the clinical signs of a downward trajectory. Nurses practicing at the expert level have mature practical knowledge about what to expect of particular patient populations. When the clinical situation unfolds as expected, the nurse responds easily and fluidly, with little conscious thought. This transformation in performance is noted as seeing changing relevance at the proficient level. At the expert level this ability continues to develop and the practitioner gains facility and satisfaction from seeing the unexpected. When faced with a situation in which the expectations are not confirmed, the nurse senses that she or he does not have a good grasp and begins to search for clinical evidence to help sort out the source of jarred expectations. For example, a charge nurse in neonatal intensive care described noticing the unexpected and following up:

> This was a term kid and the reports that we were getting was that he was nippling poorly and so what the nurses had been doing was gavage feeding the baby, which is OK, an acceptable practice. But this had been going on for a couple of days already and this kid was just really a poor nippler. So after report, I talked to the nurse that was actually caring for the baby and said that "at some point when you are getting ready to feed the baby, let me know because I want to be the one to actually try and feed the baby" and see if I could get a better idea of what was going on. It became apparent that this was not just a kid who was a poor feeder, or couldn't coordinate sucking, swallowing and breathing; not that he just couldn't put it all together, but there was definitely something wrong and I went as far as to stick my forefinger all the way down the baby's throat and there was absolutely no gag reflex . . . Neurologically this baby was very compromised. So through my actually sitting there and following up on what was just "poor feeding" was able to determine that there was something more wrong.

The above is typical of a recurring theme in the narratives of nurses at the expert level. Recognizing a clinical situation that was unexpected and/ or unnoticed by other nurses happens more often when one has experientially learned what to expect and is open to perceiving missed expectations. As one nurse described it:

> It doesn't happen everyday, but it happens enough that you get used to it—being the first to know when things are going down the drain, being the first one to notice, and get the house staff up, get them looking at what's going on, get in touch with the family, get the SICU [*Surgical Intensive Care Unit*] attending if no one's moving fast enough. Recognizing it kicks in a whole cascade of events. You can just see it. Little tiny trends and you can just follow them and you just know.

Another group of nurses discussed recognizing early pulmonary embolus, describing how they attend to early clinical signs, noticing subtle changes in the patient's appearance:

> You start picking up and you start putting the picture together and you can tell them "I think the patient's having a PE [*pulmonary embolus*]." And they go "Look at the gases. Look at the X-ray." And they look at numbers, then you say, "No the color's not right. The pulse . . ." Of course, when they come in and check the pulse, the pulse is just fine, but 5 minutes later you're right back again with the thready pulse and it fades out and it comes back. And you get a widening pressure and the heart rate goes up and down, and they wouldn't believe me until 2½ hours later.

For these nurses, then, salient aspects of the situation just stand out. They have practical understanding of what to expect for the patient population, and often know the particular patient's patterns of responses. This practical know-how sets up the possibility for noticing when things are awry, when the clinical situation is not unfolding as expected. Since they have a practical understanding of what it feels like when they have a good clinical grasp, they can sense unease when they do not. For example, one nurse described being alerted by a clinical picture that doesn't add up, and the sense of alarm she feels at the patient's distress. The patient was a young man, post-LVAS [Left Ventricular Assist Device], who was complaining of severe abdominal pain. He had been characterized by his physician as a "baby" and a "wimp," who shouldn't be having so much pain. The nurse goes on to describe how she puts the picture together:

> All right, so now I've assessed the abdomen, but I was told at report that it was firm. So OK, this has been this way for a couple of days, so maybe I shouldn't be alarmed, but I am. It bothers me. I'm seeing this weird wave form. I'm giving 5%. It's not affecting his stroke volume at all. I go back to the flow sheet. If anything, he's below the pre-op weight. Which would make sense, the LVAS would improve his kidneys because he was in renal failure and he would lose all that third spacing. But I'm also looking at the last

hematocrit, drawn at 5:00 AM that morning and it was 30.1. And I turn over the flow sheet and I'm looking and I saw he got a unit of blood for a hematocrit of 30.6 the day before. And now, 5:00 AM his hematocrit is even lower after a unit of blood. It should have brought it up at least 2 points. So I send a stat hematocrit. Meanwhile the stroke volume is dropping more, so I give him a second unit of 5%, and I'm thinking, well, this will be dilutional by the time I get done. . . . That feeling when I got him in the chair and then when I looked at him and saw that this kid is sick and got him back in bed. Just in the back of my mind I'm thinking, "This kid gave it his all and he's really sick. This kid is not a wimp."

She describes how she evaluated the overall appearance of the patient. The account demonstrates modus operandi reasoning similar to that found in detective work (Bourdieu, 1990; Benner, Hooper, & Stannard, 1995). The nurse successfully lobbied for the physician to return, and re-evaluate the patient. The patient was returned to surgery where it was discovered that he had bled massively into his abdomen. The set created by the physician was that the patient wasn't getting up because he was a "baby," and that the nurse should push him. She got him up in the chair, but knew instantly that things were not right. She felt ill at ease, "alarmed"; the clinical picture, and the patient's response to getting up in the chair, the fact that he had "given it his all" simply didn't fit the physician's account.

Knowing and reading the patient well allows the expert nurse to notice when the patient has subtle changes in clinical and human possibilities. The following story is an account of a woman who had been critically ill for months when the nurse senses a new strength and possibility for weaning her from the respirator:

Nurse 1:   We had multiple, multiple times tried to get her off the ventilator after she had finally stabilized, and she would end up going back on pressors, it was a nightmare. So I finally got to the point where she was off all her drugs, her lungs cleared, she looked 100% better than she had ever looked. And the vent sometimes popped off her trach tube and her pulmonary counts were terrible, everything was terrible for this woman. She is probably the worst person with COPD I have ever seen. Her vent would pop off and you'd have to go in and reconnect her and everything. And she did not, she could not understand why she needed the ventilator to breathe. It pops off, I'm fine. What is your problem? She just couldn't get it. So, the team came around. And the team had sort of pigeonholed her. She's a chronic patient, we're waiting for a chronic bed. She's going to hang out and when she gets a chronic bed, she'll move. But her big thing was being with her children, and being a wife and a mother and being able to go home. She did have a lot of support systems. She could have potentially gone into a home-vent program at home. It was never really discussed with the family 'cause we were sure about her vent settings. [The ventilator settings were so high that no home-ventilator program would consider admitting her.] I basically wanted to try. She said, "I can breathe without the ventilator and I want to try." But the team didn't want her to try. I was the only one that wanted to try to get her vent settings down so that at least a home-vent program would even look at her. I mean looking at her numbers they would never have touched her. I just wanted them to try, and they were adamantly against it.

Int: So they were just willing to let her stay . . .

Nurse 1: Where she would have to wait at least a year and a half for a vent bed. So on rounds I wanted them to try—I didn't want them to drop her breaths to zero and let her breathe on her own, I just wanted them to drop her vents a little bit. "No, no, no."

Int: What was the reason they said no?

Nurse 1: Because every time we tried it before she had failed.

Int: So why did you want them to try it again?

Nurse 1: Because the patient—we had tried many times before but the patient was not saying, "Let me try." She was much, much better. She was much better. She didn't have a temp. She was being fed. Her pulmonary mechanics were not great.

Int: Now did you put all this out to them?

Nurse 1: Yes.

Int: And what did they say?

Nurse 1: No. [*laughter*] 'Cause at first I brought it up and the resident said, "No." I mean, I didn't, wasn't even finished and he was like, "No, we're not going to do that." And he hadn't even listened to me yet. I said, "At least let me speak." So I went on my schpiel of how she was different, how she was being fed, she was afebrile. He said, "Well, she's still got poor pulmonary mechanics." I said, "Well, you don't know what her pulmonary mechanics were when she was at home before. These might be better than what she lived with at home. You know, she didn't fail being weaned, we never gave her a fair chance, and I think we need to give her a chance. And I think if you listen to her when you go in the room instead of going, 'How are you doing, see you later,' you know. If you listen to her, you'll realize that she wants to try." So they sort of . . . Well, they went in to see her and her attending came in. So I explained to the attending about how she was acting and how she wanted to get off the vent and about the whole home-vent program and he was very interested in her discharge. Discharge planning is his thing. So I told him about the home-vent care, explained that we would have to work with her to improve her vent settings. I said, "We have to try." He was kind of reluctant. I explained to him why they (the house staff) were reluctant. He thought that was reasonable, but I continued to press. "I think the patient wants to try and I think we should really try. So why don't you go talk to her?" He goes in and says "I hear you want to try and get off the vent." And she's going, "Yeah." And he said, "Well, maybe we'll try today."

The patient was eventually weaned from the ventilator, went to a rehabilitation hospital, and finally home. Seeing new possibilities in this situation was dependent on the particular relationship between nurse and patient and upon the nurse knowing the patient (Tanner et al., 1993). The example illustrates key aspects of moral agency available to the expert practitioner. It is relational, situated, and can express solidarity or membership and participation, but this nurse can also take a stand on the unexpected, advocating what the patient needs and wants.

AGENCY

For the expert nurse, new possibilities of moral agency are created by clinical grasp, embodied know-how, and the ability to see likely future eventualities in clinical situations. Moral action is tied to the skills of seeing, doing, and being with others in respectful caring ways. As demonstrated above, skill is not the only condition for being an excellent practitioner, but it is an essential condition for acting in the moment in very complex clinical situations.

Clinical and existential caring skills are also required for expert nursing practice. Learning to work with others and orchestrate one's actions in relation to others are central to the moral agency possible at the expert level of practice. Expert moral agency requires (1) excellent moral sensibilities (a vision and commitment to good clinical and caring practices); (2) perceptual acuity (the ability to identify salient moral issues in particular situations); (3) embodied know-how; (4) skillful engagement and respectful relationships with patients, families, and co-workers; and (5) the ability to respond in the situation in a timely fashion.

The development of clinical expertise inherently demands the development of ethical expertise. We have theoretically made a distinction between medical and nursing theory related to science and existential caring skills (see Chapter 2). Expert nursing practice requires expertise in both realms. As described in this work, learning from experience is itself a moral art and skill, because it entails having one's expectations turned around, confronting the unexpected and even failure (Gadamer, 1975). One must be able to be confronted, be open to the situation, and be able to form trustworthy relationships with vulnerable partners. This work has much in common with Aristotle's notions of phronesis, virtue and skill; however, in contrast to Aristotle, emotion is recognized as integral to openness, knowing and responding, rather than always being considered a source of error and interruption (Aristotle, 1179/1953; Dreyfus, 1979). Though anxiety, arrogance, fear, and other passions can disrupt or prevent expert performance, they are also a source of understanding and access to the self and the situation. Thus, anxiety must be questioned in relation to the situation. Others in the situation can assist in understanding one's own emotional responses and understanding. The advanced beginner, by virtue of an inexperienced grasp of the situation must depend on others' perspectives. They must dampen emotional anxiety in order to act in the situation. But as experience creates embodied narrative memories, along with immediate emotional and embodied responses and mood (e.g., a sense of dread or peace), emotions attune one to the other and to the dangers, challenges, and opportunities in the situation. Emotional attunement is central to expert clinical and ethical comportment. This implies a discipline of correcting false emotional responses and strengthening correct ones. As noted in Chapter 2, the competent driver must not feel exhilaration upon cornering on the edge of the tires. Likewise, the nurse must make emotionally toned qualitative distinctions between controlling, caring, neglecting, and being sentimental about patients. This discernment can only be made *in* the situation and *in* the relationship with the other. This does not mean that these issues are hopelessly subjective or private and completely relative or emotive; it just means that they are situated and require relating and reasoning in specific transitions.

At all levels of nursing practice, relational ethics, in the form of caring practices and relationships, i.e., being true to, recognizing, hearing, seeing, and responding to the other must guide the development of clinical and ethical expertise (Benner, 1984a; Benner & Wrubel, 1989; Lindseth, 1992; Logstrup, 1956/1971; Martinsen, 1989; Phillips & Benner, 1994). Ethical nursing practice demands that the nurse not only do things for the right reason but also *be* in a good or right relationship to the other. Expert caring practices elaborate and extend the subtle voices and concerns of the weak and vulnerable. Expert care also celebrates, encourages, and extends the strengths of the other.

Thus the expert narratives of helping most often focus on the strengths of the other, rather than chronicling heroic helping feats of the one caring (Benner, Wrubel, Phillips, Chesla, & Tanner, 1995; Hauerwas, 1981). A caring stance can place the caregiver and the vulnerable ones cared for in disadvantaged positions in a system that requires adversarial and economic power for public assertion. Therefore, expert practitioners must develop skills of advocacy, communicating their concerns and designing the system to support caring practices in order to create a supportive public space for their caring practices. This calls for self-respect and independent thinking. As Dworkin, a defender of autonomy as a key moral principle, points out, it is through an enhanced understanding of "tradition, authority, commitment, and loyalty, and of the forms of human community in which these have their roots, that we shall be able to develop a conception of autonomy free from paradox and worthy of admiration" (Dworkin, 1978, p. 170).

Experientially gained clinical and ethical expertise develops a moral voice and a morality shared by a group of practitioners. We found many examples of expert practitioners advocating for their patients and demanding that the system change in order to be more just and more caring. There were examples of solidarity, i.e., standing with health care team members and patients and families, and examples of critique and correction. Both are integral to mature ethical and clinical expertise.

Moral agency for the expert is relational and situated and constituted by experiential learning in a group of health care practitioners, patients and families. While it is not possible to fully explicate the moral agency of the expert, we can give voice to what we heard and saw in practice. This discussion will focus on three major aspects of the moral agency of the expert practitioner: (1) developing the skill of involvement; (2) managing technology and preventing unnecessary technological intrusions; and (3) working with and through others.

The Skill of Involvement

Nurses practicing at the expert level often tell stories of cases where they had a particularly good connection with the patient and where this relationship opens up possibility in the situation. The few patients with whom sustaining relationships were established were remembered. Because of their involvement, nurses understood a patient's wishes in ways that would not have been possible without the particular connection and respect. In the following excerpt, the paradigm case introduced on pages 144–145 is continued. The nurse cared for this retired physician over a 6-month period of time while he was recovering from bypass graft surgery and subsequent ARDS and renal failure. The nurse was solicited by the patient's "vitality," what she saw as his interest in living. During times that he would withdraw, he would still respond to her care and concern. She told him stories about her family, show him pictures, anything she could do to make her care "more personal." When he was discharged to another hospital after nearly 6 months, the primary nurse and another colleague visited him, wanting to assure that the nurses at the next hospital knew that he was cared for:

Nurse: The relationship we had was one of the strongest ones I've ever had with anybody in nursing. I felt like I was part of his life force, and that, if he was still depressed and withdrawn, he would do so much better if there were people there that he connected with. We were part of the force that kept him going. That goes along with my philosophy, but with him it almost becomes tangible.
Int: Can you think how?

Nurse: I try not to be illness-focused with people, and to take them someplace where they feel safer. He was very vulnerable; and he was safer where there was somebody with him that was really strong.

This nurse's involvement with this patient might be considered overinvolvement, where the nurse loses objectivity, where the patient needs are overwhelming, where the nurse is committed to the patient as a person and treatment goals are overlooked or secondary. However, at no point does this nurse overlook treatment goals. Indeed, her engagement makes it possible to continue with treatment goals. There is an imagined ideal of a "comfortable" level of involvement. But the suffering and vulnerability of patients call for a level of connection that responds to the demands of care. At expert levels of practice, nurses tell of "exceptions" to the usual levels of involvement. There are stories where skill, connection, and luck conspire, and the care is synergistic in ways that cannot be predicted or mandated. Nurses can only be open to these ways of caring and support one another in order to facilitate the time and organization of work to allow this vital caring work to occur. The general cultural assumption that there is a "right" level of involvement makes even expert nurses somewhat reticent in talking openly about the nature of their interactions, their sense of commitment to the patient, and the ways in which they personalize care. But, as this exemplar and many others illustrate, there is no context-free "right" level of involvement.

The above excerpt also illustrates how involvement creates the possibility for advocacy. The nurse described protecting him by creating a climate of safety in memories, in relationship, in familiar rituals, and in the environment. As Callahan (1988, p. 13) points out, "Emotions energize the ethical quest . . . A person who wrestles with moral questions is usually emotionally committed to doing good and avoiding evil. A good case can be made that what is specifically moral about moral thinking, what gives it its imperative 'oughtness' is personal emotional investment." This is evident in the following discussion between neonatal intensive care nurses and a pediatric intensive care nurse:

Neonatal Nurse: You have to be a little obsessive to work in our place. You have to be a little bit perfectionist. You have to be very meticulous because every "cc" [*drop of IV fluid or medication*] makes a difference. Every little movement that you do makes a difference. Half of a cm [*centimeter*] is the difference between being intubated and extubated. You can't be fooling around. You're the type of person whose going to incorporate all that you can do into your care because that's the type of person you are. You may not know how to comfort a baby but once somebody shows you, it automatically becomes part of what you do, because you are compulsive about that completeness . . .

Pediatric Nurse: That's what I think the nurses that work with preemies get their gratification from because the comfort measures work. Where in Pediatrics, preemies drive me absolutely bananas because they have no personality [to me]. I think that they don't have a personality. I don't do a lot of neonatal, obviously. But they don't smile at you, call you a nerd, or they don't act out [*in contrast to young children in pediatrics*]. You can't read them stories, you can't sit with them and watch Dumbo on the VCR, or hold her hand. I like a little more give and take. That's why I like kids. But I also expect them to whine and act like babies . . . But I also get gratification from getting the kids not to whine or not to act that way.

Neonatal Nurse: But I think that's part of why my gratification is that if I take a patient [premature infant] that everybody says is a twitty brat, and I'm able to get in there and settle him down with 30 minutes, I find that tremendously gratifying.

Second Neonatal Nurse: Yeah, because it is a response. If you take a kid who's all over the place and all disconnected and get that kid nested and see that baby relax, and really go to sleep, that is just as much of a response as some kid who invents a pet name for you, that kind of stuff.

The conversation continues with more specific kinds of gratification linked with patient improvement in different patient populations:

Pediatric Nurse: That's internal. That's the kind of gratification that's internal for you. It's like Psych nurses like to work with these schizophrenic types and every 6 months they might see a little improvement . . .

These nurses illustrate the ways that expert practice is constituted by a caring relationship with the patient and guided by the patients' responses. These nurses take for granted that their work is located in relationship, and that their skills of being with infant and children include comforting, distracting, and being with the infant or child. Their skill of involvement is guided by their "gratification" at being able to soothe, to comfort. Their action is guided by known states and outcomes. The standards are stringent. The margin for error is small; a cubic centimeter or a centimeter can make a difference. Perfectionism is called for. One must do one's best, one must be guided by patient responses and desired outcomes, and learn from the inevitable failures.

Managing Technology, Preventing Unnecessary Technological Intrusions

Managing technology and appraisal of its use was integral to many of the expert narratives. Experiential wisdom about rendering technology safe, and about when technology is harmful or futile, was shared in concrete stories. This is illustrated in the following narrative:

Nurse 1: It's even minor stuff like postoperative heart—You come on some times and the kid is 4 days post-op, extubated, is eating and the nurses are still doing every-4-hour labs. And, they are all brand new or new graduates or something and it's like: "Why don't you ask the docs when they're around if you can discontinue the kid's 4-hour lab, make them once a day, or why are we still doing this?" It doesn't connect. It doesn't. Why are you going to sanguinate this kid when he's sitting up watching T.V. eating or (laughter). It's just little stuff like that. Or, continuous calcium infusion. That's another big bone of contention. . . . Three days out and they're giving hourly calcium and the kid is eating on top of that. (laughter) Have you asked them [doctors] if we can discontinue this? What is his calcium? Is it a 6? Do we need to give it to him every hour? Is it O.K.? It's little things.

Nurse 2: Things they forget to discontinue all the time.

Nurse 1: Right, it's kind of up to you to remind them. To remember to take the stitch out of the cutdown. Or, it's like little stuff that people who are really new just are taking the things that are on the Kardex [care plan] that tell them how to take care of the patient. And, when they get a little more experienced they and their assessment skills get better. They can notice that maybe they're wheezing a little bit or that they're a little cold. They're a little blue or something. But it's like cleaning up.

Experts learn common oversights and potential technical hazards for patients, and these become sources for surveillance and training for others. In this sense, the experts are the cultural standard bearers. As one nurse said: "With [mechanical] ventilation, if you are not helping, you are almost certainly doing harm." And then this maxim was spread to other forms of technology, for example, IV's, tube feedings, et cetera.

By definition, expert mastery of technology, coupled with expert caring should provide a critical perspective on technology, and this was evident in the expert narratives. While an outsider may have an outsider's critique that may be more radical than that of the insider who becomes accustomed to the use of technology, we found a prudent and critical view of technology dependency in expert narratives. Progress was measured by the patients regaining their own powers. Technological control of the body is always suboptimal and hopefully temporary. A critical stance and counter to the technological takeover and control of the body is illustrated by the following neonatal nurse's comment:

When we think we know what the course ought to be and the baby says: "No, we're not going to do it that way. You know, I can only eat so much, or I can only tolerate so much," we find out that when we actually go with what the baby seems to want to do . . . I know that sounds strange, but letting them sort of guide their care a little bit more directly instead of enforcing them into a mold that we think they ought to follow.

She and other nurses talk about "following the body's lead" (Benner, 1994d). Response-based practice and proceeding with care and respect set limits on dominance and control through sedation, paralysis, and various technologies. These nurses struggle with sanctioning and legitimizing the necessary intrusive technology, rendering it less frightening, and recognizing when its use has become excessive:

> She had a trach and we were actively weaning her. She was fine. We put her on a mask for about 10 hours during the day and then she would be back on the ventilator at night. But they had an arterial line in her for about 50 days. They kept putting A-lines in her. I said: "Why are you putting A-lines in her?" "Well, she is vented and needs to have one." I said, "No, she doesn't need to have one. One machine does not give you the criteria to put in an A-line. We know what her gasses are . . . We know when she gets into trouble. She tells us by other parameters . . ." She was also having hematocrit problems because they had been taking such frequent blood gas samples for the past 50 days.

This shows a clinical and ethical assessment of the patient needs and responses to the diagnostic procedures. Technology assessment is often related to pain infliction, pain control, and the alleviation of suffering:

> We had a transfer during the night and I was coming on to the day shift and this gentleman was transferred because of poor ABGs. He had vasculitis and he was having hemoptysis, basically bleeding into his lungs, and he was a DNR by his wishes, and his family's wishes, but he came to us because they wanted to do everything they could up to intubation. . . . I watched this man deteriorate before my eyes. He just became so restless and tachypneic. He started to become incoherent . . . He can't breathe and he's suffocating . . . I mean, he was trying to climb out of bed, he was pulling his mask off . . . he was hypoxic and he was air-hungry. He was just trying to breathe. It was terrible. It was probably one of the worst experiences I've had . . . Because he suffered so, and I feel as though we could have prevented that, we really could have. There was no need for it. And it's really my responsibility, you know. I mean, sometimes the medical staff doesn't see that [*providing comfort, alleviating suffering*] as their priority, but I think as nurses, we do and we should.

The above narrative is told with moral courage to learn from this regrettable situation. The nurse in retrospect realizes that she should have called on her colleagues for help to perform the necessary tasks, while she mobilized a more effective plan for comfort measures and pain relief. In retrospect she realized that she should have insisted that the physicians stay in the room to witness the suffering. They were trying to follow the family's wishes to stop short of intubation, and not hamper his respiratory drive by excessive medications. These were worthy goals, but needed to be altered by first-hand witness to the patient's suffering.

Becoming practiced in a field opens one to a kind of conservatism based upon getting used to the environment and the technologies used. Critical care nursing is no exception. But on an encouraging note, these expert narratives demonstrate that the notions of excellent practice, the caring relationships with particular patients, and cumulative and collective wisdom about the qualitative distinctions between justifiable heroic care and excessive futile interventions that prolong suffering and dying offer a corrective and critical perspective.

Working With and Through Others

Having a good clinical grasp, and having interventions and responses linked with that clinical grasp, sets up the possibility for expert nurses to take strong positions with other nurses and physicians to get what they believe the patients need. Recognizing the unexpected requires persuading and marshalling appropriate responses from others. Nurses practicing at this level feel compelled to make a case when they believe that the medical therapy is inappropriate for what the patient needs. For example, one nurse described "going up the ladder" until she got the responses from the physicians that she felt were appropriate for what the patient needed.

Nurse: I went to the senior resident. First, I went to the ortho[paedic] intern, and the chief and his intern came down and evaluated it. But everything persisted still and then I called the trauma intern. I didn't care for what he said. So then I jumped up to the senior and that's where I got results.

Int: Is that a common occurrence for you to have to go to . . .

Nurse: A higher-up? Yeah. I think it's our responsibility. If you don't get a good answer you're expected to do that.

Int: Any negative consequences for doing that?

Nurse: I think sometimes the intern or the junior, whoever you jump over, gets a little upset at you for not talking to them. But if you're not getting the right answer and something goes wrong and you didn't pursue it, then the patient gets in trouble. So I can deal with someone getting mad at me. If I think it's serious enough, I'll go to the top.

This sense of responsibility for the patient's well-being is more realistic in terms of actual possibilities inherent in the situation and in the nurses' capabilities as compared to the hyper-responsibility and burden experienced by the competent nurse. This is illustrated by concrete preparation for emergencies:

> It took me from that first time when I walked into that C-Section room and found out by shock that I was responsible for that infant until 3½ years later for it to be O.K. for me to be responsible for that infant. I can take care of that baby until the doctor gets there [describing an emergency situation]. And there was an interim period in there where I didn't feel comfortable with that. I think we work with a wonderful group of doctors. I really do. I can say that of almost all of them. They were willing to let us learn skills . . . Even for my own peace of mind that may happen once a year. It may never happen again for another 5 years, but I know in the back of my mind that I've seen those vocal chords. I know what size [endotracheal] tube to put in and I can do it if I have to.

It is personally and ethically untenable to experience helplessness in the face of medical emergencies when lives are at stake. Thus expert clinical and ethical comportment require that the nurse prepare to be the first response to the crisis, since the nurse is the one who is usually with the patient when the crisis occurs.

The moral agency of the expert nurse is more fully socially embedded with better recognition of what those present in the situation can bring to it. An increased ability to read the situation allows the nurse to step in and step back as the situation demands. There is a more realistic understanding of limits, and this is a corrective to hyper-responsibility, as one nurse explains:

> My feeling is you can't make things all right for families. You're never going to make something that is horrible all right and that it's a fallacy when we try to approach it that way. [*She goes on to give an example of a tragedy that was beyond expectations and interventions.*]

Experiential learning allows the practitioner to come to terms with boundaries, limits, and possibilities. Thus, the expert demonstrates taking a moral stance, in the case of the exceptional and unexpected, at odds with convention and others' expectations. The expert also demonstrates prudence in recognizing the strengths and weakness of others. Nursing practice, like all caring practices, cannot be done in isolation. It is not a heroic solo performance, therefore, part of nursing expertise lies in strengthening and working with others so that no one is overburdened and all possible resources are brought to bear in difficult situations.

SUMMARY

Clinical and ethical expertise are inextricably interrelated. And in nursing practice, both are made possible in the concrete relationships between nurse and patient and families. The development of expert practice is dependent upon having expert practitioners show the way by their response-based practice in concrete situations.

Educational Implications

Expert practitioners in any field embody the practical knowledge, and the extant dialogical understandings, of how to integrate practical and theoretical knowledge. Articulating expert practice as we have tried to do in this chapter is crucial for designing our formal organizational work and accounting systems in ways that do justice to and facilitate expert practice. Too often, the stories of expert practitioners reflect Herculean efforts to overcome organizational impediments to their practice. We must find ways to bend our formal systems to the best of our practice, rather than inhibit expert practice by organizational policies uninformed by examples of excellence. Typically organizational structures and policies are geared to minimal expectations, pushing excellence to the unacknowledged and unaccommodated margins. Gearing organizational structures and policies to the minimal standards of performance covers over the very examples of excellence that we would like highlighted and extended in practice. It also handicaps organizational leaders by making them focus on shoring up deficits rather than designing the organization for excellent practice.

It is impossible to spell out all the implications of any expert practice, just as it is impossible to completely formalize expertise. The most notable implication is that we should study and learn from expert practice. We must become more attentive and skilled at giving voice and public sanction to the difficult work of meeting and recognizing others in times of vulnerability. We will attempt to live up to the vision of excellent practice offered by these experts in the remaining chapters.

Chapter 7

IMPEDIMENTS TO THE DEVELOPMENT OF CLINICAL KNOWLEDGE AND ETHICAL JUDGMENT IN CRITICAL CARE NURSING

Jane Rubin

This chapter describes a type of nurse whose practice falls outside the normal developmental trajectory of beginner-competent-proficient-expert. It falls outside the trajectory both in the sense that this type of nurse never seems to perform at any of these specific levels of practice, and that the type of practice that characterizes these nurses has no developmental trajectory of its own. From the beginning, these nurses seem to be stuck in an unchanging form of practice that severely restricts the development of their clinical knowledge and their ethical judgment. In this chapter, I want to describe the practice of these nurses and attempts to demonstrate how their lack of development of clinical knowledge forms the basis for an inability to recognize ethical issues in their work.

The nurses described in this chapter were primarily the 25 nurses who were identified by nursing supervisors as being experienced, but not expert, practitioners. All had worked in ICUs for at least 5 years, and thus their practical experience paralleled that of nurses in this study who demonstrated expert practice. However, qualities of their practice led knowledgeable supervisors to mark these nurses' practice as safe but not expert, despite years of experience.

The concern in designing the study was to capture a range of nursing practice, from exemplary to problematic. The aim was to capture this variability in the practice of new and intermediate nurses by leaving open-ended the criteria for selection in this level of experience. That is, no quali-fiers were placed on the kinds of practice new and intermediate nurses demonstrated other than the duration of experience. With nurses who had practiced more than 5 years, head nurses were asked to name nurses who they considered to be outstanding or superb practitioners, as well as those they considered to be safe, but not superior practitioners. It is note-worthy that the majority of the narratives described in this chapter were drawn from the group identified as experienced but nonexpert nurses, but that was not always the case. In some instances, head nurses identified practitioners as expert, and in examining their narratives, we saw characteristics of their practice that evidenced less than expert prac-tice. Head nurses may have identified some nurses for this group based on different understandings of expertise than we employ, or they may have been more distant from the nurses' particular ways of work-ing than we were able to become in the course of gathering detailed narratives.

In order to describe the way these nurses understand their work, I em-ploy a paradigm case of one nurse, who without much deliberation or clar-ity, administers medication to a dying patient that ends the patient's life. I have chosen this case because it seems to exhibit many, if not all, of the essential ways in which the nurses in this group take up their work. A longer paradigm case is used here (as it was in Chapter 1) because the full story of care of a particular patient is needed to demonstrate the nature of these nurses' work. Multiple brief examples provide insufficient context for understanding the complex issues that arise in the work of these expe-rienced but not expert nurses.

I want to emphasize from the beginning the importance of the notion of practice in this analysis. As we will see, it is tempting to attribute the defi-ciencies of the nurses in this group to individual idiosyncracies, such as psychological problems. It is also tempting to attribute them to underly-ing social problems, such as the overly litigious society that causes these nurses to be concerned with the legal consequences of their actions at the expense of moral considerations.

It is not my intention to discount in any way the importance of psy-chological and social factors as impediments to the development of clini-cal knowledge and ethical judgment in the nurses in this group. I want to argue, however, that these nurses share a common structure of prac-tice that stands in relation to, but cannot be reduced to, psychological and social factors. While this kind of practice does not always produce the ethical blindness described in the paradigm case, it often does produce inadequate care. It is my hope that identifying the structure of the prac-tice can help to prevent both blunted ethical perceptions and the inad-equacies of care.

STRUCTURE OF PRACTICE

When I began studying these nurses, one of the first things that struck me was that they could not remember very much about their patients. Not only could they not describe a critical incident that had made a difference in their practice; most could not even remember the specifics of a particular case, even the most recent. When asked to talk about a patient, one of these nurses, who worked in a neonatal intensive care unit, replied, "The last kid that I took care of had something else going on and I can't . . . I would have to look it up." Another nurse, when asked to describe in more detail a patient who, she had indicated, had made a difference in her practice, said, "I can't remember him. I'm worried about my memory now." A third nurse, after listening to an expert nurse's moving description of her work with dying patients, was asked by the interviewer, "You said earlier that you thought things might get triggered for you. I wondered if anything did?" The nurse replied, "All that gets triggered is death and dying. There's no specifics. It's like all mish mash."[1]

The paradigm case I will discuss in this chapter fits this pattern. At the beginning of the interview, the interviewer asks the nurse to describe "a clinical situation that's vivid to you, that you remember." The nurse responds:

> I'll tell one that I'm sure you've heard before about someone who . . . was admitted on a Saturday and had a chronic illness and was elderly and had lost her home and was being asked to move into a nursing home and she had to give up her pets and so on. And by Sunday, she . . . had changed her mind, was ready to die and was dying and there wasn't a lot that could be done to prevent it anyway unless she wanted to be intubated and have a long course and probably die anyway, and opted not to be intubated and to take—what did she take?—some minor Valium or something. I've forgotten what, and stopped breathing, basically. That to me was vivid.

The nurse's lack of memory for the specifics of this situation is quite striking. She has administered a medication that, while relieving suffering, has hastened the death of her patient and she does not remember what medication she administered. She also does not remember the patient's medical condition or her age. Asked by another nurse, "What did she come in with?" she replies,

> "I think it was MS or something, some long-term neurologic."
> **Int.:**   About how old was she?
> **Nurse:**   I would say 75, maybe 80.

The lack of memory is especially noticeable since this was the first time this nurse had ever administered a medication that may have contributed to an earlier death. She continues: "It was the first time I actually delivered a medication that I knew was going to cause this woman to become hypoxic and then stop breathing." It is highly implausible that all of the nurses in this group are suffering from organic forms of memory loss. And it is almost equally unlikely that all of them have nonorganic clinical syndromes, such as depression or substance abuse, that can cause memory loss. I want to suggest, therefore, that their lack of memory has less to do with their individual biology or psychology than with their common way of practicing.

As I indicated above, these nurses' form of practice is one in which clinical knowledge and ethical judgment play no meaningful role in the experience of the practitioners. In other words, while these nurses often make clinical and ethical judgments, they do not experience themselves as doing so. Their inability to experience themselves as making clinical and ethical judgments in their practice differentiates them from the nurses in all of the other groups in this study and is responsible for their peculiar form of practice described in the introduction above.

In order to make this claim plausible, it is necessary to describe what I mean by clinical knowledge and to show how it is absent from these nurses' experience of their practice. I will then go on to describe how their inability to experience themselves as making ethical judgments derives directly from their inability to experience themselves as making clinical judgments.

CLINICAL JUDGMENT

In the next section of the interview, the nurse in the paradigm case describes her understanding of how her patient came to the decision to end her life:

Nurse: She had lived up until that time in her home and was very active in the community, and had a lot of friends and support, but over the years that just sort of dwindled. And I was just struck with the rapidity of how quickly she changed her mind, but how at the same time she remained trustworthy, I guess, in her decision.

Int.: But when you say, "changed her mind," she changed her mind from what to what?

Nurse: She changed her mind from struggling with the issues of how to live in her new setting without her furniture, without her pets, without her former support group, uh, to deciding not to live.

Int.: Do you know how she came to go through that transition? Did she verbalize to you at all or did she talk to anybody else about it?

Nurse: No, I don't know how she came to it. I'm sure that it was not news to her that she was chronically ill and had to make some decisions. And I wasn't there, I don't think I was there when the actual change occurred. I mean, one day she was wanting to struggle, could barely breathe and so on. You know, frequent blood gasses and all the treatments and she was, you know, frustrated that she couldn't rest and the next day she had pretty much decided. So I guess it happened when I wasn't there. I don't think I had a lot to do with it. I think she had everything to do with it.

The first striking fact about this nurse's account is that she admits to having no direct knowledge of the patient's having made the decision to discontinue the treatments that were keeping her alive: "I don't know how she came to it. I wasn't there." She does not even seem to have indirect knowledge, such as reports from others who were present, that this was, in fact, the woman's decision: "And I was just struck with the rapidity of how quickly she changed her mind, but how at the same time *she remained trustworthy, I guess,* [emphasis mine] in her decision."

In addition to this nurse's not knowing what and how the woman decided to discontinue treatment, she also does not know if the woman's physician complied with her request. She seems to take the fact that the physician complied with the patient's request for a sedative as evidence that he was complying with her wish to die. In addition, she seems to take the patient's acknowledgment that she will die when the medication is administered as constituting informed consent:

Int.:   How did she get her way? I mean, how did she communicate with the physician and with the nurse that this is her decision?
Nurse: I don't remember anything about that except that I did at one point call her doctor and ask for a sedative, per her request. And that's about all I remember. And I knew when I gave it that it was going to be an important step and I also said that to her. "You know when I give you this injection that your breathing's going to slow down and you will, you will die." And she said, "I know."

Despite her lack of indirect knowledge of the patient's decision, this nurse makes two very important assumptions about it: (1) that the patient has decided not to struggle with issues of living in her new setting; and (2) that she has decided not to struggle with the frustrations of breathing. It is in these two assumptions that this nurse's lack of what I am calling clinical knowledge is revealed.

Apropos of #1, this nurse makes no attempt to find out the meaning, for this specific patient, of leaving her home, her support group, her pets, and so on. Instead of getting to know her particular patient, she sees her as a kind of stereotype: *"I'll tell one that I'm sure you've heard before* [emphasis mine] about someone who had a chronic illness and was elderly and had lost her home and was being asked to move into a nursing home and she had to give up her pets and so on." While the nurse indicates that, at the time of her admission, the patient was "struggling with the issues of how to live in her new setting without her furniture, without her pets, without her former support group," she seems to make no effort to try to understand how the patient experiences her conflict about moving into a nursing home. Instead, she seems to see the struggle as already having been decided and she experiences none of the usual professional mandates to clarify these issues.

Apropos of #2—the patient's struggle to breathe—this nurse does not acknowledge, either to the patient or herself, the anguish of the patient's situation—namely, that, with the discontinuation of respiratory treatment, the only way to ease the patient's breathing and make her more comfortable is to administer a medication like morphine or Valium that decreases her distress but also hastens her death. Instead of presenting the treatment options to the patient, the nurse simply announces to her that she is going to administer a medication that will cause her to stop breathing and die, apparently assuming that the physician has worked out the treatment options with her.

In the remainder of this section, I want to expand upon the above comments by demonstrating the similarity between this nurse's responses to the patient's struggle with the issue of moving from her home and her struggle to breathe. I hope to demonstrate that similarity resides in this nurse's—and this group of nurses'—inability to make meaningful—or, as the 19th century philosopher, Soren Kierkegaard, and the 20th century philosopher, Charles Taylor, call them "qualitative" distinctions.[2] I hope to show that the ability to recognize qualitative distinctions is what we mean by clinical knowledge and that the absence of this ability in this group of nurses accounts for their lack of clinical knowledge.

What qualitative distinctions are missing from this nurse's account of her experience with her patient? First of all, this nurse makes no meaningful distinctions between different patients. Presumably, a nurse with this number of years in critical care would have taken care of many elderly patients who had been in situations similar to that of this patient. One would expect that, on the basis of this experience, she would recognize that patients experience this situation in many different ways. Her recognition, for example, that other patients have been able to find their lives worth living despite their having to undergo such a major upheaval, might allow her to see her patient's current despair as one possible response, rather than the only possible response, to her situation. This would both allow her to empathize with the patient's perspective and to offer alternatives.

I am not suggesting that continuing this patient's life was necessarily the right decision in this case. I am suggesting, however, that it is impossible to know what the best decision might have been because we do not have enough information about the patient—in this instance, specifically, information about how the patient was experiencing her situation, and how she came to experience it in that way.

I am also not suggesting that this nurse was necessarily the best person to elicit this information from the patient. However, if she were consciously aware of her limitations in this area, she would presumably consult with her colleagues or order a social work, psychiatry or clinical nurse specialist consult in order to more fully determine both this woman's mental status and her knowledge of the practical alternatives available to her. Because the understanding that this woman's situation might have more than one meaning is absent from this nurse's experience, however, she does not do this.

Thus, one way in which nurses in this group fail to make qualitative distinctions is in their failure to make distinctions between their patients. Another way of putting this is that the idea that their patients have individual, subjective experiences of and understandings of their situations seems to be completely unavailable to them. Instead, they assume that the objective features of the situation—being elderly, losing one's home, etc.— have only one meaning and that that meaning is the same for everyone: death would be preferable.

It is important to emphasize here that this habit of assuming that a particular experience has the same meaning for all patients is not limited to situations where the meaning is assumed to be negative. These nurses make the same assumption in situations where meaning seems to be positive. For example, one nurse in this study reported working with a patient who, after experiencing expressive aphasia following surgery, recovered his speech. The nurse assumed that the patient's experience of recovering his speech should be an unambiguously positive one. She had no tolerance for, let alone understanding of, his fears and anxieties:

> He could say his name. He was thrilled to death at saying his name. But during the time when he was having great difficulty talking you couldn't get him to go to sleep. He was very frustrated. He wanted to call his wife. We're like, "No, we're not calling her at 12:00 to tell her you can't talk. It's going to be okay." So this morning when his speech came back, *all I said to him* [emphasis mine] is, "Look, it's back, you're getting better. You need to rest. It may go away again, but remember it will come back." Because it will!

Related to this inability to make meaningful distinctions between their patients is the inability of these nurses to make a meaningful distinction between themselves and their patients. Insofar as they do acknowledge a realm of individual, subjective meaning, they assume that their patients will find the same meaning in the situation that they, the nurses, imagine they would find if they were in a similar situation. Indeed, these nurses seem to be able to establish a relationship with a patient only to the extent that they can imagine that that patient's experience is the same as their own. When the nurse in the paradigm case of the patient refusing further respiratory support reflects on her experience with her patient, she says:

> I think that's how I'm going to do it. That's why I felt that. I mean, I think one day I'm just going to decide, that's enough. You know, that's how I want, I hope that someone's there for me when I'm ready, basically, so I had no qualms about what I did, and I admired her so much for what she did.

We can recognize a similar response in the actions of another nurse in the study. When she heard that an alcoholic patient had been admitted to the emergency room, this nurse left the ICU to spend time with the patient in the emergency room. She subsequently spent a great deal of time with the patient on the medical floor. The nurse, in this case, was herself a recovering alcoholic. She describes the reasons for her unusual involvement with this patient as follows:

> I know that when I first saw this woman, I, I, there was, I just developed a relationship of sorts, on some level. I mean there was some kind of a connection. And it's not that she said anything . . . And so, uh, I am a recovering alcoholic and I have been sober for 4 years and I think that that's part of the process that I went through *to look at people in, that are specifically alcoholics, a more humane way* [emphasis mine] . . . But having come to terms with the disease of alcoholism in my life *and knowing what it means in my life* [emphasis mine] and how it's affected me has given me the insight to be able to take care of these people more compassionately.

At this point in our discussion, it should no longer be surprising that the nurses in this group have no memory of their patients. Because of their inability to make distinctions between patients, and between themselves and their patients, these nurses never come to experience their patients as individuals. Because they have no experience of the particular patient, they have no one, in particular, to remember.

The first kinds of qualitative distinctions that are missing from the practice of these nurses, then, are the kinds that differentiate individuals from each other. There is another kind of distinction that is also missing, however. These nurses also lack the ability to make distinctions between clinical phenomena. A return to the interview will clarify this point. The nurse continues her discussion of how her patient came to her decision to end her life:

And by Sunday, she had changed her mind, was ready to die and was dying and there wasn't a lot that could be done to prevent it anyway unless she wanted to be intubated and have a long course and probably die anyway.

I mean, one day she was wanting to struggle, could barely breathe and so on. You know, frequent blood gasses and all the treatments and she was, you know, frustrated that she couldn't rest and the next day she had pretty much decided.

One of the most striking features of this passage is what is missing from it. As the nurse presents the situation, there are only two alternatives—either the patient will struggle with her breathing or she will die. Completely absent from her consideration is the idea that she might be able to make the patient more comfortable as her physical condition deteriorates.

In the practice of these nurses, the idea that there is only one issue in patient care—improvement or lack of improvement in the patient's physical condition—continually recurs. What is missing is any qualitative distinction—what I want to call genuinely clinical knowledge. This can be illustrated by contrasting an expert nurse and a nonexpert experienced nurse.

The nonexpert nurse describes a situation in which a woman comes into the CCU with chest pains. This nurse is trying to determine what is causing them by trying a variety of medications. Nothing, from Mylanta to blood pressure medication, works. There is nothing unusual about this technique; it is standard practice in such a situation. However, at one point in the interview, the question turns from what this nurse did in the situation to how she recognizes different clinical pictures. In this instance, the interviewer asks the nurse what she would expect to see if a patient came with a clear-cut case of angina:

Int.:   Could you talk about what, if somebody came in and they had angina and it was a real clear cut case, what you would expect to see?

Nurse: Well, it depends on how bad the angina is. Sometimes what you try and do first is try and control it on nitrates. You give them some nitroglycerine and you give it to them a couple of times. Then you try a little bit of morphine. And then if that doesn't work the patients get put on nitroglycerine drips. And then you have to titrate according to their blood pressure. You have to keep their blood pressure usually greater than 100. And hopefully that will control the angina.

And you're also going to have . . . They'll be monitored and EKG will show if there's any ST elevations, which would tell us that we're getting or having a true MI. And then sometimes a little nitropaste will help. Some procardia, nyphetapine, some of the calcium channel blockers, are not immediate, but they're the ones that will take care of the pain in the long run . . .

And if nitroglycerine doesn't work, I've seen people put on balloon pumps. And that's usually when I'm up at the Medical Center. You go to the nitro and if that doesn't work they go on the pump. And they come here. Because we don't take care of pumps. Usually they need surgery or something like that. We'll take care of a balloon pump overnight. But that's the progression. You start simple. You start with some nitroglycerine. Then if that doesn't help, or if it's helped some and hasn't totally taken it away, then you might give them a little morphine, and hopefully by then it will take it away. And you're also checking the pressures 'cause sometimes you just can't give all that stuff. And then eventually, after the nitrates, morphine, if nothing's helping, a nitroglycerine drip, and then to the balloon pump. That's the progression I've seen.

What is striking about this account is that, in this entire lengthy description, this nurse describes a typical protocol, but never describes angina. She refers to blood pressure and ST elevations and she mentions the patient's pain. Near the conclusion of the interview, she refers to these factors again:

Int.:   If you had to choose or try to sort out, was it the Mylanta, was it the decreased blood pressure, how would you sort that out?

Nurse: I have a feeling it was because her pressure went down, because I gave her drugs at midnight, at 2:00 AM, I checked her pressure, and it was like 110 over 70, and she said to me "My pain is gone." And I really think it was her blood pressure coming down. That's what made her feel better.

My point here is that this nurse has no meaningful way of distinguishing between angina and, for instance, G.I. [gastrointestinal] problems, which she also suspects in this case. For her, clinical phenomena are differentiated on the basis of quantitative differences between the *same* objective measures, such as vital signs. In other words, this nurse never sees patient responses to angina or G.I. problems; she sees vital signs and other objective measurements. Her conclusions about the patient's improvement or lack of improvement are based upon these objective measurements and on the patient's subjective reports of pain.

At first glance, there may seem to be nothing unusual in this practice. It could be argued that the objective measures provide a more refined means of diagnosis and treatment and that the objective measures make elaborate differentiations among clinical phenomena unnecessary. In order to recognize what is missing from this practice, it is helpful, therefore, to contrast it with the practice of an expert nurse.

This nurse is recognized in her unit for her unique skills in working with dying patients and their families. A great deal of her practice involves the use of medications. She is asked how she makes decisions about medicating patients who are dying. In her answer, she makes it clear that the comfort of the patient and his or her family is her criterion for making these decisions:

If you give too little the only concern is that the patient and the family will be uncomfortable. I don't worry about giving too much. They're going to die, and as long as they die comfortably, that's the only thing that really matters. There's hardly such a thing as too much at that time. If they were viable . . . I worry about too much on patients who are going to live. I always am concerned about drugs and that we overuse them in an ICU, but not at that time.

As she discusses her medication practice further, it becomes apparent that the distinction between comfort and suffering plays a major role in structuring it. Despite her statement that there is no such thing as giving too much of a drug when it is being prescribed for reasons of patient comfort, she goes on to say that, even in these cases, there is an optimum amount of a drug to be given. However, she does not describe this optimum amount either in terms of quantitative measures of patient comfort and suffering, such as vital signs, or in terms of quantities of medicine. She does not equate creating comfort with administering a particular quantity of morphine:

> With some patients you might not need any drugs. With other patients you need a lot of drugs. It depends on who they are. Sometimes 2 mg will do what 70 mg will do . . . And so you just have to give what they *need* until she looks comfortable, looks asleep, and everybody else feels at peace. And there's sort of a peacefulness when they're not air-hungering and scared.

We can now see more clearly what is missing from the practice of nurses who lack qualitative distinctions between clinical phenomena. The nurse in our paradigm case cannot talk to her patient about the ways she can make her comfortable while she is dying. All the nurse can do is tell her that the medication she can give her will make her stop breathing. Furthermore, this nurse does not seem to be able to produce the kind of comfort that the expert nurse can. We have no evidence that the nonexpert nurse is able to recognize the signs of comfort or to correlate doses of medication with them. The inability to recognize clinical qualitative distinctions, then, has far-reaching consequences for nursing care.

ETHICAL JUDGMENT

When the nurse in our paradigm case is questioned about the ethical implications of her administration of the medication to her patient, the exchange is as follows:

Int.: That dying process can be really agonizing; and working with them to give them enough sedation to make them comfortable but not enough that you would call it mercy killing . . . Did you feel like you were in that grey zone?

Nurse: Well, I wondered if what I was doing was legal. And I think I must have found a way to, uh, make it okay in my mind. I mean I don't want to get sued.

This nurse's answer is representative of the ethical perspective of the nurses in this group. These nurses have no clear conception of the existence of the ethical *per se*; instead, they consistently, if confusedly, reduce ethical considerations to legal ones. For these nurses, the distinction between right and wrong is constantly being replaced by the distinction between legal and illegal.

In this section, I want to illustrate how the lack of clinical qualitative distinctions—in both of the senses of these distinctions described above—is responsible for the lack of ethical distinctions in the practice of these nurses.

The interview continues:

Int.: If we're talking about the ethics and legality of it, the alternative would have been what?

Nurse: For her to be very uncomfortable . . . She was clearly, you know, legally not a code so it was not an issue, but, yes, she would have died shortly. I never say when.

Int.: But with a fair amount of distress because she was having . . .

Nurse: A lot of difficulty breathing . . . She was extremely short of breath; she was cyanotic; she was using her head to breathe and her neck to breathe, and her belly to breathe; and she was contracted such that there wasn't a lot of motion to begin with. So every word was an effort . . . It was sort of the respiratory treatment that was supporting her through Saturday. So as soon as she quit and made that decision to stop that, then she started getting really uncomfortable and deteriorating even more quickly. And I think that's another reason why I felt comfortable.

Because her patient has elected to terminate ventilatory support and not to be intubated, this nurse sees death as the only alternative to extreme discomfort. Thus, the ethical choice is clear for her. Because the patient is going to die soon anyway, it is better to hasten her death with medication than to let her suffer. The only problematic issue is whether the obviously ethical choice can be legally justified.

To state the matter in another way, this nurse seems to have no place in her practice for the goal of making the patient comfortable. Instead of experiencing the hastening of her patient's death as the consequence of her providing her patient with comfort, this nurse seems to take the patient's death as the goal of her intervention. The patient's "comfort," if it can be termed that, is the cessation of her suffering in death.

The relationship between this nurse's lack of awareness of the ethical implications of her decision and her lack of clinical qualitative distinctions should be evident from this example. However, it can be made more explicit if we again compare this nurse's decision in this case to the practice of the expert nurse described in the previous section. For the expert nurse, when a patient is going to die, the overriding concern is to make the patient comfortable. She is able to describe the comfort she attempts to produce in a great amount of detail:

> And then when a patient's going to die, and we know they're going to die, and they're going to withdraw support, we usually give morphine. That's usually what we use and what we want to do is keep them from gasping, keep them from looking uncomfortable, keep them from opening their eyes and looking frightened if they're awake after that decision's been made.

Insofar as she knows the distinctions between gasping and breathing comfortably, looking frightened and looking calm, and so on, the expert nurse is able to recognize and articulate the good that she is attempting to realize in this particular situation. As a result, she is spared the moral confusion of the nurse in our paradigm case. Thus, for the expert nurse, comfort is the goal that results in death; but, for her, comfort is not equated with death. Indeed, the time between the patient's initial experience of extreme discomfort and the patient's death is a time that is uniquely significant for this nurse. For the nurse in our paradigm case, in contrast, this time seems not to exist. For her, there is only the time of suffering and the time of death.

One of the most disturbing consequences of the lack of clinical knowledge exhibited in these sections of the interview—and in the interviews of this group of nurses as a whole—is the complete deferral of responsibility for clinical decisions. On the one hand, these nurses cannot experience themselves as doing what is good in critical clinical situations; on the other hand, they clearly have moral qualms about their actions that they cannot effectively articulate to themselves or others. As a result, they can consistently attribute the responsibility for their decisions to other people.

One especially frightening consequence of these nurses' need to impute responsibility for their actions to someone else is that they take statements and actions that could have several meanings as unambiguous authorizations for their actions. The nurse in our paradigm case takes two other people—the patient's physician and the patient's friend—to have authorized her administration of the medication to her patient. As we see in the following quotations, in the absence of her own ability to make ethical judgments, this nurse is both desperate to have this authorization for her actions and anxious that it is not completely trustworthy.

With respect to her encounter with the patient's physician, the nurse in the paradigm case reports that the fact that this particular physician is ordinarily conservative in his prescription of medications gives her a "clue" that her administration of the medication was, as she says, "okay" in this case. Her reliance on "clues," as opposed to first-hand knowledge, reveals both her need to believe that her action was justified and her uncertainty about this:

> The other thing that occurs to me is that her physician, not only did he say, "Okay, give her that." But he's a physician that's sort of not free with medicine, so I knew that if it was okay with him to do that, that it was okay. That was another thing, another clue I had.

A similar deferral of responsibility informs this nurse's relationship to her patient's friend. She has no clear memory of this friend. In fact, she does not even remember the friend's gender. Yet she takes the friend's not protesting her action to be an endorsement of it:

Int.:   You said in this case there was a friend that sort of, and that was more evidence for you to [think] you were doing the right thing in this situation? Can you talk a little about that?

Nurse: I really don't remember. The friend was very supportive of the woman, no matter what she wanted to do, she would be—I can't remember if it was a she or a he—she just listened to the woman while she talked about being ready to go and she was supportive of her and she didn't give her a hard time and she didn't try and talk her out of it, she just, it was okay with her. And that's about all I remember.

And I, she was there when I gave the injection and she heard me say this is, this is going to cause you to stop breathing eventually. You're going to get sleepy, and she, she was, she didn't jump up and say, "Oh, no, you can't do that." She just sat there calmly and I think she held the woman's hand, it was very, it was a pleasant end, and I was happy to have participated in it.

Rather than acknowledge their moral uncertainties, then, the nurses in this group defer the responsibility for their decisions in critical clinical situations. Because these nurses do not recognize and cannot articulate clinical qualitative distinctions, their moral confusion leads them to rely on extremely questionable "objective" evidence to assure themselves that they have made the right decision. The deferral of responsibility characteristic of this group differs from that seen in the advanced beginner group. Advanced beginners tend to "delegate up"; they are awash with anxiety, and believe that they lack the knowledge to make the judgments called for by the situation.

A similar point can be made about the relationship between these nurses' moral confusion and their lack of awareness of the qualitative distinctions that could allow them to understand their patient's subjective experience. For the nurses in this group, the ultimate arbiter of the morality of a particular clinical decision is what the patient wants. This is illustrated in the following section of the interview. The nurse is asked about her feelings about being in such a morally ambiguous situation as the one she experienced with her patient:

Int.: Giving the drug put you in a grey zone. How would you have felt if you would not have given the drug?
Nurse: Had she, if she had asked for it?
Int.: She'd asked for it and it was . . .
Nurse: And the physician refused like I thought he would.
Int.: Right, the physician refused—let's do it both ways. Let's do it if the physician refused and let's do it if you refused because . . .
Nurse: Didn't feel comfortable doing it . . . One will be easy to talk about because I've been in that situation before where the physician, something happens and the patient doesn't get what they want and they're wanting to die and can't. And that's frustrating . . .

I would feel determined . . . I would work hard to get what the patient wants. If all those indicators where that, yes, it's okay with everybody except for this one glitch, it's clearly just a glitch and not a reasonable fear . . . the other I don't, I don't know.

Several things are apparent from this exchange. First, for these nurses, patients' "wants" are taken as constituting the unchallengeable foundation of psychological life. The idea that patients might be confused or conflicted about what they want; that the meaning of what they experience themselves as consenting to might be different from what the nurse experiences them as consenting to; that what they want might be influenced by depression or anxiety, etc.—none of this enters into these nurses' clinical or ethical considerations. These nurses don't see desires as having meanings; they don't have distinctions between the various kinds of desires and the different ways they are expressed.

Second, and perhaps even more important, these nurses do not experience themselves as influencing the patient's desires in any way. Instead, they see themselves as simply the means to the fulfillment of the patient's ends. They do not question their role in influencing those ends by their presentation of treatment options or other matters. With respect to our paradigm case, it does not seem to occur to this nurse that her presentation of the options as suffering or death instead of suffering or comfort can affect her patient's experience of her death—that there is a qualitative difference, in other words, between experiencing one's death as an escape from intolerable suffering or experiencing it within the context of the provision of comfort.

Finally, it is important to note how these nurses respond when they are unable to get authorization for administering the drugs that would end their patients' lives. They express genuine indignation at this situation and cannot imagine how anything other than what the nurse in our paradigm case calls a "glitch"—a purely technical obstacle—could be responsible for it. The idea that there could be genuine clinical or ethical objections to hastening the patient's death is not expressed:

> Where there has been a glitch that seems reasonable to me, if that glitch gets resolved, then things sort of move toward the end that the patient wants. But it's usually some person or some thing that, some family member or some one doctor or some issue—I don't think it's ever a nurse—some person needs to let go . . . settle whatever issue it is, legal issue or whatever it is, then once that gets settled, then things move along the way. But I can't imagine being that glitch.

One final way of highlighting the absence of the qualitative distinctions that would allow these nurses to make ethical sense of their practice is, again, to contrast the nurses in this group with expert nurses. One of the most striking differences between expert nurses and the nurses in this group is that expert nurses speak a language of needs rather than wants. Unlike the language of wants, the language of needs implies evaluation and judgment on the part of the nurse. This becomes especially clear in several statements from the expert nurse whom we quoted earlier in this chapter. This nurse describes a woman whose husband is about to die. She is asked if she experienced any difficulties in working with this family. She replies:

Nurse: He was transferred to this hospial for a liver transplant. He was relatively young, a man in his late 30s. He had liver disease, but was septic and so sick that they finally had decided that he wasn't going to get a liver. And if he wasn't going to get a liver there wasn't anything anybody could do for him. But they did come here with high hopes. He had been awake talking and wasn't out of it. But he'd quickly gone into encephalopathy, renal failure and had some infections. His wife was fighting for him, wanting the liver and wanting everything to be done. She was a really strong young woman, had children, one son about 9 years old. . . . But when they finally told her that he wasn't going to get a liver, she sort of went hysterical for awhile . . . [I] just put my arm around her and asked her if there's anything she needs. And right away she started telling me what she needed was to be able to get in bed with him. First she went and talked to the doctor and called her family and had them bring her 9-year-old son in. And then she came back in and I had already moved him over.

I didn't do very much . . . I asked her if she would like to have the tubes taken
out of him and she said yes. So we disconnected all the IVs except one and
took almost everything apart, moved him over, put a blanket there for her to
lie on. They came in and extubated him while she was there and she got in bed
with him and held him for about an hour until he died. . . .

Int.: What sort of problems had they had?

Nurse: Her resisting withdrawal of support for the patient and not wanting to
give in to the fact that there wasn't anything that anybody could do for him
anymore. She just *needed* [emphasis mine] more time, I think.

This nurse gets unneeded equipment out of the room and makes a place
for the woman to lie in her husband's bed until she is ready to accept her
husband's death. The nurse doesn't try to hasten the husband's death. Eventually, the husband dies peacefully and the wife gets up from the bed.

In a more general account of her work with dying patients, the nurse
continues:

You sort of assess what that particular family *needs*. And when you come
into a room, and if you're working with them for a long time, it just sort of
is happening, what they *need* [emphases mine].

What is most striking about this nurse, however, is her willingness to
place the patient and the family's comfort above all other concerns, including her own professional security:

I'm not afraid to create a peaceful death if that *needs* to be done. Most people
are afraid. They're afraid they'll lose their license or they're afraid of . . .
usually that's what they're afraid of. I don't understand. I always say, "I
would rather lose my license than be part of a patient's frightening death, *if
I can have the ability to change that at that time*" [emphases mine].

In contrast to expert nurses, whose use of the language of needs is an
indication of their ability to engage with their patients, the nurses in this
group use the language of wants as a way of disengaging from their patients. On those rare occasions when they speak of a patient needing something, they invariably speak either of asking the patient to tell them what
they need or of the patient's need to control their emotions or behavior
without help from the nurse. One nurse's use of the language of wants demonstrates both the distancing function of this language and the seemingly
unbridgeable gap that separates the practice of these nurses from the practice of expert nurses:

I was thinking about letting people die in the CCU. A patient had chest pain
and I think she had breast cancer and stuff . . . And we were not to do any

extraordinary measures for her . . . So she came up to the CCU and we just let her die. And it took her a good 2 hours to die . . . It was awful and *you couldn't do anything.* The guys up in [the hospital] are real anxious about giving drugs and stuff like that. But I just spent time saying, "It's okay to let go. If you *want* to go, go ahead. It's fine. Everybody's here [*emphases mine*]."

This same nurse, who was quoted in the previous section when she was unable to diagnose a woman who came into the hospital with chest pain, sums up her impression of that patient in a manner that convincingly illustrates the distancing function of the use of the language of needs in this group of nurses:

They *need* to take control. You know, the doctor doesn't go home with them to live with them? They *need* to be able to take control of their lives and know what to do so they stay healthy, whatever it is.

CLINICAL AND ETHICAL AGENCY

One of the most common themes in the interviews with these nurses is their feeling that they are not very important. This was expressed quite poignantly by another nurse in this group:

I was sort of overwhelmed when I first considered this [participating in the study]. I thought, Great, I can volunteer. And then when I found out what I was supposed to do, I thought, Ha! What difference do I make? I do the same thing every day.

Given the analysis of this chapter, this response should not be totally surprising. I have argued that the lack of qualitative distinctions in these nurses' work prevents them from recognizing or achieving those goods that characterize expert nursing practice. This same argument suggests a way out of the difficulty expressed by the nurse in this quotation. While there is an unmistakable tone of depression and even despair in this nurse's view of herself and her work—and in the interviews with these nurses in general—this does not appear to be exclusively the result of their individual psychological dynamics. Instead, it seems to be inextricably related to their inability to recognize the good they could be doing.

Indeed, in some cases, it seems to be related to an ability to recognize the good that they are doing. One nurse in the study, who works in a neonatal intensive care unit, describes how an infant in her unit was gradually showing remarkable signs of improvement. As his condition improved, the infant needed a particular kind of bed that the hospital did not have. He was transferred, at great cost, to another hospital. Only as she was questioned by the interviewer did this nurse seem to recognize how much good her unit had done for this child and only then did she realize that she should, and could, have requested that the bed be brought to the child rather than the child to the bed. The interchange is as follows:

Nurse: I had sort of said, "Look, if we can't have a crib, we can't have him have some kind of developmental input here, it would be better to send him away." I didn't want to send him away. But, when I realized that we weren't going to be able to do what we really needed to do, you know, we started pushing for him to go.

Int.: I'm not clear. Was the main reason he had to be transferred to [the other hospital] was just for the sake of getting him into a larger crib?

Nurse: The fact that we couldn't meet his developmental needs.

Int.: It wasn't that he was acutely deteriorating or anything of that nature at all?

Nurse: No, he was getting better.

A return to our paradigm case will further illustrate this point. Near the end of the interview, the interviewer returns to the issue of clinical judgment. The specific issue is the kinds of clinical judgments that contributed to this nurse's decision to use the type and amount of medication that she did with her patient:

Int.: That was kind of a judgment you were making, that in this situation any amount of sedation—valium's not that strong.

Nurse: It wasn't valium, but it was something . . . innocuous. It was not a . . .

Int.: It wasn't morphine?

Nurse: It was a librium or, I've forgotten.

Int.: Yeah. But it was a tranquilizer rather than morphine or something that is sort of notorious for driving respiration down?

Nurse: Right.

Int.: And yet even though it was mild, relatively . . .

Nurse: I knew.

Int.: You knew that it would be enough to stop. Now, how, how did you come to get that knowledge? See that's a very interesting judgment, isn't it? You were right about it . . .

Nurse: I guess I was so shocked that the doctor said okay, but I don't know how I knew that. I just knew it. I knew by looking at her. I mean, there wasn't anything, unless, unless she was intubated . . . there was just nothing, no place for her to go. She was going anyway. She was, she just didn't have to be so uncomfortable.

Int.: So it was really that recognition of how close to death she was and that you know . . . that just anything could tilt her over?

Nurse: As soon as she even fell asleep, I knew it. As soon as she even, if she just got tired and fell asleep on her own, I knew that would be the last time she fell asleep. She just looked terrible.

The interviewer's question has to do with how this nurse knew that this particular amount of this particular medication would be enough to make the patient comfortable and hasten her death. The first remarkable feature of the nurse's answer is that she does not remember either the specific type or amount of medication she administered. Her lack of memory makes it extremely difficult to believe that she actually made the kind of clinical judgment that the interviewer would like her to have made. If she had, she would presumably be able to provide a description of how the medication she had administered works, as well as a rationale for using it. Instead, she immediately invokes the physician's authorization as the basis for her decision.

The most revealing part of this section of the interview, however, is the nurse's account of her own thinking in this situation. At first, it sounds as if she was trying to make the patient comfortable as she was dying. However, the nurse immediately calls this interpretation into question when she says that the woman would have fallen asleep and died without the medication. From her perspective, in other words, the administration of the medication made no difference. The patient would have died whether she received the medication or not.

It is impossible to know from this account whether the medication did or did not make a difference in this patient's condition. What is clear is that this nurse feels very uncomfortable saying that it did make a difference when the only difference she can conceive of it making is that it hastened the patient's death. This nurse's feeling that she made no difference in this situation, in other words, is directly related to her lack of knowledge of clinical qualitative distinctions and the practices that support them. If, like the expert nurse, this nurse knew how to recognize and produce comfort, she could have made a positive difference in this situation.

Critical to a person's ability to make a difference, of course, is her willingness to take responsibility for her actions. We have seen that the nurses in this group have great difficulty doing this. They seem to find responsibility frightening.

We are now in a position to see why this is the case. If taking responsibility means taking responsibility only for negative outcomes such as a patient's death, it is no wonder that these nurses are constantly looking for other people to take responsibility for their actions. However, if responsibility also means responsibility for the good outcomes, there is presumably much greater motivation for being responsible. We can see the nurse in our paradigm case struggling with just this issue at the very end of the interview:

Nurse: How much does it have to do with power? That just occurred to me. I was in a very powerful situation and I never thought about that before. But I don't remember feeling powerful at the time. And really I wasn't, so, ultimately, I was not.

Int.:   How would you have known that you weren't imposing your power on the patient, and in the way that you told the story and presented it to us, already we have a strong sense that it was very important to you to be clear that it was the patient's wish and that even her limited community, her friend, was clear that this was her wish, and that all of that was very clear for you. So it wasn't a power trip or, you know, but yet it was, it was a very, a very present and responsible sense, and powerful in the sense of, uh, taking responsibility and owning, uh, owning your ability to make the judgment and to take the action in behalf of the patient. So it's that kind of power, right?

Nurse: I am just saying from a cause and effect . . . I mean what you said earlier about moving up the time of death, for example, from one point to an earlier point. That's all I mean . . .

Int.:   And that was the power you were thinking of?

Nurse: Yeah.

Int.:   Not power relationships.

Nurse: Not I have it over her or anything . . . I keep hearing this being played back in the courtroom and wondering.

In the previous section of the interview, this nurse had asserted and then denied that her administration of the medication made a difference to her patient. Here she asserts and then denies that she was in a position of power with respect to her patient. There is clearly a connection between these two assertions and denials. The interviewer would like to believe that this nurse made a judgment about what was best for the patient based upon her clinical knowledge. If she had done so, she would, as the interviewer says, have been acting responsibly. She would have acted out of a sense of responsibility to the standards of care in her practice.

To state the matter another way, if this nurse had acted in the way this interviewer wishes she had, she would have acted with authority. She would have felt authorized by the standards of her practice to do what was best for her patient—in this case, to make the patient comfortable while she was dying. However, because this nurse is lacking the knowledge of these standards—of these qualitative distinctions—she cannot experience herself as acting with authority. Instead, she experiences herself as acting with power, as imposing her will, unmediated by any conception of the good, on her patient. Because this idea is intolerable to her—as it should be—she reduces the idea of responsibility to the idea of "cause and effect."

She did not make something happen for this patient that would not have happened without her intervention. She just caused something to happen more quickly that would have happened anyway.

The shift from the notion of responsibility to the notion of cause and effect is a shift from a personal to an impersonal form of discourse. A machine, after all, can cause something to happen, but it can hardly be seen as a responsible human agent. If, as we saw above, these nurses lack the conviction that they make a *difference,* they also lack the conviction that *they* make a difference—that they are human agents whose capacity for clinical and ethical judgment differentiates them from automatons.

At the beginning of this chapter, I suggested that the structure of the practice of the nurses in this group is responsible for the inadequacies of the care they provide. If this is the case, the general form of the remedy for these inadequacies is clear. Whatever the psychological difficulties or moral shortcomings of these nurses, their fundamental problem is their lack of knowledge of the qualitative distinctions that are embodied in expert nursing practice.

As we have seen, these nurses are at least somewhat aware of this problem. Their awareness manifests itself in their wish to make a difference and to have a genuine sense of agency. The solution to this problem, then would seem to be neither psychotherapy nor ethics courses—important as these are in other contexts—but a form of nursing education that is governed by the goal of improving clinical and ethical judgment by focusing on the goods specific to nursing practice and the skills that allows nurses to achieve them.

NOTES

1. There are two interesting exceptions to—or variations on—the lack of memory for specific patients on the part of the nurses in this group. The first is the memory of a negative experience with a specific type of patient. One nurse in this group, when asked to talk about a critical incident in her practice, says, "J. is definitely the worst BPD [broncho pulmonary dysplasia] I've ever had. I've had other kids that had BPD but they were never as difficult." J. is not seen as a person but as a type of patient.

The second variation is what I call a negative paradigm. This is the memory of a negative experience with a patient that colors all of a nurse's subsequent experiences with her patients. One nurse in the study describes a difficult experience with a patient on an involuntary psychiatric hold. She concludes her discussion by saying, "I also probably learned a bitter lesson, as well, which is sort of a hardened attitude towards patients that I might not have had the day before."

The similarity between both of these types of memory, of course, is that they reduce the individual patient to a general type.

2. Soren Kierkegaard. (1962). *The present age*. New York: Harper and Row. Charles Taylor. (1985). "What is Human Agency?" In Charles Taylor (Ed.), *Human agency and language: Philosophical papers I*, pp. 15–44. Cambridge: Cambridge University Press, 1985.

Chapter 8

THE SOCIAL EMBEDDEDNESS OF KNOWLEDGE

T his chapter focuses on the social aspects of clinical and caring knowledge. Both entail engaged practical reasoning in transitions. Though clinical knowledge draws on science and technology, it is historical and dependent upon shared understandings among clinicians and patient/ families. Caring knowledge also requires community and occurs in dialogue and relationship with the other. Both clinical and caring knowledge require qualitative distinctions and are best understood through observation and narratives about the transitions from the participants (see Chapter 2). The accuracy and fidelity of clinical and caring knowledge are clarified through scientific knowledge, clinical outcomes, and personal and social understandings as they become available. Thus, clinical reasoning and caring practices are socially embedded, in that they require reasoning in transition, occur in relationship, and can never get beyond consensual validation (Benner, 1994d; Taylor, 1989). Even post-hoc clinical reasoning, based on clinical outcomes, relies on social memory and group attentiveness to examine the clinical trajectories and outcomes.

Clinical and caring knowledge are viewed as less legitimate than criterial scientific reasoning, but this is only because we have an idealized vision of objective knowledge and unrealistic expectations of our ability to approximate scientific ways of knowing in everyday life. Scientific knowledge, too, is embedded in the background practices of scientists (Kuhn, 1970; 1991). However, the confirmatory procedures of rational empirical science are based on the idealized model of static criterial reasoning, static appraisals of two situations frozen in time and made explicit (see Chapters 1 and 2 for a critique).

Caring for one another is social through and through. Both clinical and caring knowledge require the identification of salient situations and knowing how and when to act. Actual concrete clinical situations and dialogue are required to call forth (i.e., bring into consideration, make visible) knowledge and skill related to the relevant risks, opportunities, and distinctions of particular clinical states. Clinical states are recognizable by expert clinicians within certain degrees of accuracy and are confirmable by objectifiable physiological data only within certain limits. And, of course, some clinical situations are so complex or novel they go beyond extant clinical knowledge.

One soon reaches limits in trying to make all the relevant scientific, technical, clinical, and human concerns inherent in clinical situations explicit. New graduate nurses are keenly aware that they cannot find out everything that they need to know from textbooks and scientific articles for their clinical practice. Even if they could, they would not have the time to find the information quickly enough to respond in a timely manner. But even more troubling is the fact that due to lack of experience, beginners suffer from secondary ignorance. They do not know what they do not know, and they may not see a situation or know when action is needed. They must rely on other practitioners to call their attention to what they cannot yet recognize, and they offer their observations and data to more experienced clinicians for interpretation (see Chapters 3–4). The reliance on others is different in kind and extensiveness for more experienced clinicians; however, they too are dependent on the multiple perspectives and the pooled experience of other clinicians for clinical and caring wisdom (see Chapter 11 for a discussion of negotiating clinical knowledge with physicians).

The small group interviews and observations are replete with examples of the ways that clinical and caring knowledge are socially embedded: The nurse must relay the clinical and caring knowledge she has gained in taking care of a patient to the next nurse taking care of the patient. Lapses in attentiveness by one practitioner are shored up by another and an ethos of collective attentiveness. The inability to see a salient clinical sign or symptom is corrected by others' experiential wisdom and skill of seeing. Lack of practical experience with particular technology and its peculiarities is alleviated by asking someone who has experiential knowledge with the equipment. Ambiguous difficult clinical problems are approached by pooling memories, past clinical examples, and clinical expertise. Difficult finesse and technical and human skills are learned by watching others who demonstrate the embodied skillfulness. The style and habits of a social group shape what knowledge is valued and determine what perceptual skills are developed and taught. The style and habits of a social group also determine the extent of teaching and learning from one another. Collaborative and cooperative teamwork allows the pooling of expertise and creates a climate of support and possibility that can combat the threat of helplessness in the face of grave, critical situations.

The socially embedded nature of clinical and caring knowledge is explored in this chapter in relation to the following major social aspects of knowledge:

1.   Pooled expertise and the power of multiple perspectives refers to the ways that knowledge is dialogical and collective, i.e., it occurs in conversation and relationship with others, and is collective in that shared understandings create a whole larger than the sum of the parts;

2.   modeling embodied skills and ways of being refers to teaching by demonstration and example that occurs in a social group;

3.   sharing and shaping a collective vision of excellence and taken-for-granted practice refers to the notions of the good and the unexamined practices shared by the social group's culture; and

4.   the social emotional climate refers to the qualities of trust, mood and sense of possibility within the group.

These complex aspects of the lifeworld are best defined by example and, of course, do not exhaust all the ways that knowledge is received, transmitted, and created. They do offer a correction to the Cartesian vision of the private subject possessing and creating knowledge in isolation, and to the technical vision of knowledge created by theory and science and applied directly to practice without interpretation or direction from the situation.

POOLED EXPERTISE AND THE POWER
OF MULTIPLE PERSPECTIVES

Expertise is both deliberately and informally pooled. Knowledge is produced not by private individual knowers, but in dialogue with others with different vantage points and perspectives (Taylor, 1985; 1989). Pooled expertise, dialogue, and multiple perspectives are possible because of shared taken-for-granted background habits, skills, and practices, and because of differences in practical and theoretical knowledge and experience. There were six pervasive examples in the interviews and observation notes of how pooled expertise, dialogue, and multiple perspectives create and transmit clinical and caring knowledge:

1.   learning what counts as a sign or a symptom;
2.   knowing the patient, learning particular patient's responses;
3.   gaining practical knowledge about how equipment works;

4. pooling wisdom through identifying clinical experts;
5. pooled attentiveness to sustain adequate powers of noticing;
6. learning from other's experience through narrative.

These six examples illustrate the social nature of knowledge in a practice but cannot provide an exhaustive account.

What Counts as a Sign or Symptom

As noted in Chapters 3 and 4, advanced beginner and competent nurses are engaged in learning the practical manifestations of signs and symptoms, e.g., fatigue, withdrawal, depression, cyanosis, pitting edema, breath sounds, body stylistics, et cetera. It is only with the context created by skilled experts that these practical manifestations can be pointed out to and/or validated for less experienced and skilled nurses. In nursing school, students have difficulty imagining what a sign or symptom looks like from lectures and textbook accounts. They tell of learning to recognize cyanosis in patients (Benner, 1984). Central to developing clinical know-how throughout practice is the development of perceptual acuity. Typically, the beginner turns to more experienced clinicians for the interpretation of signs and symptoms and the identification of trends and deviations from the normal. At the competent stage, nurses use past experience to compare current appraisals of signs and symptoms, and they may analyze whether or not these constitute a pattern or trend. Nurses practicing at the expert level may just see trends in the patient's condition and make complex qualitative distinctions about patients' concerns and conditions. For example, one nurse asked: "Is he actively withdrawing, or is he less alert due to sepsis?" (See Chapter 6). Other expert nurses commonly evaluate the cause of a low central venous pressure by determining whether it was due to lack of blood volume, poor vasal tone, or pump (heart) failure. These are crucial clinical distinctions that can only be sensibly made in the concrete historical situation with particular patients and particular patient populations. Nurses readily call on the perspectives of their colleagues to clarify and confirm their perceptions.

Nurse: With neonates, I think there are so many other factors involved, in blood pressure, for instance, besides those drugs [*vasopressors*]. I think with older cardiac patients those drugs are their blood pressure. But with our kids, it's just not the case. Their hydration and their fluid status and how many blood cells they've got running around in there, and whether or not they've bled or whether or not they have central nervous system involvement. All those things matter and it isn't just the drugs. So you have to assess all those things every time you start messing with something. You can't just turn the drug up. That may not be the problem.

Int: It's much more complex?
Nurse: Well, it's much more likely that you need volume or you need a colloid or something besides more drug.

This excerpt illustrates the sensitizing information that nurses pass along to one another, to prevent single-factor thinking, or tunnel vision. Expert critical care nurses who care for cardiac patients will make their own qualitative distinctions based upon knowing a particular patient within that particular patient population. These distinctions are experientially learned and passed on by the dialogue, questioning, advice and conferring about specific patients. Nurses were commonly heard giving cues about the multiple meanings of signs and symptoms and possible interactions between therapeutic responses.

The socially embedded web of perspectives and distinctions is most effective when unit culture is collaborative and when the staff is relatively stable, and the nurses come to know what other nurses know and on whom they can rely:

Well, certainly, there are 3 or 4 nurses on my unit that are excellent and I look to them as far as where I kind of guide myself in that way. I apply their level of expertise on my unit and the shift I work on now, the PM shift. There are a lot of very good nurses on that shift.

Knowing the Patient, Learning Particular Patients' Responses

Being able to care for fragile, inarticulate, or silent patients requires that any experientially gained knowledge is preserved and passed along to other nurses, since the conditions for gaining the particular understanding may not occur again. For example, we observed nurses demonstrating to one another what they had learned about suctioning a particular infant. What infants will tolerate varies significantly. Some infants are so labile that they require two people to assist with airway clearance and suctioning in order to keep adequate oxygenation. As the expert clinicians talk about it, infants "like" different things, meaning that they tolerate different blood levels of oxygen due to suctioning the trachea. Whenever possible, the successful (trial-and-error-learned) suctioning technique with a particularly fragile infant is demonstrated to the oncoming nurses.

> **Observation Note:**[1] *I first ask about the baby with the patent ductus arteriosus that I observed the first time when he was a "fresh post-op open heart." This is a lovely baby, who looks better today. He is less edematous.*

Observer: Tell me about the rest of the night.

Nurse: He did well. He had one little episode where they were suctioning him and he was desaturating and he became bradycardic and his PA [*pulmonary artery*] pressure went up and his systemic went down. But we were able to sedate him, and hand-ventilate him out of it. It's kind of funny, because the nurse at the bedside . . . He was running lower than what was running normally on his [oxygen] saturations. I said "Well, maybe it's because he is getting a little pulmonary edema, or maybe it's because he needs to be suctioned. I don't know, he has a little ET (endotracheal) tube in and sometimes they plug up." She said, the nurse who took care of him on days said, "Don't suction him because we had a bad time with him with his blood pressure dropping." I said, "Well, how long ago was he suctioned?" She said: "About 5 hours ago." I said I wouldn't do it by myself, but I would try it. And she tried it and it happened just like it did on day shift. So I said, "Well, it is just one of those things, you are damned if you do and damned if you don't." Because if you didn't and he plugged his tube, you would be in trouble. She was a little bit nervous because the person who gave her report had said: "Don't suction him unless you absolutely have to." Well, this kind of judgment call is six of one and a half dozen of the other. You may have to, although it may be that he is desaturating for another reason because he is getting pulmonary edema.

Observer: Did you ever figure out why he was desaturating? It wasn't because of the tube . . .

Nurse: He was just getting to the point where he was third spacing more. He was getting more pulmonary edema. And they just had to go up on his PEEP. I just said, well it is a judgment call.

Observer: Well, it is scary not to suction a small tube . . .

Nurse: Then if you waited until the next day and it plugged, then it would be someone's fault. I said to her before, what you can do to keep from getting into trouble is to get him very well sedated and make it a two-person job so that you can hand ventilate him really well. And she did all those things, and you still got into a little bit of trouble, but it wasn't as bad on the day shift where they had to hand-ventilate him for about 15 minutes, whereas for us it was about 2 minutes.

Observer: Because you were prepared?

Nurse: Yeah, We knew what he would do.

This is an ambiguous situation, but the second suctioning episode, while still difficult, is better than the earlier one where the infant required 15 minutes of additional respiratory support. The advance through historical experiential learning is incomplete, but it is still an advance. The instructions are necessarily detailed and practical. The performance is necessarily guided by the infant's respiratory response and the reading of oxygen saturations. With increased experience, the nurse gives more elaborate detail closer to the patient's own experience, as illustrated below:

[*This patient had suffered a stroke after cardiac surgery.*] The worst feeling is to have air hunger and not feel that you are breathing properly, so we first made him comfortable by improving his respiratory status. To make this patient comfortable has made a difference in the rest of his care. He was very withdrawn; he has some very strong physical weaknesses but he's not flaccid; he has some motor ability; he has sensation. He has definite reha-bilitation potential, but by making him comfortable through his respiratory system, making him stable that way, his other activities have come on.

This nurse describes the way the patient looks, how he moves, responds to air hunger, and what his muscle tone is. Her description comes from a web of comparison with other patients so that it is concrete and historical and she assumes that we know what she is describing. This narrative dem-onstrates learning to make more refined distinctions about signs and symp-toms. Learning this skilled perceptual acuity continues in the clinician's development of clinical know-how throughout practice, and is refined by comparing one's own assessments with other practitioner's assessments.

Recognition of trends and patterns are added to perceptual acuity over time. As Merleau-Ponty (1962) points out, seeing is an integrative mind/body skill. In the following interview excerpt, a neonatal critical care nurse describes her perceptual acuity in recognizing changes in infants:

In neonatal critical care units, you can look at a kid and say: "He doesn't look right." You know that he is getting a little sour and that something is going on that should be addressed. Then you go on and do more of a com-plete assessment and figure out from his history clinical information what's going on with this kid. Whereas with adults you might have to have the numbers first . . . Adults don't seem to bite the dust as rapidly as kids. The kids look dusky and just not well perfused before they are going to crash.

This nurse's perceptual acuity is based on knowing both how neonates in general should look and how a particular neonate usually looks. Learning these assessment skills is greatly influenced by having others point out subtle distinctions, having observations confirmed by others and eventu-ally by how the clinical situation unfolds.

Knowing signs and symptoms from the pathophysiology books does not guarantee that the clinician will be able to recognize the practical manifes-tations of the textbook accounts of an illness. The leap between the flat, sin-gular descriptions of the textbooks must be made by more experienced cli-nicians who can directly point to the various manifestations in practice. Like the connoisseur, the practitioner must learn to discern the variega-tions of signs and symptoms in practice. We have noted the following three ways that knowing a patient goes beyond formal assessments:

First, because the nurse knows the typical patterns of responses, certain aspects of the situation stand out as salient, others recede in importance. Second, making qualitative distinctions, comparing the current picture to this patient's typical picture is made possible by knowing the patient. And third, it allows for particularizing prescriptions and abstract principles . . . Nurses in their narrative accounts in this study show repeatedly how clinical judgment requires particularizing formal prescriptions and abstractions, through understanding how *this* patient responds under *these* circumstances. Knowing the patient is the nurses' basis for particularizing care. (Tanner et al., 1993, p. 278)

Knowing a patient/family is central for advocating for a patient and for guiding the use of technology. However, the abilities to "know a patient/ family" must be demonstrated by other practitioners and learned directly from patients and families. Experienced nurses talk about "following the body's lead" (Benner, 1994) by which they mean close observation of what the person can tolerate in terms of activity, stimulation, feeding, et cetera. Following the body's lead counters the temptation to control the body with excessive technical and pharmacological interventions. In the case of caring for infants, drugs must not be completely substituted for human comfort measures, since the infant must be able to respond to human connection and soothing (Benner, Wrubel, Phillips, Chesla, & Tanner 1995). Following the body's lead requires that the nurses read the patient's responses accurately and pass on their knowledge of the patient's responses to others so that the knowledge becomes cumulative, open to confirmation and dis-confirmation. The notion of "following the body's lead" is a good example of socially embedded clinical knowledge that has not been articulated in textbooks, and even after it is articulated nurses will continue to rely on expert clinicians for the transmission of this knowledge.

Gaining Practical Knowledge About How Equipment Works

In our imagined ideal versions of reality, equipment is mere means, an invisible and unobtrusive tool that supplies information or action. But in real life, technical equipment has a practical reality all its own. The history of common failures or inaccuracies becomes a part of the social lore on its use. This informal experientially gained wisdom is seldom written anywhere, so people become identified as being "experienced" in troubleshooting certain equipment. In fact, we observed a remarkable casualness and lack of attentiveness to training people in the use of the equipment. We observed nurses asking questions about highly technical equipment such as cardiac assist devices that demonstrated inadequate conceptual and practical training in the use of such devices. A second pervasive problem was that the purchasing department often ordered incompatible and inconsistent supplies of disposable equipment. So it was hard for the staff to keep up with the array of multiple brands, each with their own characteristics. The problem was compounded by hiring temporary personnel even more unfamiliar with the array of supplies and equipment:

> Observation Note: *Judith is called in to examine the proliferation and mixture of intravenous lines by a temporary nurse new to the unit. One of Judith's strategies is to simplify the lines so that there are no stopcocks on CVP lines because of the increased chance of infection, in what Judith calls a place with a lot of infection. Two nurses ask for advice on setting up the lines appropriately. There are multiple lines for medications that are being administered and titrated simultaneously. And there are lines with transducers for venous, and arterial monitoring. This strikes me as an area ripe for some simplification and innovation. Also, it is an area of applied technology with not much scientific investigation on interactions, effects, et cetera.*

The technology is rendered safe only by a community of experienced practitioners who keep track of the common mistakes and problems with the equipment and who find ways of simplifying its use for safety. The use of intravenous therapies and monitoring devices gets inordinately complicated and was described as an "IVAC forest" by one nurse referring to the multiple intravenous infusion pumps.

Accurate assessment of physiological parameters depends on the skilled use of technology and socially embedded experiential wisdom. For example, pulse oximeters are notoriously variable, and when assessing oxygen saturation the clinician has to be able to interpret the validity of the pulse oximeter reading. This knowledge is carried in anecdotal or story form, with the clinicians drawing on the memory of their colleagues for the variations. The following detailed narrative memory reveals the significance of the event for this new graduate, and is typical of this form of mastery:

> I remember one time the Pulse Oximeter [*brand name given*] Representative was here with all her stuff. They were Pavulonizing (giving Pavulon, which causes complete muscle paralysis). They wanted him completely paralyzed, not even diaphragmatic movement, which is what they wanted to completely avoid. When you come off Pavulon, the diaphragm is the first muscle to return and the eyes. I was hand ventilating this child for suctioning purposes and I started watching the O_2 sats and they were dropping and I was looking at the transcutaneous monitor. She had a control *Oximeter [again a particular brand name is used]* and I was watching that, and she was looking at it saying: "That can't be right." She was looking at her Oximeter site and

I was looking at mine and I started bagging faster to get the O_2 sat up and the $CO_2$2 down. And the more I bagged, the more steady the $O_2$2 sat would be, and I am going, "This is very strange." I thought that's got to be wrong. So I started looking at hers and hers was saying 69 too. And I am going, "This is not?" And my hand is going (she gives the motions of using the hand held respirator). At that point, I said "Forget it, I'm hooking back up to the vent and see what happens. Maybe I'm bagging too fast or the way I'm bagging." The sats went right back up to 95–96. What was happening was that the Oximeter was so sensitive, and she had this fancy monitoring equipment, the Oximeter was picking up from this kid's toe where the probe was, how many times I ventilated as an actual O_2. So the pressure from the lungs was exerting pressure on the capillary bed which was pushing the red blood cells through the capillary at a rate that I was bagging and it was coming up as the O_2 sat. So I was bagging at 69–70 times a minute and that was what was showing up. And we knew that only because of this monitoring equipment that she had. The Oximeter was picking up from this kid's toe where the probe was, how many times I ventilated as an actual O_2. So the pressure from the lungs was exerting pressure on the capillary bed which was pushing the red blood cells through the capillary at a rate that I was bagging and it was coming up as the 0^2 sat. You'd look at the monitor and the bagging would go like this. And you had to blow it up to see that each big wave had a bunch of little waves in it. So it would go like this [hand demonstration]. That's how we finally figured it out. The Oximeter representative had heard of this happening, but she had never seen it before. And if she weren't there with her monitoring equipment, I'd be looking at the O_2 sats thinking they are in the high 60s, and it was really the rate of my bagging.

This excerpt illustrates the ad hoc practical reasoning required for skillfully using technical equipment. Since the nurse is a new graduate, we do not get a story of how the infant looked or responded, because the advanced beginner does not yet have enough of an experiential base to discern the infant's responses, such as subtle color changes and restlessness, in comparison with a range of infant's responses. He depends on the monitors and the sales representative's anecdotal knowledge of the equipment's peculiarities. This is in sharp contrast to the expert neonatal nurse saying that she is "better than any Hewlett Packard monitor for detecting changes in an infant." The above detailed account of learning to troubleshoot equipment failures and peculiarities demonstrates modus operandi thinking (i.e., similar to the way a detective solves a mystery). While deeply involved in the situation, nurses try out various explanations and their ramifications, attempting to get the best read on the situation as it unfolds.

Examples of equipment failure were common in most of the interview sessions. In our observations, we found that expert nurses frequently engaged in troubleshooting failed equipment or teaching others how to work with a particular piece of equipment. This knowledge about equipment quickly goes into the background habits, skills, and expectations and is not typically discussed by more expert nurses.

However, mastering the practical workings of equipment is a major pre-occupation of new graduate nurses. A second example of a different new graduate from a different hospital further illustrates the modus operandi reasoning used to master the practical workings of equipment, in this case a hand-held respirator and a pulse oximeter:

Nurse: I was taking care of a 26-year-old man who was dying. He was fighting for his life. But we needed to suction him. So the clinical nurse specialist came in and she was going to assist me. We got everything ready and I was going to do the suctioning and she was going to do the bagging. She grabbed the Ambu bag and started bagging him. I hadn't even started to suction him. I had just put my gloves on. I had the suctioning catheter and I was ready. His heart rate was just dropping down. And she's bagging him more. She's going, "Hold on . . . he's not ready." And we were watching his heart rate going down and down and down. And I'm going, "Something's wrong and we don't know!" And the respiratory therapist came in and we were all looking and she was still bagging him. Well, the second respiratory therapist came in and this is like, it seemed like hours, but it was within only a few seconds. Like 15–20 seconds. But his heart rate was really dropping down and he was going down! And I was just standing there with my suction going, "Oh my God!" And I told her bag him faster—he's not—his O$_2$ sats, you know. They were OK—99. It had gone down. I think the lowest was like 95 but it was still OK. But his heart rate was just dropping real fast. Another respiratory therapist came in and found that when she took the Ambu bag off the valve was off. She was bagging him on room air. But it was so scary. I will never, ever, ever take the Ambu bag off without making sure that little tiny ball drops. But it was scary. She was like: "What's going on?" I don't know. I don't see anything." And she was bagging with room air, and she was bagging him pretty quick. He went from tachycardia to a bradycardia. But what was really weird was that his O$_2$ sat—you know, the monitor on his finger was still reading above 95.

Int: It takes a while before it catches up . . .

Nurse: Catches up with the blood . . . You can see the heart and the blood pressure. There were just definite changes and he was on Dopamine and we were just like: "Keep the Dopamine up!" [laughs] But it wasn't doing anything to the heart rate. So it was scary.

The learning is laden with import. The patient's life is at stake. The salience and workings of the "pop off" valve are experientially learned. The learning is situated and dialogical. The detailed reflection yields a better understanding of the equipment and the danger. The new graduate again gives little information about how the patient looks and responds during this episode. She notes the changes in the heart monitor rather than the color of the patient. But the example reveals the way that experiential knowledge about equipment is passed on to others.

Pooling Wisdom Through Identifying Clinical Experts

Beginning with new graduates all small group interview participants talked about whom they trust to give reliable clinical consultation. Upon observation we found that nurses who were assigned to be resource nurses for the other nurses. These resource nurses assessed the patients and the clinical knowledge of the nurses on that evening so they would know which patients to check on more frequently. It is common knowledge among the nurses which nurses are expert. For example, in talking about running smooth codes the nurses refer to their practical knowledge about the level of expertise available during a resuscitation:

> It depends on who is on. If you have one person like Jennifer (expert) and six people who have been there for 3 months you're in trouble, and you have to give a lot of directions and they still ask questions back. What do I do about this? What do I do about that? It just makes a lot of difference in the level of experience you have.

At another point in this interview, the nurses say that if Jennifer is taking care of an infant, it would not occur to them to check the infant, but if someone new is there, they will check:

Nurse 1: If we have a lot of people just off orientation and half of the staff is brand new and you are in charge, and you have a lot of sick kids, you'll end up policing 36 people.

Nurse 2: Absolutely. And sometimes it's really scary. You said you tried not to give them the sickest patients, but a lot of times you won't give your inexperienced person a fairly stable patient, thinking they're safe with that person, because those are just the kind of kids that go bad on you. Whereas, if you give them [the inexperienced nurse] a really sick kid, you're there watching them, you know the House Staff are watching them. There is a little more awareness of their limitations. I think with a kid like that, they are more likely to ask. But if you have a lot of them sometimes I find it's worse to give them all of the less sick patients and give the experienced people the more sick ones, because you have to distribute them [*referring to the location of the experts dispersed in the room*].

Nurse 1: Sometimes it's nice to give the experienced people less sick ones and then they can get everybody whipped into shape in 15 minutes, and then they're free for the next hour.

Nurse 2: Common practice. [laughter]

Expertise is dispersed in the unit, and various strategies are used to maximize the wisdom of the experts for all the patients. The newcomers figure out who is and who is not a reliable source of clinical wisdom:

Nurse 1: We are all so new on nights in the nursery. There is not a whole lot of experience on nights. There are a couple I know. When I arrived, they said "Linda, the charge nurse, has been there 5 years." You know pretty much who to go to. But I also know who not to go to.
Int: How did you learn that?
Nurse: Just from asking them questions before and having them look at me like, it's just as foreign to them as it was to me. And then I just moved on to the next person and asked the same question again until I found somebody that did know, then I would usually go back to that person. I figured if they knew the last question they're going to know the next question.

This informal network about the location of expert knowledge on the unit is not foolproof and is continually upgraded and amended. When units have some stability and better social integration, people become known for areas of specialized knowledge. The following is a discussion by competent level nurses:

We have sworn we are going to get T-shirts with our specialty on the back "v-tach" because each of us have our own specialty and so we will have some who specialize in acute MIs [*myocardial infarcts*] and different things with heart patients. [*Some are specialists*] with Swans Ganz catheters. We pump them [*for information*] and say what's going on? Why are these numbers this way? Before we call the doctor: "His wedge [pressure] is 5, his RA is 20, what do you think we'd better be doing here." so we all—there's a lot of us that are new up there on nights and more of us coming. And we all try to figure everything out before we start calling and getting yelled at by the doctors.

Pooling expertise and gaining multiple perspectives about a clinical situation helps to limit tunnel vision and snap judgments, but these are also powerful strategies for maximizing the clinical knowledge of a group. Individual nurses work 8 to 12 hours, so they must be able to pass on their clinical knowledge about a particular patient to the next shift, e.g., what wedge pressure signals impending pulmonary edema; how sensitive the patient is to nipride and other vasopressors, et cetera. Nurses must be able to pass on their clinical learning about a particular patient if the patient is to be advantaged by what they have learned.

It was common for nurses to consult with each other about their clinical judgments: "I had five other people come over and assess the baby to see what they thought and they all felt that the baby had a lot of fluid in his lungs." This pooled expertise is a powerful and taken for granted strategy among nurses:

Observation Note: *This was my second observation of Judith. She was Unit Educator today, which means that she troubleshoots, floats between all patients and offers information and guidance. She is a walking resource person. This seems to be a cost-effective use of an expert nurse. The practice of everyone is enhanced, and clinical knowledge development is fostered. She is literally setting the standard for the practice on the unit. She offers comparisons and perspectives for the clinical situation when the practicing nurse could not possibly have had the first-hand exposure to the particular clinical issue.*

The nurse manager on the unit where Judith worked had responded to high turnover and an influx of new staff by placing her expert clinicians in the role of Unit Educators, filling in clinical wisdom, updating information, coordinating resources on the unit. On observation, it was hard to imagine that safe nursing care could have been delivered with the available staff without this flexible expert skilled judgment to fill in the gaps.

Pooled Attentiveness to Sustain Adequate Powers of Noticing

Patients in critical care units require constant vigilance. The units are generally designed for multiple access to monitors and for easy observation of patients. This is especially true in the neonatal intensive care units. Sustained vigilance is a cooperative, community-based effort. The professional ethos is to respond to any situation warranting immediate attention, whether or not the nurse is assigned to care for the patient, as illustrated in the following clinical narrative:

Last week this kid [premature infant] has an ET [endotracheal tube] taped in her mouth, but she is extubated. But she looks like she is intubated. Her belly is like this big and her saturation is 60 and her CO_2 is 80 and she is going ahh, ahh, ahh, [grunting] and the ventilator is just going along 10 breaths a minute. She is going ahh, ahh, and retracting and everything. And I'm not working in the unit. I'm just kind of walking in and I go and see the CO_2's going up and the oxygen saturation going down and I think: "She needs to be suctioned." So I start to hand-ventilate her, and the nurse comes over and says "I think she is extubated," and I say "You do." She says, "I think it has been going on for a couple of hours. I just called somebody." I say: "Get a face mask please. I'm going to take out the ET tube and then we're going to intubate this baby." It's like "Get a clue!"

The nurse caring for the baby clearly had not responded appropriately. It was a situation that should not have gone unattended for 2 hours, and fortunately the baby survived this suboptimal care. The nurse caring for the infant was counseled and given more clinical instruction.

The critical nature of the patients' condition requires collective attentiveness and responsiveness. When a critical situation is seen, all delegation and "assignments" are abandoned in favor of the most effective and expedient urgent action. Collective attentiveness creates a measure of essential redundancy. This is illustrated in the following common example of clinical teaching, supervision, and back-up provided by clinical preceptors:

Int: What tipped you off to stay in contact [with the new nurse]?

Nurse: Just because, she was hovering around the bed, looked so unsure of herself. This happens to me, if somebody is kind of hovering. Let me see what's going on. So, I said, "What's going on?"

Int: But there wasn't anything particular about the patient outside of report?

Nurse: I was tipped off by the patient's very large heart and his pressures, so I kept an eye on him. Plus, I thought it would be a very nice case for my preceptee. We were supposed to go over him that night and discuss his case. There was another exciting guy who had been throwing all these premature ventricular contractions on whom we decided to start a lidocaine drip.

Expert nurses notice when patients have a potential for problems as a habit of being prepared. Patients who are particularly unstable will be noted in report. This information is taken into consideration in relation to who is assigned to the patient. Opportunities for learning are noted for orientees. This is the kind of clinical teaching in the situation required for learning clinical judgment. It also illustrates the needed staff support for the new nurse. One of the dangers of short staffing or staffing with inexperienced nurses is that the reliability created by this redundancy is lost.

In addition to collectively attending to and observing patients, nurses monitor many details of patient care endemic to institutional care. Nurses call this "cleaning up"—the everyday maintenance that assures that patients' care progresses as it should. For example, nurses check on obsolete orders that are still being carried out:

Nurse 1:   Sometimes you find that the kid is 4 days post-op, extubated, sitting up eating, and the nurses are still doing every 4-hour lab tests. And they are new grads or brand new so you say: "Why don't you ask the doctors when they're around if you can discontinue the kid's 4-hour labs and make them once a day?" Or, you ask: "Why are we still doing this?". . . It's just little stuff like that. Or, continuous calcium infusion. That's another big bone of contention. . . . The kids can have total calciums of 8, 9, 10, 11, 12 and still be getting hourly calciums. . . . 3 days out [after open heart surgery] if they are still giving hourly calcium when the kid is eating? "Have you asked them if we can discontinue this. What is his calcium? Do we need to give it to him every hour? Is it O.K.?" It's the little things.

Nurse 2:   They forget to discontinue all the time.

Nurse 1:   Right, it's kind of up to you to remind them to remember to take the stitch out of the cutdown. Or, it's like little stuff that people that are really new just are taking care of the patient. They're doing the things that are on the Kardex that tell them how to take care of the patient. And, when they get a little more experienced they and their assessments get better. They can notice that maybe they're wheezing a little bit or that they're a little cold. They are a little blue or something. But it is like cleaning up.

This conversation continues with many more details about "cleaning up" that refer to forming a socially embedded web of attentiveness to details, and to looking out for the patient's best interests. This dialogue demonstrates a socially embedded ethos of collective vigilance and collective responsibility for following through on the myriad of details and predictable changes in critical care. It offers further evidence for the importance of maintaining the before mentioned "redundancy" of clinical expertise.

Learning from Others' Experience: The Role of Narrative

The practice of storytelling extends hard-won experiential knowledge. The oral tradition is effective in setting up salient memories. Stories are more memorable than lists of warnings that must be memorized out of context. Narrative memory sets up identification with the storyteller, creates an emotional response that causes the warning to become salient. Narratives also create sensibilities and imagination that enhance the clinician's perceptions and responses. The ethos of attentiveness, of treating mistakes as a prod to do better next time and allowing others to benefit from your expensive mistakes, is often what shapes the storyline:

Nurse 1:   I think things out of the unusual get talked about for days and days. But that's a learning experience, because if you can say what you did wrong in that situation and allow somebody to learn from it, it makes it an OK situation, provided you didn't really screw up. If you could have done something better, not necessarily wrong, but you could have done something better or more efficiently, by talking about it—

Nurse 2:   You can learn.

Nurse 1:   Everybody else can listen. It also lets you live through it enough to where you can let go of it.

The following exchange is similar and occurs in response to overlooking urine output on a patient for 2 hours. The new graduate felt badly because absence of urine could have indicated that the patient had hemorrhaged.

Nurse 1:   You only have to make a mistake once. And then, when you tell the other nurses, I felt so bad and they always have something better to tell you. One of them said: "Oh, I had a UA [*umbilical artery*] line and they don't put babies here on their tummies, and they do at Children's, and they decided to give it a try. She didn't put plastic wrap underneath the baby and the UA line came out and the baby hemorrhaged. They saved the baby, but she didn't realize the baby was hemorrhaging because it was all seeping into the blankets and it takes awhile before it goes out this way . . . But I still feel bad. Well, I don't feel as bad.

Nurse 2:   Whenever I see a baby with a UA line or if they're going to put in on its tummy, I've got the plastic wrap out and set it down to make sure.

Int: If someone tells you a horror story like that—

Nurse 2:   You remember it . . .

Nurse 3:   Everybody is real young on nights. So they all remember what it was like when they first got there. So they have some pretty good stories.

Narrative memory sets up identification with the storyteller, and creates an emotional response that causes the warning to become salient and thus more apt to be remembered. Narratives also create imagination that enhances the clinician's possibilities. Corrective narratives evidence the ethos of attentiveness in nursing. We had many stories that urged unflagging vigilance in responding to "erroneous" monitor alarms in order not to miss the accurate ones. These were stories that emphasized an ethos of collective vigilance through the frightening and sometimes tragic story of the missed alarm. But these corrective narratives also help the practitioners cope with and gain perspective on the risks of their work. Hypervigilance and guilt interfere with realistic vigilance and adequate grasp of the current situation. So nurses must find a way of letting go of past mistakes. Stories weave the social fabric together, strengthen learning, and, when they go well, yield forgiveness and shared experiential learning. A young nurse recounted a tragedy told to her by an experienced nurse to warn her and other new graduates to pay attention to heart monitors:

Nurse 1:   The baby had been really active and it was really diaphoretic. And the electrodes kept coming off. So one day she saw an "asystole" [*straight like on the monitor indicating no heart beat*] and knew that the baby was moving around and the electrodes were off again. So one would eventually go in there and put the electrodes back on. Well, what they finally decided to do after seeing asystole so many times, was just go ahead and turn that baby's monitor off. Well, they came in and the baby was dead.

Nurse 2:   It was a baby?

Nurse 1:   Yeah, it was a baby. So she told me whenever she sees a rhythm, she will never ever turn the alarm off. So now, when she sees an alarm, she really focuses on that alarm. You can watch, she focuses and she wants you to go check it. If the alarms are going on the IVs and she doesn't see anybody moving toward it, she will tell you, "Go over there and check that IV, or go over there and check that patient." Even though you are real busy.

The experienced nurse spends the rest of her career honoring the tragic experiential lesson she learned. She tells other nurses so that they will not have the same tragedy she has experienced. She no longer can ignore alarms; they have a powerful sense of salience and urgency that does not require thought. Stories of missing clinical cues, or missing the mark in taking care of patients, are told as a means of instruction and correction. The following observation note was taken in a between-shift report. The tone was one of correcting a flawed vision:

> **Observation Note:** *There is a discussion of the staff meeting that was just held. The bone marrow transplant patients were discussed. The nurses and one physician present complain that it seems as if the bone marrow team is so fixated on the bone marrow and cell condition that they overlook that the patient may be in sharp decline, and the child may die while the "bone marrow" is doing well. A visiting fellow brings up a discussion that occurred in staff meeting about a recent child's death (bone marrow transplant) where the parents weren't adequately prepared for the death because the transplant was doing well while all the child's systems were failing. They note the recent research out of USC that links a high mortality rate with ventilation assist. Putting a bone marrow transplant child on a respirator condemns them to a respiratory infection. The research matches these nurses' and physicians' practical knowledge from the limited experience with bone marrow transplant patients at this medical center.*

The stories told in the small group research interview sessions create a vision of good ways of being with patients. We specifically asked for memorable situations where things went well, as well as those situations that went poorly. Our instruction to tell stories where things went well, ran counter to the more naturalistic experience of telling corrective narratives. Yet creating a public space and time for telling stories of excellence can extend clinical excellence. Nurse participants looked forward to the storytelling sessions, and frequently told us that the experience made them feel proud of their work and the work of their colleagues and that the sessions had given them new ideas for their own practice.

In summary, the pooling of clinical and caring knowledge functions in at least four major ways to create knowledge:

1. Clinicians engage in dialogue and pool experiential knowledge gained about particular patients at different points in time.
2. Clinicians consensually validate their clinical understandings with one another.

3. Nurses ground their understandings and clinical perceptions of patients through consensual validation with other nurses over time, and this creates a socially embedded set of distinctions and connoisseurship within a community of practitioners.

4. The pooled expertise and multiple perspectives foster the development of clinical expertise of individual nurses.

Because narratives are so central in learning expert clinical and ethical comportment, this topic will be taken up more extensively in Chapter 9.

DEMONSTRATING EMBODIED SKILLS AND WAYS OF BEING

Much in skillful clinical and caring knowledge can only be exemplified by practitioners who have embodied skills and ways of being with patients. In this way, the knowledge of skilled experts is both embodied and socially embedded.

Gaining Embodied Knowledge

Physical assessment, body care, positioning patients, comfort measures, monitoring labor, delivering a baby, therapeutic interventions, and managing technology all require skilled know-how or embodied intelligence (Dreyfus, 1979; Dreyfus & Dreyfus with Athanasiou, 1986). These skills are learned through demonstration and observation. For example, the skills for comforting premature babies are indeed complex and learned by observing other nurses, and through being trained over time by the infant's responses. Nurses describe the development of their "small baby protocol" which describes ways to "nest" the premature infant so that they feel secure. While this skill can be described on paper, it requires demonstration and learning the practice from particular infants, as demonstrated below:

Nurse 1:   Preemies never really like being handled. They almost never do. They just desaturate, they cannot handle any kind of stimulation. So, I start out, first of all, I get into the isolette quietly. I don't bang the portholes, and make them jump a mile. I put a hand on the baby's back and just let her get used to the idea that I'm there and that I'm not hurting her. I always try to touch them, put my hands on and leave them there. Let them kind of squirm around and then figure out what they want to do with themselves. I usually stick their fingers in their mouths first thing. So that if they decide they want to cry and be upset they'll have something in there to suck on. And, usually they do. And I can't really think of anything else specifically.

Nurse 2:   You're prepared when you go in, you have everything lined up that you need to hand, so that you're in there for the shortest possible time.

Nurse 1:   Try to do everything, get everything done, and then close the door and do your charting.

Nurse 2:   Handle one part at a time and contain the other parts while you're . . .

Nurse 1:   Turning them. You just don't turn them over, you bring their knees into their chest and hold their arms at their sides so that they don't, when you sort of pick them up off the bed they turn their back on you. It's reflexive, that when you startle them they're going to do that. It makes them very nervous. So you get them contained when you go to turn them. In fact, a lot of times when I first go to do vital signs first thing I'll do is put the kid's feet inside his diaper to get small enough. You just pamper them entirely up to their waists and get their legs inside then you don't have to worry about them anymore. They can't kick around and it makes them much happier. A lot of times I'll wrap a diaper around them or a blanket for the entire vital signs as much as I can, so that they don't flail around and they feel secure. It's just, it's making them feel secure that's all it is. It's so easy. (laughter)

Nurse 2:   It's easy if you think about it. And, if you think it's important. It's hard to . . .

Int: Look at all the know-how involved in that easy thing that you do.

Nurse 1:   I try to teach people to do that. If I go to help somebody asks me to help them suction, you know, I'll go over there and I'll start doing these things to the kid. People always laugh at me, I'm always sticking these fingers in their mouths they say, "There goes Linda again." Or else I give them my finger, or if they have IVs or something I'll let them suck my hand, which is not terribly sanitary but it's not bad if you wash them. But it makes such a difference in how upset they get. But people don't really seem to pick up on it.

Nurse 2:   I think you don't realize how much things have changed. You very rarely see a kid these days who isn't nested, or people at least have carried through with what other people have started.

Nurse 1:   Well, in the last year or so, we've got a developmental committee now, and they've got this small baby protocol with things like "Keep them in a flex position, keep blanket rolls around them so that they're in the nest, and not sort of lying there flat on the back."

Nurse 2:   And shading the isolettes. Almost every isolette at least has a blanket over it.

Nurse 1:   Yeah, we cover the isolettes, and we can't really do day and night up there, but we just keep their isolettes covered all the time except when we're in there.

For expert practitioners skilled at comforting premature infants, handling premature infants is easy, habitual, and response-based. But a complex response-based skill, such as comforting premature infants is quite difficult to learn without watching experts. The beginner must learn touch, pacing, and attunement. The skills of handling a fragile premature infant are subtle and more difficult than the newcomer or outsider might imagine:

Nurse 1: We had a new nurse just a couple of weeks ago. She was already flustered anyway and she was already sort of being watched, so she was really nervous. She had the baby's head turned to one side and I told her to turn the baby over on its stomach. She went to turn it the wrong way like the head would have been turned 360 degrees. I yelled "Stop!" She had it almost all the way over. I said: "Put him back. Look at the baby, you can tell the front from the back." She realized what she had done. That was a horrible moment. I can't believe, people had told me about people doing that, but I'd never seen anybody do it.

Nurse 2: I think you have to make these people [referring to those in the small group interview] understand that the fronts and backs of these babies don't always look all that different. And, that you really have to pay attention. They're very bony and their ribs go all the way around . . . Interns do that too [*referring to interns inexperienced in handling premature infants*].

Learning response-based skills requires learning a repertoire of skills that can be adjusted to the particular infant and situation. Over time the repertoire itself becomes associated with successful and unsuccessful response patterns. With the focus on technology, diseases, and therapies, it is hard to keep the basic issues of comfort care, working with fragile injured bodies, in the forefront of people's attention. Yet these skills are as central and life-preserving as any of the more intrusive technical procedures. These are human ways of being with and touching and must be modeled to be safely learned. When done well, these skills look deceptively simple. Preceptors provide much demonstration and also create an embodied standard for practice. For example, a new graduate talks about the difficulty he had calming an infant with Down's Syndrome:

Nurse: I was paired with somebody and somebody else had him and I just watched what she did, and that was really instructive.

Int: What did she do?

Nurse: She left him alone. (laughs) It was like, "Oh, that's O.K.!" And what she had said is a lot of kids with Down's Syndrome that she has worked with, what she tries to do is group her activities, get in there, do it, and then stop touching them, that the stimulation sometimes is too much. And people have different approaches. Some would get in there and swaddle him and that works sometimes, too.

Neonatal critical care nurses are convinced that their own tensions or insecure, nervous handling of infants create tension and irritability in the infant:

Nurse 1: I think that there's something to the fact that they [the infants] know when they're being handled by somebody who knows what they're doing and when they're not. . . . I think it must make them nervous. It certainly would make me nervous.

Nurse 2:   Or if you're at the end of your fuse, if you had a really bad day and you're real crabby, they pick up on that too.

Nurse 1:   They get real crabby right along with you.

Nurse 2:   They know when your hands are tense.

Nurse 1:   Sometimes in our unit you can tell who the twittiest nurse is because the patient she's taking care of is being the twittiest.

Nurse 2:   Really, I think that the kids pick up on that stuff.

Nurse 1:   Yeah, it's like the kid that never settles down all shift. It's because the nurse can't take her hands off the kid and is really uptight for whatever reason.

Nurse 2:   Which is why everyone laughs at me. I don't feel any qualms about going over and saying: "This is what I do and it really works well," and calm both of them down. Because you have a much better day after that.

In the above excerpt, the socially embedded and modeled skills of comforting are sustained by the group's comforting practices and their shared expectations around comforting infants. The nurses notice the infant's responses to the nurse's embodied skills of handling and comforting infants . . . they also notice the lack of these skills. Comforting practices are salient to neonatal intensive care nurses. These skills are transmitted by demonstration in concrete situations.

Technical skills such as inserting IVs, doing arterial sticks for blood gasses, running an extracorporeal membrane hemo-filtration oxygenation system (ECMO), putting in endotracheal tubes, inserting feeding tubes, suctioning patients, et cetera, also require learning the craft with a range of patients from expert clinicians. Principles and procedural descriptions are not sufficient for skilled performance. For example, in learning to insert IVs, with practice, there is a bodily takeover so that the end of the needle feels like an extension of the body and one feels the wall of the vein and the way the needle feels and the skin looks when the needle slips out. This is similar to Merleau-Ponty's (1962) description of the blind man's use of a walking cane. Initially he feels objective pressure in the palm of the hand, but with experience he feels the edge of the curb. Learning to hand-ventilate a neonate is a similar perceptual embodied skill, guided by patient response and the nurse's comparisons within a field of experience:

[*Upon discovering that a respiratory therapist is not effectively hand-ventilating a neonate, the nurse describes her response:*]

Nurse 1:   "If you have something else to do, I can bag [hand-ventilate] this baby up for you." I'm sure he's got to change some tubing or something. Because they are driving you crazy, and you know that you are going to be there a half an hour because the baby's totally . . .

Nurse 2:   That's the thing, once the kid reaches a certain low point.

Nurse 1:   That's the point.

Nurse 2:   It takes a long time to get them back and you don't want them to get to that point. But at the same time you don't want to be rude.

Nurse 2:   But how do you explain that [how to hand-ventilate] to somebody is beyond me. It's just so many times doing it over and over.

Int: Do you have any rules of thumb?

Nurse 1:   I tell people, when people are hand-ventilating, that there are several patterns that they can use. You can use long deep sighs which is what the attending likes. You can use short fast puffs which is what the respiratory therapists tend to like. Or you can do a combination and I find that works the best. A 4–1 ratio [*short and long*] or else try the slowly . . .

Nurse 2:   It's funny we've arrived at the same kind of pattern without discussing it.

Nurse 1:   Like I said, you watch the kid, you try whatever is your pet way and if it doesn't work within 5 seconds, switch to something else because that isn't doing it for this kid and every kid is different.

Much is learned by observing other practitioners and by observing the infants' responses. In the above excerpt, the nurses cannot be explicit or definitive about the knowledge they have in their hands and skills of seeing, but they can demonstrate it and they can have their experiential wisdom called forth in the particular situation. Because we lack rich language for skilled know-how and for the skilled social body (Benner & Wrubel, 1989; Dreyfus, 1979) this kind of knowledge tends to be excluded from academic teaching. Bourdieu points out a similar problem with structural accounts of practices (see Chapter 6; Bourdieu, 1980/1990). The clinician must learn to respond to the patient responses and to the skills and responses of the health care team. For example, a group of experts describe running a "good" code as one of teamwork where everyone knows what they are doing and require little or no instructions.

Int: Help us understand what makes a code smooth and what makes a code not smooth.

Nurse 1:   Well, not smooth is generally the way it runs when you're not expecting it, or when you are short-staffed because there are a lot of preparation in terms of getting the drugs out, getting them drawn up, and handing them to the person who's going to be giving them. Mixing the drips which takes a little time, also when you're putting in chest tubes and you're running around looking for extra suction and things like that. When you're prepared and all those things are in easy reach and it's just you do your task and you can do it in a timely way, then it runs smoothly. And, it's not smooth when you don't have enough people and you're being pulled in 4 different directions. You feel like you are not doing anything well, trying to do too many things at once.

Nurse 2:   And also, I think it's the less you have to talk about it the better it goes. So if everybody has a job and everybody knows what they are doing and (several people talking) everybody knows what to do now, and you don't have to

be talking a lot. . . . it makes a lot of difference in the level of experience you
have . . .

Nurse 1:   In a good code everybody can see you and you see them looking at
you and looking at them, but there isn't a lot of talk, but there is a lot of eye
contact . . . people know that you just got an IV line in and someone is handing you a drip.

Smooth codes are orchestrated with all the team members understanding
what needs to be done and doing it. This skilled know-how includes being
set up with all the equipment and drugs ready to hand in advance. This
practice can only be learned with team members and in response to clinical responses from the patient.

Nurse 1:   Somebody just went bad and we had to intubate him. We had four
people in there and we had all worked together and so everyone knew what
they were doing and we were all just cooking, and the doctor said, "You guys
really work well together. I've never seen anything like it." Because we were
just . . . everyone was on top of everything.

Nurse 2:   Yeah, we admitted this patient in what? Less than an hour.

Nurse 1:   Oh yeah, you get everything done. (voices overlap) Because you have
someone to do all your stupid piddly stuff and then you, if you are the nurse,
you get report—so you can see what's going on instead of worrying about how
much urine he has out or something.

Nurse 2:   And that's a big difference on days and nights. I rotate to days, too.
But, on days you're pretty much on your own. It's too busy for you to—uhm.
The only person that you can really depend on—it depends on who your charge
nurse is—is your charge nurse. But other than that, I mean your patients could
be almost dead, literally—and you will be there on your own. And I've been
caught in those situations. But at nights, I think it's a lot quieter and you have
time to talk to your co-workers and you develop a better rapport with them so
that when a patient comes, it kind of stands out if you're sitting in the corner
just doing something, as opposed to getting up and helping someone admit.
And it's just second nature for you to get up and go change an IV dressing. Go
change an IV tubing, go change—uh, start a care plan . . . start this. So you can
actually admit a patient in an hour or two.

Int: As opposed to on days, when it might take you . . .

Nurse 1:   . . . 4 or 5 hours—and not get the care plan done. [*The nurse refers to the
lack of teamwork and the number of interruptions on the day shift.*]

Functioning well in a code is enhanced by working well together in
nonemergency times. In the example above, nurses contrast their experience of working as a team on nights versus working as individuals on the
day shift. Markedly different possibilities for clinical practice and clinical
knowledge development are created by the social structures of the two
shifts. The teamwork itself is experienced as a resource that sets up a climate of possibility (see pp. 226–230).

An expert group discussion of caring for post-cardiac surgery patients demonstrates group expertise and transmission of clinical knowledge about fine-tuning a patient. A nurse describes teaching a new nurse how to recognize hemodynamic recovery transitions in open heart patients, and to set the monitoring parameters to capture changes. The excerpt demonstrates recognizing patient transitions during recovery, being prepared, and playing the "nipride game" as a signal that the patient is highly unstable or that the interventions are not on target. The game metaphor, commonly used by critical care nurses, captures actions taken to anticipate and respond to patient changes.

Int: Are these things that you try to tell a new nurse that's going to take care of a heart patient? . . .

Nurse 1: A lot of times you just have to help them figure if they need to go on nipride . . . A lot of times they need help figuring out, which stage of the game they have to go to. Because patients go from one extreme to the other extreme. They go from cold and clamped down to dilated with these huge volume requirements, and one minute you're pouring fluid in them. You need to help them [patients] reach transitional stages of their recovery a lot of times.

Nurse 2: I think when you're teaching new people about nipride, that's one of the things you talk about, maybe setting your alarm parameters a little bit tighter. If you are titrating it, it's a real fast-acting drug, so you can set your alarms tighter so if the patient's blood pressure drops, you're going to know if it's too low, and conversely, if you're titrating upwards and they're waking up, you may want to set their high alarm a little bit lower so you can increase the nipride.

Nurse 1: I think it takes a while for a lot of them to get that fine-tuning down. That's really fine-tuning, and it takes a long time for them to get that.

"Fine-tuning" is a response-based experientially learned skill. The skilled know-how for playing the nipride game is socially embedded and embodied. There are many tips, sets and expectations that cannot be found in the procedure book (Hooper, 1995). Often the skilled know-how has to do with timing and organization. For example, the patient's blood pressure readings are not just discrete facts but interpretations of the patient's responses:

Nurse: Sometimes when you're with a person working closely with a patient, you know, like you said, when you give sedation. It's O.K. if it [blood pressure] hangs at 80, because it will come back up, and you're not going to adjust the drips up just for a pressure of 80 for ten minutes. You know it's going to come back up, whereas somebody covering [*standing in for the nurse during a break*] won't necessarily know that you can tolerate a pressure of 80. You have different tolerance levels, I guess. (Laughter)

Int: What had his pressure dropped to, do you recall?

Nurse: Yes, it was like 75 or something. It didn't crash; it just drifted.

The nurse makes a qualitative distinction between a sudden drop ("crashing") and a blood pressure that "drifts" in response to pain medication. This is a good example of practical engaged reasoning during transitions. Timing must be taught. The prior example illustrates learning to organize and orchestrate responses. The nurses counsel new nurses to always have at least 2 liters of lactated Ringer's in the room in advance for when the patient warms up after open heart surgery and requires additional fluid quickly. They continue to describe predictable patient events that allow the nurse to plan ahead:

Nurse 1: "When they are coming in to do the chest x-rays, you have the syringe and sedation ready because they wake up with a bang and they're wild when they come to."

Nurse 2: Yeah, and their pressures will go sky-high and they'll get real tachycardia which is just what you don't want them to do. So you get your little syringe and give them a little bit and you talk to them, "We're going to put you on this hard plate," and watch for eyelid response.

These expert nurses complete one another's instructions in one accord, indicating that this is the common wisdom on the unit for taking care of open-heart patients, so new nurses will not have to learn this knowledge from trial-and-error learning.

Summary

Demonstrating embodied skills and ways of being include emotional and physical responses, comportment, organization, and pacing in particular and typical situations. Acting in a situation demonstrates practical reasoning and skilled know-how. Imitation of others allows the newcomer to enter the situation with enough safety and imagination to learn from it. The expert practitioner accomplishes what no instructional aid can adequately do—i.e., respond in particular situations with effective action and appropriate responses. Fluid, reliable responses create an essential vision of excellence for other practitioners.

SHARING A COLLECTIVE VISION OF EXCELLENCE AND TAKEN-FOR-GRANTED PRACTICE

The culture of the unit carries a vision of what is excellent and ordinary, taken-for-granted practice. These practices and visions determine what kinds of expectations the advanced beginner and competent level nurse will learn. Competent nurses have mastered the task world, but unless they take up a new focus for their clinical learning, they may imagine that clinical learning is limited to learning new types of procedures, and caring for new patient populations, they will not easily shift their focus to knowing a patient and learning about particular patient populations. An extreme form of this technical approach to clinical learning is evident in the following excerpt:

> I'm concentrating on learning the congenital anomalies . . . I'm taking classes and reading and that is just increasing my knowledge base. I'm always interviewing at different places where else I can get more stuff from. Everyone teases me, "Oh, you've been here a year, where are you going now?" But I've gotten a lot of knowledge and I personally think it's helped me to change and work in things that I don't get stagnant and I don't know a lot about everything, but I know a fair amount about a lot of things.

While "mastering new technology and techniques" is essential in a rapidly changing field such as nursing, when expertise is viewed as a form of counting how many things one knows how to do, gaining expertise as a socially embedded, historical practice may be overlooked. The focus on mastering an array of technical skills may inhibit focusing on patient responses and gaining synthetic understanding of the patient's condition, since elemental tasks become the definition of knowledge-skill acquisition. The tension between mastering the technical demands and refining the art and skill of working with particular patients and families can show up as a deliberate choice:

Nurse 1: It sounds real cruel, but I'm not a real good primary nurse. I don't do primary nursing even though I know it's real important. I don't do it.

Nurse 2: You don't take the same assignment every time?

Nurse 1: I usually keep the same assignment if I am working 3 days in a row, but if there's a kid that's more critical, I'll take that child.

Nurse 2: You're the only one who does that?

Nurse 1: No, I think there are a couple of other nurses probably on evenings that are like that, but most of them are really into primary care which I think is wonderful, but I can't deal with it.

Int: Help me understand that. What is the trade-off?

Nurse 1: I get really attached to the kids and I guess to separate myself from them, that's how I do it. I just take the sickest kid and then go on to the next sickest kid. Where some of the nurses can handle that attachment and the detachment when they leave and they really get involved with the parents. I mean some of them become best friends, and they see each other on the outside. I think that's great.

Int: Have you ever done that?

Nurse 1:   Once or twice I have gotten close to families and to kids and stuff like that. But, no, not nearly as much as the other nurses. I guess I always felt, in the last few years, I'm not too young, but, I'm too young in my profession to do primary nursing. It sounds terrible. There's so much to learn! There's so many things I want to learn and to do primary nursing, but the actual clinical technical stuff, I wanted to learn very well, and that's why I do it and I've just kind of stayed in it.

Int: Do you think that will change? It may or may not, huh?

Nurse 1:   Not as long as I'm hungry for new stuff and doing new things. I mean, maybe in 20 years when I'm burned out, you know, if I get burned out, maybe . . . Some of the nurses are learning to intubate now. You know, the charge nurses and relief, and I really want to learn but they're not going to let me, because they know I'll probably start doing that all the time, too. Yeah, it's just the way I am.

Doing primary nursing focuses on the relationship with the particular patient/family and working through clinical and recovery issues in ways that allow for knowing the patient and planning continuity in the care. But these caring practices may not be as valued as highly technical skills. In the interview above, the nurse is asked to compare herself with other nurses on her unit and she responds:

> My charge nurse is a real good clinician. She's not a good primary care nurse, either. I mean, she really gets into the technical stuff and the nurse that trained me before I even became a nurse, when I took my preceptorship through school, is the charge nurse on day shift and she is an excellent cli- nician. So I guess I've kind of had those two role models that have shown me where I want to be, plus I also want to do this.

When she talks about being an excellent "clinician" she is referring to mastering technical skills and handling emergency clinical situations, rather than doing highly technical care in relation to particular patients/families, i.e., integrating clinical reasoning in transitions with caring knowledge such as teaching, coaching, and comforting patients and families. This is evident in her discussion of what a "slump" in practice is:

Nurse: Lately, it's like I'm in a slump in IVs. I can't get IVs in kids and that's very frustrating. It's like there are some nurses that can just find a vein and put it in and, you know, I try twice and that's it. You get up to three times and I've tried twice, and then someone else will come along and just put it in.

Int: Do you have a sense of what you are missing?

Nurse: I think sometimes I'm just in too much of a hurry. A lot of those nurses who are really good just take their time. I'm always in a hurry. I think if I just slow down a little bit, I could probably be a little better at it. I just think some- times you're tired.

Mastering the techniques of inserting intravenous catheters is only one skill, an important one, but it does not yet constitute a practice (see Chapter 9). Indeed, to become proficient, the competent nurse must begin to focus on patient responses and develop a beginning understanding of particular patients within a general patient population. In the same small group interview session, a nurse on another unit presents a different role model of excellence in response to this discussion:

Nurse: There's one nurse on days that I really admire. I think that she's an excellent nurse. She's a very good clinician and she's very good with the families too, with the social aspects. I would hope to be like her in a few more years in time.

Int: What is it that you've seen her do that really impresses you?

Nurse: Well, she has a very good knowledge base as far as physiology and disease process are concerned and she's able to anticipate what problems a patient is going to have 2 days down the road or two hours down the road and I think that that's very important. I'd like to be able to develop that better. She is very good at giving comfort and reassurance to families. She develops a very good rapport easily and right away with families. And I think that is also very important. Families are in crisis when they are in the ICU, it's very important to be able to nurse them as well as their loved one.

Early on, new nurses select role models, nurses who embody their notions of what it is good nursing practice. In this example, we have contrasting visions of holistic primary care and highly technical care that devalues primary care. One nurse has the vision that "clinical" and "caring" can be integrated, while the other nurse feels that the two represent a mutually exclusive choice.

Influence of Unit Culture on Clinical Learning and Judgment

Unit cultures develop distinct approaches to learning. For example, different critical care units have distinct patterns of collaboration and competition. A nursing unit may develop an elaborate culture of teaching, support, and collaboration, or it may emphasize individual achievements and treat knowledge as the private possession of the individual. Both cultural self-understandings are present in most social groups. The following interview excerpt illustrates a strong unit culture for learning. Experiential learning is viewed as a common good to be shared with the caring community, rather than an individual possession or a source of individual advantage or power:

Nurse: Anytime you are faced with a new situation, you have to review it after. Run it through your mind, relive it and learn from it. I must run through new situations 100 times in my mind—what can I do better next time, or different.
Int: And you are able to do this?
Nurse: Yeah, I can pull things out and can talk to other staff and reiterate it. I talk about it for several reasons. One, it is a teaching tool for myself; it can also be a tool for other nurses to prepare them for situations. To do this has really helped me to set priorities about what absolutely has to be done. What is really nice is to have a staff to do this with. The PM shift is overall very good. They are a lot of clinically sharp people that I learn from also. I don't have to know everything, there are other people who know more. Plus we work as a team. Most of us have worked on PMs [*the evening shift*] for a few years, so we know each other, plus the docs know us and what we know and what we can do. It is hard for new nurses because they don't have a lot of confidence, so even if they know something or don't understand something, they won't say it to the doctor. So I also tell them it takes awhile to get their confidence and just keep going to deliveries and keep doing it and then they will get it. I will keep working with them. The first couple of times I am right there, then I begin working back a little bit to the point I am in the room but I don't say anything unless they ask. That kind of thing. And then we can discuss how things went afterwards. I also do this same sort of thing with staff that haven't worked a lot with ventilator babies. On a quiet evening, I will put someone who hasn't worked a lot with vents [*ventilators*] with one of those babies and then really spend time with them. At the bedside. I like to teach staff, I enjoy it so whenever I can I do it. I try to put people into situations where they can learn. I want people to be confident they can do it. Push yourself a little.

Teaching and learning are social, and the social expectations and practices for sharing scientific and experientially learned knowledge determine the development and pooling of clinical and caring expertise within a work group.

The unit subculture also has taken-for-granted ways of thinking and being with patients that get transmitted. In a very distressed hospital nursing system, undergoing great change and chronic high turnover and staff shortages, we found a "tough nurse culture." We heard stories about patients and families that distanced the nurse or evidenced an external or outside-in and therefore more judgmental impressions of the patient and family. From this hospital we heard almost exclusively "war stories" instead of narratives of learning. We did not become acquainted with patients/families as persons with specific concerns and life histories in these nurses' stories.

This was contrasted for us by a unit that had developed exquisite shared recognition practices so that the whole unit came to know directly or indirectly silent patients with grave illnesses and difficult communication problems. There was a shared practice of communicating to others any new understanding gained about a chronically critically ill patient so that cumulative understanding was achieved. On a neurological unit, we observed a cultural norm of highly specified objective reporting of fine distinctions about patients' physical capacities and level of consciousness. This well worked-out shared language conveying the patient's specific capacities and level of consciousness created a collective possibility of recognizing and transmitting subtle changes in behavior and sensorium that could convey critical neurological changes. This socially shared skill made early warnings of neurological changes a collective possibility.

In a highly effective trauma critical care unit, we observed a shared ethic for direct patient observation and involvement. This was supported by the head nurse, the attending physician, and staff nurses who "kept informed" and "knew" their patients, and was supported by the design of the monitoring system. There was no centralized monitoring on this unit, and this increased the nurses' responsibility to know their patient and be at the bedside. On some units there were taken-for-granted meanings about allowing the family as much access to their loved ones as possible, whereas on other units, allowing the family access was told as exceptions in stories (Chesla, in press). Each unit culture sets up patterns of practice, relationships, surveillance, and transmission of clinical and caring knowledge. Examining these patterns can open new avenues for enhancing the clinical expertise of the health care team.

Collective Wisdom and Rapidly Changing Technology

Continuous technological development is culturally expected in a highly technical field. What was impossible this year is expected to be possible in future years. This common premise is often borne out in clinical practice. When a new technology is introduced, there is usually a high failure rate because the technology is not yet worked out. This is most evident in neonatal intensive care units, in cardiac surgery, and transplantation:

Nurse 1: We are saving babies now that we weren't saving 5 years ago with ECMO.
Nurse 2: And the cardiacs we're doing now. We have only been doing newborn cardiac surgery in the last couple of years.

Because of the cultural press to extend the technology and science, the clinician must temper current clinical expectations with what will be possible with emerging science and technology. In small group interview sessions where nurses were describing futile cases and excessive heroics, stories were told about the patient who survived against all odds; or in the expert group, nurses would offer examples about having been fooled in the past and express the need to keep an open mind. The tension for expert clinical and ethical comportment is to offer neither too little nor too much technology. The goal is to be prudent and realistic in the treatments offered so that futile death-prolonging treatments are avoided, while continuing to be open to new possibilities available in science and technology. This was one of the major fields of risk that came up in almost every interview session. The danger of offering too little or too much was ever present in the nurses' narratives:

> We discontinue support a lot in the nursery. I mean that's just a way of life because we have a lot of little preemies who have very poor lungs, and have head bleeds and all these other things. And it's, you know, just a way of life, and you learn to deal with that. And sometimes I think, sometimes I'm ready to give up too soon. Especially on the preemies who are 24 weeks gestation, and they've got big head bleeds and they have terrible lungs, and you know that if they have a life at all, it's going to be just horrible. You know, after all these years, it's become easier for me to say: "I think it's time to stop." But here was a full-term baby. She was beautiful, she was alert. There was nothing else wrong with her, and I think, I don't know, it's purely emotional I think, because I have a hard time thinking of lungs as a vital organ—I know it is strange to say, but I have seen them recover.

For all its ambiguity, this expert nurse narrative illustrates the tension of offering too little and too much. She struggles to be true to an infant who may have a chance to survive with a high quality of life. Living with this tension and being solicited by the particular infant's life and possibilities is an essential and rich moral source provided by prudent and committed critical care nurses.

Social Patterns of Ethical Tension and Silence

Cultural traditions unwittingly create some clearings (i.e. habits, practices, skills, understandings of being, and questions) that make some things, issues, and human beings visible while rendering others less visible or even invisible. As illustrated in the above example, there is much ambiguity and controversy over the end of life. Critical care units are set up to save lives. By design, dying patients are not supposed to be in these units. If further treatment is futile, the belief is that patients should be treated at home or admitted to palliative care units. Yet the units have high death rates, and patients stay in the units after Do Not Resuscitate orders have been written. The realization of futility comes unevenly to nurses, physicians, patients, and families. In all of the hospitals studied, the "slow code" was mentioned as a way of dealing with inadequate medical and familial consensus and where the health care team had come to believe it was a futile situation:

Nurse 1:   Slow code, but that's not really . . .
Int: That's not really cricket, the slow code? But that seems to be . . .
Nurse 1:   Sort of that un-talked about . . .
Nurse 2:   "Don't do anything until you call me first and by then it's too late anyway."
Nurse 1:   Yeah.

The slow code is illegitimate and not morally or legally acceptable. It is an ad hoc corrective response to stop futile treatments that have become torturous and death-prolonging. There is a tacit social agreement not to talk about "slow codes" because ideally the ethical choices will have been made clear, having been openly discussed, so that a patient will receive either a full resuscitation effort or no effort at all. In practice, the situation is far more fraught with ambiguity and the preferred clarity is elusive. Neither historical, experientially learned knowledge nor statistical data from science is infallible or can offer definitive answers in all situations. Prudent judgments call on both experiential clinical and caring wisdom in concert with statistical data. Attempts are being made to develop objective prognostic systems such as the APACHE III system designed by William A. Knaus (Guest, 1993). While such systems can clarify the extreme situations, they do not replace practical reasoning in transitions. Astute clinical and caring judgment are required to identify the salient situations where the system should be used, and for all the middle-range scores where the predictive value of the scale is limited. Given the life-and-death ethical stakes, the demand is to understand the situation as fully as possible in order to be with the vulnerable person in caring ways that respond to the possibilities inherent in the patient's capacities and concerns. Nurses talk about "keeping open" and being willing to be surprised because they have witnessed radical changes in patients' clinical possibilities even within the past 5 years. This ethos of keeping open contributes both to the tensions and clarity about judgments of medical futility. For example, two nurses joined with the parents' fight to have a baby extended on ECMO until they could improve her nutritional status. The delay was successful and the infant was weaned from ECMO and the respirator and was discharged home. This learning may be overgeneralized, but it serves to keep the nurse open to the possibilities of survival in the most extreme cases:

It was a tough call, but I'll never be as easy going about giving up on a baby and saying this kid's not going to make it. Why are we doing this?

The exceptions and near-miraculous recoveries spur the health care team to stay open to the possibilities of new treatments and technology. The progress theme is sometimes at odds with past experience. There is both a technological imperative (Koenig, 1988) to keep improving and using available technology in these units, and an ethos to stay open to the possibility of survival in all cases. Ethical practice demands that this taken-for-granted technological imperative be overridden only when the suffering is too great and the possibilities for survival too small. There is also a strong ethos to avoid false hopes and futile treatments that heighten suffering and prolong dying. This is a judgment call that must be schooled by clinical and caring knowledge as well as science. This is an area where more articulation research such as this must be done to describe the everyday ethical practices and issues that occur in diverse organizational contexts.

Regardless of the clinical and caring issues with a particular patient, the tension about technology transforming the impossible into the possible is inherent in scientific medicine. New possibilities must temper historical and experiential knowledge so that clinical knowledge doesn't become too fixed or rigid. Practical clinical and ethical reasoning based on past cases allows practitioners to know how to be with patient/families and how to advocate for them. The statistical and objective guidelines from science provide useful parameters and correctives, and sometimes clarity. Most often, the situation is underdetermined and evolving and requires that clinicians be willing to struggle with the tensions of competing goods, possibilities, and concerns to make the best possible clinical and ethical judgments. Clinicians who use the dialogue, contrasts, and ethical tensions created by experiential and scientific guides offer an essential middle ground between rigidly following the mandates of past experience or blindly following statistical guidelines or abstract rules.

Styles of Medical Practice

The oral tradition of telling stories as well as educational background, habits, practices, and institutional structures, including financial incentives and accounting practices, contribute to a style of medical practice. For example, the nurses in the next interview excerpt compare two different medical groups. This discussion illustrates the strong influence of the style of medical practice on nurses' shared vision of excellence and taken-for-granted practices.

The nurses have said earlier in the interview that they do not like to take care of postoperative heart patients who are being supervised by a particular ICU team of anesthesiologists. This discussion about the specific medical teams cannot be generalized; indeed, on other units, the anesthesiology medical team was preferred. The point of the interview excerpt is to make the style of medical practice visible in the way it is relevant to nurses' clinical judgment and caring practices. These nurses compare two different medical groups:

Int: Why the ICU team?
Nurse 1:   Because they are learning doctors and they are anesthesiologists.
Nurse 2:   It really makes me nervous when you have a sick heart—
Nurse 1:   And they sit in there the whole time and you can't make any decisions on your own. Like the other doctors give us parameters and we give the patients fluid, change the respirator, wean them as tolerated, and can make the changes within what they do not want to be called on.
Nurse 2:   It's the surgeon who has allowed this other team to take over for him, so it's not the surgeon. Sometimes I'll say to the surgeon: "You know, it's time to make rounds on this patient and say you don't want them to give him anymore fluid."
Int: How does that work?
Nurse 1:   It usually works but you do it under, I mean it's like going over their head. But I feel like I'm saving the patient another day of grief because it doesn't make any sense while they are practicing . . .
Nurse 2:   At the expense of the patient.

It is beyond the scope of this work to capture all the ways that the style of medical practice influences nursing expertise and taken-for-granted practices, but pervasive in our data were also examples of the impact of the not-so-hidden role nurses play in the education of physicians and the differing clinical possibilities offered during the day and night:

Int: Did the resident listen to the lungs? Did the stethoscope come out of his pocket?
Nurse: No, he didn't. We told him, "His lungs are wet." Even though the patient didn't really need it, I said: "Would you like a chest X-ray?" [*Here the nurse is acknowledging that she was playing the doctor-nurse game, hinting at but not giving a diagnosis*]. He said: "Well, I am unsure." He is so unsure, because it's July. (*Laughter*) [*Residents are new in July after graduating from medical school in June*]. I'm sorry to say, it's July and they are so new, and they're so scared to write orders. We understand, but we have to tell them, "Why don't you call the Resident Three?" I asked him that finally: "And see if we are doing the right thing."
Int.:   You sort of coached the Resident One to call his Resident Three?
Nurse: Yes, because I know he is very nice, and he's very receptive. He listened to us. . . . Anyway, those are the things, working nights can be frustrating, because you don't have the resources. It will take you hours to get the Resident Three, and so basically you are dealing with Resident Ones all the time. Sometimes they say: "My R1 (Resident One) is there. What are you doing? Why don't you call him?" I said, "I will call him if he knows what he is doing." It's just so hard, a lot of decisionmaking. This is very hard at nights.

The art and skill of negotiating clinical judgments with physicians are taken up more fully in Chapter 11. Suffice to say here that the cultural vision of excellence and taken-for-granted practices of nurses are developed in relation to the styles of medical practice and medical education. Explicating these styles can do much to improve clinical knowledge development and assist in critically evaluating both excellent and poor clinical judgment in nursing practice.

THE POWER OF TRUST AND MOOD

The social level of trust, cooperation, and expertise can create a culture of expectation and hope. The mood or ambience of a unit sets a tone for sense of possibility, trust, and support within the culture of the work group. For example, one unit was known in the larger surrounding area for the nurses' expertise in weaning patients from respirators, and patients who were very difficult to wean were sent there from the surrounding geographical area. In the following small group interview, nurses from this unit describe the mood and culture of the unit:

Nurse 1: It's an attitude. It's like, we are going to get this patient off the ventilator, whereas, I can see sometimes a patient that you predetermine that he is going to [be weaned] and the treatment tends to run in that direction . . . so you work real hard doing whatever it takes.

Nurse 2: It's tough for these guys so it's a thrill to get them off. They are so dependent and then to get them used to activities of daily living and convince them that they are going to get better.

This community of nurses has developed many skills and practices for coaching and encouraging patients to take up life again after losing the strength of their respiratory muscles and being dispirited by prolonged helplessness and dependency on the respirator. Stotland (1969) has written about the psychology of hope in the care of psychiatric patients. It would appear that a sense of possibility and expectant mood and high levels of confidence is working in this unit. They have developed many innovations in their practice, but the nurses credit their own expectations and prior successes to their good patient outcomes. Attitudes and skillfulness reinforce one another.

The power of social expectation is strong. As noted above in interview sessions where nurses were describing futile cases and excessive heroics, stories would be added about the patient who survived against all odds, or in the expert group, nurses would insert examples about having been fooled in the past and express the need to keep an open mind.

A climate of expectation and hope sets up a web of social expectation and group identity. Experiential learning and successes create a sense of possibility within the practicing community. Poor outcomes with particular patients/families can be contrasted with better outcomes and better care with the goal of preventing future breakdowns and improving care. The strong ethos for doing "postmortem" examinations and conferences to confront errors, as well as narratives of learning, are done in the spirit of doing better next time if the morale and identity of the group is positive and supportive:

> As charge these are all people I have worked with for a number of years, so it is very pleasant. It is amazing how your environment can really be changed by the personalities on a given day. We are all used to working together and as a team, it seems to come natural. We had an interesting patient rhythm this morning so I xeroxed her 12 lead EKG. It only seemed natural to do that. Because we all looked at it and gave our opinions. We all saw it as a learning experience.

In the above example, a culture of learning is supported by a mood of enthusiasm. However, as Stotland (1969) documented, the mood can go in the other direction. In the face of chaos, staff cutbacks and staff turnover, the level of competence can decline and the mood can become one of despair and helplessness:

Nurse 1: We have had three really bad codes lately; only one made it to the unit. Some codes could have been run better if the residents would have known what they were doing. Some stand there and say: "Well can we have a rhythm?"
Nurse 2: Or does anyone have any ideas? (laughs)
Nurse 3: Yes, that's a good one.
Nurse 1: But the last code I went to, I swear there were three doctors on an extremity apiece, looking for intravenous access. And I say: "The patient has a central line."
Nurse 2: Is that true?
Nurse 1: That's all they could think about.
Nurse: That happens a lot. Oh sick.

On this unit there was a distrusting, contentious relationship between nurses, nurses and physicians, and between the health care professions and patients and families. When errors occurred there was talk of blame and defense rather than troubleshooting and shared responsibility. The climate of blame rather than correction is clear in the next excerpt, where a nurse is telling of erroneously directing another nurse to put an oral medication into an intravenous line:

I said [*to the other nurse*] I did tell you to do that and it's all my fault. It's my fault. And I was just hysterical. It was just awful and so everyone knew of course, because they were all trying to find out who did it. It was talked about throughout the whole staff and finally, I was the one and I was on vacation. I couldn't defend myself. I mean there was nothing to defend except for the fact that there was an unmarked port. So I really remember that, and in the end, the patient was O.K.

While sources and causes of errors must be found to allow for correction and prevention of future problems, a climate of shame and blame disrupts the knowledge work of the social group. In the grave situations caused by errors in critical care, self- and other punishing styles do little to prevent future problems, yet they effectively prevent a climate of openness and trust that allows for the identification of problems. In an emotional climate of distrust, shared clinical lessons, memories, and consensually validated clinical distinctions diminish. The group loses much of its collective capacities and their ability to focus on strengthening one another's practice. The possibilities of pooling wisdom and shared vigilance as well as flexible assignments based on strengths and learning needs diminish.

Implications

Much has been written about the importance of morale and social climate for reducing absenteeism, stress, and turnover. But the level of clinical expertise, knowledge development, and caring knowledge are drastically reduced when the subculture of the unit focuses on questionable visions of excellence, or when the mood of the group becomes one of despair and hopelessness, adversarialism and blame, rather than support and improvement. Skill acquisition and the development of clinical expertise are dependent on the social ecology of the work group. Team-building that focuses on improving performance and shared visions will improve the level of expertise in an organizational setting (Mohr & Mohr, 1983). In highly complex tasks where the risk of error is great and high reliability is required, managerial strategies that break the task down into the smallest units and assign them to the least skilled personnel diminish the level of understanding required for troubleshooting and recognizing early changes in patients. Breaking the tasks down for multiple staff members may disrupt the focus on synthesis and clinical learning. Or as Borgmann (1984) points out, we do violence to our human practices when we radically separate means and ends. Such separation sets up an insidious devaluation of the "mere" means.

Summary

The goal of this chapter is to capture aspects of the ways clinical and caring knowledge are socially embedded. Concepts of culture, dialogical understanding, clinical reasoning in transitions, historical understanding, and practices, skills, and habits of a group of practitioners have been illustrated by the nurses' practice. The fact that knowledge is situated historically and worked out in a particular community does not render it hopelessly relativistic or meaningless. Narrative memory and multiple perspectives of skilled practitioners in concert with science and technology can create clinical and caring knowledge that is reliable and cumulative, if not ahistorical and timeless. Scientific theories and information become knowledge and judgment only in the hands of skilled practitioners who have the opportunity to clarify, and extend general explanations through understanding particular situations.

NOTE

1. "Observation Note" refers to field observations of nurse's practice. See Methods, Appendix A.

Chapter 9

THE PRIMACY OF CARING AND THE ROLE OF EXPERIENCE, NARRATIVE, AND COMMUNITY IN CLINICAL AND ETHICAL EXPERTISE

E thical and clinical knowledge are traditionally separated in academia. This serves to allow a separate and analytically important distinction and focus on the two areas of knowledge. Yet, for the practicing clinician, ethical and clinical knowledge are inseparable. Ethical principles and notions of the good provide an essential guidance for clinical decisionmaking. When nursing students learn clinical skills, they also learn how to be with and take care of patients. Ethical principles relating to patients' rights, autonomy, and beneficence must be translated into everyday ethical comportment. Indeed, it is the everyday ethical comportment that makes the learning of ethical principles understandable in action. The goal of this chapter is to take up in more detail the role of narrative and community in learning ethical and clinical distinctions. If the nurse is not in conversation with other practitioners who share similar concerns and qualitative distinctions in caring for patients, these distinctions will be lost or, at least, not refined. The nature of narrative in learning and remembering practical reasoning in transition is considered.*

---

*This chapter was originally published as an article: Benner, P. (1991). The primacy of caring, the role of experience, narrative and community in clinical and ethical expertise. *Advances in Nursing Science*, 14, 1–21.

This book assumes that in order to examine notions of the good life, what is worth being and preserving, one must study everyday ethical expertise and narratives embedded in the practices of communities. The practices and stories told within a community provide the necessary background understanding for everyday ethical comportment and for formal ethical judgments. Quandary and procedural ethics depend on everyday skillful ethical comportment and practical moral reasoning that is formed by embodied knowers. Quandary and procedural ethics focus on breakdowns in everyday ethical comportment and on the adjudication of rights. Procedural approaches to ethics that adjudicate rights and principles focus on what is "right to do rather than what it is good to be, on defining the content of obligation rather than the nature of the good life"(Taylor, 1989, p. 3).

Procedural approaches to ethics that adjudicate rights and principles cannot stand alone because they cannot provide a positive statement of the good, and yet they are dependent on an everyday practical knowledge of the good to sustain them (Sandel, 1982; Taylor, 1989).

In nursing, the dominant ethic found in stories of everyday practice is one of care, responsiveness to the other, and responsibility. Care is defined as the alleviation of vulnerability; the promotion of growth and health; the facilitation of comfort, dignity, or a good and peaceful death; mutual realization; and the preservation and extension of human possibilities in a person, a community, a family, or a tradition (Benner & Wrubel, 1989; Gordon, Benner, & Noddings, in press; Tanner et al., 1993). As pointed out in the last chapter, an ethic of care must be learned experientially because it is dependent on recognition of salient ethical comportment in specific situations located in specific communities, practices, and habits.

"Experience" refers to the turning around, adding nuance, and amending or changing preconceived notions or perceptions of the situation (Benner, 1984a; Gadamer, 1975). The development of skillful ethical comportment is experientially learned and transmitted by a group of practitioners. The term "ethical comportment" is used to refer to the embodied, skilled know-how of relating to others in ways that are respectful, responsive, and supportive of their concerns. "Comportment" refers to more than just words, intents, beliefs, or values; it encompasses stance, touch, orientation—thoughts and feelings fused with physical presence and action (Benner & Wrubel, 1989; Benner, Wrubel, Phillips, Chesla, & Tanner, 1995). Experience occurs when one encounters a practical situation in such a way that one's understanding of the situation is altered. Experience is gained when one actively learns to recognize to do and be better and worse in practical situations and to see and feel salient ethical distinctions. Experience, then, is considered the active history of a tradition, a working out of a tradition that can be captured in everyday skilled practice and notions of excellence and breakdown in narratives of practice. A practice is defined as skilled actions that have notions of good embedded in them because they are lodged in concerns lived out in a community of practitioners.

In nursing practice, everyday ethical comportment and practical moral discourse are most often concerned with protection of vulnerability and fostering of growth and health, or a good and peaceful death. The term "ethical comportment" is used to refer to the embodied skilled know-how of relating to others in ways that are respectful and support their concerns. Abstract reasoning or generalizable, decontextualized principles cannot influence practice if situations relevant to these principles go unnoticed, or if the practitioner does not have the skill to act ethically (Benner, 1984a; Benner & Tanner, 1987; Benner & Wrubel, 1982; H. L. Dreyfus, 1979; S. E. Dreyfus, 1982; Dreyfus & Dreyfus with Athaniasiou, 1986).

As noted in previous chapters, through experience within a socially based practice, stories and concrete first-hand experiences build narratives and memories of salient clinical situations so that one moves from a novice to a skillful practitioner. This process of membership and participation creates a socially embedded knowledge of the good in the practice. As expertise is gained in the practice, the abstract is supplanted by the concrete. With experience, the concrete situation becomes coherent and the practitioner develops a narrative sense of doing better or worse, of recognizing similarities and differences, and of participating in common meanings and practices and others' practice narratives that allow the practitioner to recognize common clinical entities and issues. Abstract principles, after all, are never completely matched by reality and must be extended and clarified in real-life experience. Problem-solving can only occur if problems are recognized and actions can only be taken if salient issues are noticed (Benner & Wrubel, 1982; Vetlesen, 1994).

In this and other studies of the practical knowledge of nurses, we have examined the notions of good and the knowledge embedded in the practice of nursing (Benner, 1984; Benner & Tanner, 1987; Benner & Wrubel, 1989; Benner, 1989, 1990). Narrative accounts of actual clinical examples of excellent practice, breakdown, or a paradigm case (a situation where the nurse gains a new clinical understanding that alters future practice) are examined for their everyday clinical and caring knowledge. First-person narratives of practice provide texts for interpretive phenomenological studies of ethical comportment, practical moral reasoning, and ethical distinctions. The concerns, fears, hopes, conversations, and issues are disclosed and preserved in telling and discussing the stories. A story allows for less linearity, more parentheses or asides, and an easier flow from initial to later concerns than a clinical case study or accounts of diagnostic reasoning that leave out the agent's perceptions and concerns. Narrative accounts uncover meanings and feelings in ways that shed light on the contextual, relational, and configurational knowledge lived out by the author in the practice. Narrative accounts stand in sharp contrast to the typical codified, cryptic, efficient exchange of professional assessments about a patient's condition. The interpretive goal for other practitioners hearing or reading the story is not to get beyond the stories but to understand the know-how, meaningful patterns, and responses that they depict. As noted by Rubin (see p. 172), experienced nurses who are disengaged from their practice do not offer rich narrative accounts of encounters with particular patients. These experienced nurses present technical accounts of events or general statements of what they consider typical of their responses, but lack stories rich with qualitative distinctions and ethical concerns (see Chapter 7).

Examining the notions of good embedded in narrative accounts of actual practice using an interpretive phenomenological approach (Benner, 1994a, d) stands in sharp contrast to casuistry (Jonsen & Toulmin, 1988). Casuistry uses case studies to exemplify a particular ethical principle, whereas a first-person narrative approach is inductive and uses naturally occurring situations to explicate ethical concerns and the good and worthwhile in relation to particular persons, communities, and situations. In naturally occurring narratives, new issues and innovations are introduced as the situation demands, rather than reducing the situation to the preconceived ethical issues.

In practical ethical reasoning, clarity rests in a situated knowledge of the person and his or her relevant reference groups. Furthermore, this particular knowledge reflects practice-based understandings of the good and its violation (Taylor, 1989; 1991). For example, we have found that nurses have an elaborate practical discourse about "knowing a patient," and knowing a patient comes prior to assessing a patient (Tanner et al., 1993; Tanner, Benner, Chesla, & Gordon, 1993). Knowing a patient is central to the ethics of care and responsibility (Benner, Wrubel, Phillips, Chesla, & Tanner, 1995; Gilligan, 1982); often this moral art has to do with knowing the patient and family as persons in extremely deprived, extenuating, and highly vulnerable circumstances. This engaged knowledge of the patient and family can yield wisdom and attuned caring because knowing the patient calls the nurse to respond to the person as other, worthy of care with no expectation of reciprocity.

Embodiment provides a common human circumstance that allows for understanding, compassion, and the protection of vulnerability that objective rational calculation cannot provide. The common experience of embodiment acts as a moral source in everyday ethical comportment (Taylor, 1989). It is in disembodied and conceptual distance that normative ethics fails to grasp essential embodied human distinctions of worth, such as honor, courage, suffering, and dignity (Taylor, 1989). Ethical deliberation devoid of engaged historical understanding may provoke thoughtful consideration of ethical principles and unnoticed issues, but it does not provide the best understanding of the notions of good offered or threatened by the situation. Framing the situation as a problem or dilemma based on abstract principles or rational calculation can bypass a wise framing already lodged in the stories of those engaged in the situation. Framing the issue without direct access to embodied suffering blocks accurate understanding and empathy. Therefore, disengaged reasoning should not be given a privileged status over engaged reasoning in the particular situations (see Chapter 1; Taylor, 1989; Taylor, 1993). At most, disengaged ethical reasoning should enrich and correct the dialogue about the possibilities and constraints in the situation.

Skillful ethical comportment develops over time by doing better or worse, where "better" cannot be strictly rule-governed or procedural, because it must be guided by situated understanding of particular human concerns in particular contexts and transitions. On the other hand, doing worse means creating impediments, contributing to breakdown, limiting possibility, or violating the notions of good embedded in the particular caring relationships.

NARRATIVE THEMES

From cumulative research on nursing narratives, two major types of commonly occurring narrative themes or plots are pervasive. They are presented here to illustrate the function of narrative in excellent practice:

1. constitutive and sustaining narratives; [1]
2. narratives of learning.

Subthemes of constitutive and sustaining narratives include:

1. Narratives of healing and transcendence;
2. the heroic saving of a life through skillful, quick action and the appropriate use of technology. These are characterized by nurses as a "real save," in which the person returns to a full life. The opposite of a "real save" are lives saved inappropriately so that prolonged dying occurs;
3. fostering care and connection between patient and loved ones or patient and nurse (often this occurs with premature infants in neonatal intensive care units, but also with families of adult patients who are extremely compromised); and

4.   stories of presencing or not abandoning patients. These stories depict the difficulty of fidelity in the midst of suffering. A dramatic example is the communication, touch, and connection with a patient suffering from a "locked-in" syndrome where there is conscious awareness but no motor ability to communicate, except perhaps by blinking the eyes.

This list may be extensive, perhaps infinite, but this should not detract from the exploration of commonly held constitutive and sustaining narratives. Constitutive, sustaining narratives are usually linked to larger cultural stories, and notions of good embedded in the larger culture. The only constitutive and sustaining narrative explored in depth here is that of healing and transcendence, though there are examples of all the constitutive and sustaining narratives throughout this book.

Subthemes of learning narratives include:

1.   learning the skill of involvement;
2.   being open to experience;
3.   narratives of disillusionment;
4.   narratives of facing death and suffering; and
5.   liberation narratives.

These two major narrative themes and their subthemes or plots illustrate the function of narrative in a practice in revealing and creating social memory, skilled ethical comportment, and the role of first-person narratives in community and culture building.

Constitutive or Sustaining Narratives

Constitutive or sustaining narratives depict situations that constitute the person's understanding of what it is to be a nurse. They capture the significance of the practice and demonstrate meaning-laden clinical episodes that convey the worth of the work. These narratives often speak to the sustaining power of the memory during the difficult times. One can usually sense a relationship between the lived story and larger cultural narratives, whatever the tradition (Jewish, JudeoChristian, Islamic, et cetera). The following narrative by Kimberly Baird demonstrates a constitutive, sustaining narrative, as well as other themes and story lines. The way the story is told will demonstrate that it functions as both a constitutive and sustaining narrative.

"Sammy"

Kimberly Baird, RN

"Sammy," I'm sure I will carry his face, his name, his story with me for a very long time; maybe forever. Sammy was a 6-year-old Amish boy who had the misfortune of being on the bad side of a particularly nasty mule on the family farm. The injury he received when the mule's foot met his cranium left him with a skull fracture the neurosurgeon described as a "jigsaw puzzle of slivers," brain lacerations/contusions, and profound cerebral edema.

Sammy had spent days in Pediatric Intensive Care Unit after his craniotomy for the repair of his head injury. He was ventilator-dependent much of that time. He was transferred to the floor at the end of my shift on Friday with a Keofeed tube in place and a horseshoe-shaped incision on the right side of his head. Like most head injury patients, he was extremely combative and needed constant restraints to prevent injury to himself or dislodgment of his tube. "Great weekend ahead," I thought grimly, eyeing this latest addition to an already busy group of patients.

Unfortunately for Sammy and his family, the damage done to his brain tissue was extensive. The physician had told his parents the best they could hope for was a child who could take food orally. Sammy would never walk or talk. He would always be completely dependent on them.

Saturday morning began auspiciously enough. As I made walking rounds with the 11 P.M. to 7 A.M. nurse, we found Sammy's mother already dressed, knitting quietly at his bedside. Sammy had somehow wiggled out of his restraints and had pulled out his Keofeed—it lay next to him in bed. "Nice start," I thought to myself—confirming my fear of what the weekend would hold. The Amish, as a group, are a quiet, reserved sect, not given to emotional outbursts. Although I feel I usually handle parents well, particularly in a time of crisis, I found it difficult to spend any extra time in Sammy's room—not because of him, but because of the quiet, accepting, *waiting* manner of his mother. Having a daughter myself, I found it difficult to reconcile her seemingly passive acceptance of their tragedy and what I was positive would have been certifiable lunacy on my part, had I been in her shoes.

Except for the predictable diarrhea so common in patients with bolus nasogastric tube feeds of Ensure, Saturday passed without further incident. Sammy's mother did much of his care, changing his diaper, bathing him, helping me turn him without letting his free hand grab his tube. Her touch was always gentle and loving, but her quietness continued to disturb me.

Sunday started out better. Sammy's mother explained that the family would be going to church but that Sammy's older sister would stay with him. The sister, she explained, spoke English and Dutch and would be able to translate if Sammy needed anything. The fact that Sammy hadn't made an intelligible sound in *any* language didn't seem to figure into her thinking at all.

Just after lunch, the call light over Sammy's door went on. The voice of his sister over the intercom confirmed my worst fear—"Sammy pulled his tube out." As I walked to his room, I mentally tallied the people who might be available to help hold Sammy while the resident replaced the Keofeed and during the subsequent X-ray to check tube placement. In his room, it was just as I had anticipated—the tube lay in his bed and his sister was vainly trying to prevent him from shredding his diaper—a lost cause.

I talked to him as I began to untie his remaining restraints and change his diaper. What I said is not important, probably something trivial like "Sammy—what are we going to do with you?" But, as I spoke, I looked at him and felt for the first time since I'd been caring for him, that he was looking at me—not the vacant wild-eyed look I'd grown accustomed to, but an understanding, "with-it" gaze I had not seen before.

I thought about the standing order on his Kardex: "May try P.O. fluids." We had all laughed about that—Sammy had no swallow or gag reflex at all. As I looked at him, remembering the struggles of replacing the tube the previous days, I thought: "Why not?—let's give it a try." I told his sister I was going to try to give Sammy a drink by mouth. She looked somewhat skeptical, but didn't say anything. I cranked his bed up, left his restraints hanging at the sides and filled a Dixie cup with water from the sink. I cannot describe the feeling that came over me as that child *gulped* down that 60 cc of plain old tap water—the fluttering of my stomach, the pounding of my heart, the shortness of my breath. And, when I went to refill the cup, Sammy spoke.

Even if I could pronounce or understand what he said, I could not reproduce it here because Sammy spoke in Dutch. But, even to my ignorant ear, it was evident that this 6-year-old was demanding something. His sister's eyes opened wide as she looked from him to me and said: "He would rather have iced tea." To this day, I think I flew to the kitchen to get Sammy some iced tea. After an additional 150 cc went down without incident, I decided he was ready to advance. I called his resident to ask if he could have some ice cream. I am reasonably sure the resident thought I'd lost my mind or was chemically impaired—they all knew Sammy had still been a "neurologic nothing" on the morning rounds. But he said I could try—"Just don't let him aspirate, he goes to the rehabilitation center tomorrow."

I returned to Sammy's room and (unthinkingly) asked his sister if vanilla would be all right. I was only two steps up the hall when she came after me. "He says he'd rather have chocolate." It was only a short time afterwards that Sammy's family returned from church. In that time, I was just thrilled at the progress he made—even *walking* to the bathroom with minimal assistance to void in the toilet. I wondered how his mother would react when she returned.

Not only his parents, but grandparents, siblings, aunts and uncles came to see Sammy that day. The reserve they have never lifted—as Sammy's grandfather said: "This is God's way"—but the excitement in the room was palpable. And, the two tears that glistened on his mother's cheeks when Sammy spoke to her in Dutch told me that inside, Sammy's mother was shouting her joy from every rooftop.

The conclusion to Sammy's story is that several weeks later, after a stay at a nearby rehabilitation center, Sammy came back to see me—walking, talking Dutch with his family, and shy, as many 6-year-olds are with people they don't know that well. His mother thanked me for the care Sammy had received and said how wonderful all the doctors and nurses had been. Her praise made me feel more than a little ashamed. After all, we were the ones who had pooh-poohed the oral fluid order. I had mentally cringed at the idea of letting Sammy's sister be at his bedside as an interpreter because we all "knew" he would never speak again. But these people with their quiet faith, despite what must have been a terrible heartache for them, had believed in their God, in Sammy, and in us.

The significance of this event in my professional life is multifaceted. First, it made me examine myself and the way I deal with others—particularly the quiet parent. Even though it may be uncomfortable, I make myself take extra time to talk to that quiet mom or dad. Often that reserve is a facade of their inner terror. Although they appear to be coping, a few gentle, non-threatening questions about the kids at home, their jobs, or some trivial chitchat can open them up, allowing them to express their fears, thoughts, and questions.

The second area of significance has to do with labels. Although we are taught as nursing students that labels such as "slow" or "retarded" can become self-fulfilling prophecies, I do not think that concept fully impacted on me until that day. So now, even though I do not always succeed, I make the extra effort to orally feed a baby with a gastrostomy tube looming in her future or extra hard to teach a mom who has difficulty grasping the importance of Digoxin and Lasix therapy for her child. Labels, as I found out, can be misleading and can dull good nursing sense.

Finally, this event is most significant because I regard it as something of a miracle. Having worked on pediatrics for 6 years, I know physicians give the parents an optimistic but realistic prognosis, if possible. To hear their pronouncement for Sammy signified that this was indeed a sad situation. I've since heard other parents talk about their "miracle baby" or the "miracle" that happened to their child and I have to think there is an intangible something in human beings—faith in the God of their choice, the essence of the human spirit, an inner drive's obvious source. This is what keeps me at this difficult, wonderful job—helping these children physically, hoping that their "miracle" will come through for them. On those long days when every IV is blown and every resident is in a foul mood, the miracle and triumph of Sammy can still make me smile.

This is an ethical discourse. Central to the story are notions of the good and ethical concerns that exceed a deficit normative account, or a procedural concern about meeting minimal standards of conduct for rights and justice. Iatrogenesis, or the possibility of a lawsuit, do not loom in the background; rather, the discourse is propelled by how "true" the nurse is to the particular demands of the human situation. A dialogue on how to be true to the ethical demands of this situation and its moral instruction is taken up in Baird's subsequent nursing practice. But it is more than mere instruction; it provides a source of moral imagination, a sense of possibility that gives integrity and value to her work. The narrative memory actively engages her embodied skilled know-how, complete with feelings that allow her to recognize similar situations. Feelings allow for the perception or identification of similar situations without necessarily creating the ability to articulate why one recognizes or notes the situation as similar. Strategic language takes a back seat to significance language (Taylor, 1985, pp. 97–114). The "experience" doesn't turn the nurse into a believing Amish, but it does enlarge her moral imagination to include the possibilities she now recognizes in the Amish community. She translates their "faith" experience into her secular world, but leaves room for the somewhat incommensurable world she has encountered.

The concrete example of the Amish community of transcendence and healing sustains her in difficult times, "makes it all worth while, and can bring a smile to her face." No doubt future clinical situations are interpreted or understood in light of this paradigm case (see Benner, 1984a), which functions as a constitutive and sustaining narrative.

NARRATIVES OF LEARNING

Narratives About Being Open to Experience, About Turning Around, Being "Upended"

Kimberly Baird's narrative could also be classified as a narrative about being open to experience, although this category alone cannot exhaust the meaning of Baird's story about Sammy. Had the story a different outcome, she still might have had a turning around of her preconceptions about a quiet mother, and perhaps the story would have only fit into the "upending" plot characterization without becoming a constitutive, sustaining narrative.

The narrative shows every evidence that Baird is engaged morally and personally. For example, she is disturbed by the mother's differentness. It troubles her, and she is confronted by her own agitation over confronting the *other*. She now knows what it means to live out the moral injunction (the principle or norm) not to exclude human possibility through labels. The exemplar sets a new vision and possibility for excellence in Baird's practice. She has the moral courage to allow Sammy and his family to teach her, to turn her preconceptions around. Thus, from a phenomenological perspective, this situation counts as experience (the journey and process of change are included) and it is publicly accessible because it is lodged in a practice and a tradition. Though it is personal, it is not wholly subjective and therefore private. The good Baird discovers is brought forward in concrete practices and distinctions. The lesson encompasses an active moral dialogue in which theory on the problems of labeling is enriched, because it includes relational skills, exposes her blind spots, and creates new possibility for ethical comportment.

Being upended or open to new experience implies learning from failure. These stories are related to maintaining vigilance, paying attention, and noticing, and they often resemble the moral of the story of the little boy who cried wolf. They are "war stories" that warn the nurse and her or his colleagues to take potassium levels seriously, be meticulous about intravenous flow calculations, watch for drug reactions, and not to become immune to the warning of frequent, erroneous monitor alarms so that the alarms are ignored (see Chapter 8 for a discussion of an ethos of collective attentiveness). Often these stories are about the nurse's learning to do emergency medical interventions so that she or he is not helpless if there are no physicians available in time to help the patient. The narrative about Sammy can also be considered as a corrective narrative, because Baird learns to pay attention to "neurological nothings" in a new way and learns to patiently feed patients to avoid more technical interventions. The narrative functions to integrate feelings, thoughts, perceptual recognition, and memory so that the story represents a way of noticing salient ethical issues and comporting oneself ethically.

Narratives of Learning the Skill of Involvement

Learning to be a nurse means learning the relational skills appropriate to the practice of nursing. The kinds and levels of involvement for physicians, nurses, teachers, lawyers, dentists, ministers, counselors, and social workers are all different (Phillips & Benner, 1994). In our culture, the skill of involvement is too often considered a talent or trait rather than skilled knowledge developed over time through experience. Narratives convey and preserve knowledge about the skill of involvement (getting the right level, and kind of interpersonal involvement and distance to fit the situation) because relational skills always involve the concrete other and are always context dependent. These are stories of gaining personal knowledge (Polanyi, 1958). Biases and exclusions are encountered so that new possibilities for connection are discovered. Narratives about the skill of involvement often describe learning to be open to the person as concrete other, with an entitlement to freedom to be who they are, rather than to comply with the nurse's vision of optimal "care."

Nurses have an elaborate discourse on the right kind, level and amount of involvement with patients and families (see Chapters 5 and 6; Benner, Wrubel, Phillips, Chesla, & Tanner, 1994). They talk about being over-involved, or overidentified, so that they lose their ability to offer alternative perspectives, or even offer support as an interested "other." This is clearly "getting it wrong." They also talk about leaping in, taking over, and making the patient/family excessively dependent (Benner, 1993; Heidegger, 1962). This is also getting it wrong. Getting it right (being in a good relationship) is, however, typically told in terms of being in tune with the patient family needs and wishes, recognizing early warning signs of harm or danger, facilitating the next step in recovery, understanding and coaching, and being able in some situations to just be present in silence and tears (Benner, 1984a; Dyck & Benner, 1989; Magnan & Benner, 1989). These summary statements are not objective criteria that can be used without reference to particular concrete situations. They only point to situated understanding and action that require a particular situation to demonstrate what these practices look like. Baird depicts her level of involvement with Sammy's mother as distant and initially rejecting. This experiential learning causes her to change her relationship to quiet mothers in the future. Nurses also talk about those who have lost their ability to care, to be involved. These are the wounded ones, who by community consensus are truly no longer nurses, no longer practitioners, no longer standing within the meanings commonly held by the community.

In such complex human relationships and practice, there is no way to do well without sometimes doing poorly. Doing well requires skill and moral vision that comes only from moral dialogue and engaged confrontations within particular clinical situations. One can be placed in the situation with the best preparation for noticing qualitative distinctions about involvement and caring, suffering, hope and recovery, but the learning occurs in actual situations. And one's skillful ethical comportment is based upon a continued dialogue with doing better and doing worse in specific situations. Unless the dialogue is taken up in actual practice with actual situations, it simply will not augment and extend the notion of good represented by shared ethical norms. Abstract principles are necessary for orienting and alerting one to the appropriate regions of concern and for clarifying the public discourse, but they cannot guarantee that one will recognize in practice when these norms might be relevant nor will they guarantee that the ideal can be actualized. As one Intensive Care Unit nurse explains:

> [I]t's just a gut feeling you have to know how to handle families, what to do and how close to be and how far away to stay. And there's no way to explain it. It just comes from being around and sometimes making mistakes

and finding out: "Oh, she didn't want me to do this." As I go on in nursing I become more verbal asking: "Would you like me to . . . ?" "Would you rather I . . . ?" "I'm here and I'm here for you and whatever you want I'll do. Do you want me to call a priest? Do you want the doctor? What can I do to help you?" And that's what I think nursing is for to a large extent. That's what it means for the nurse to really be there for the dying patient and the family.

In a particular community of nurses, one finds a whole historically developed set of stories that demonstrate concerns, know-how, and caring practices for preserving dignity, mobilizing hope, and preserving illusions of control and autonomy. A rich tradition of practical know-how, developed over time in many concrete situations and in dialogue with patients, families, and colleagues sets this human skill in motion, complete with feelings that trigger recognition and engender satisfaction with success, and disappointment or sadness with failure.

It is impossible to bypass the skilled know-how with formal explicit statements of principles or rules for action. Norms and principles may give clues about the importance of timing, but historical knowledge of concrete situations is required to learn issues of timing (Bourdieu, 1980/1990). Timing is based on conversations with patients and families, but it is also based upon recognition of familiar patterns. Attending to patient and family readiness cannot be free of the risk of imprudence, paternalism, or misunderstanding. Skillful focused attention, listening, and ethical comportment that seeks to be faithful to the patient and family concerns are the only correctives available to the practitioner. This stance of realistic risk and humility makes it more likely that the caregiver will develop skills for noticing possibilities as well as infractions, rather than simply relying on a formal system of rigidly following rules that predetermine what rights and issues of justice are at stake (Benner & Wrubel, 1989).

Skills develop in understanding patients and families. Concrete past situations offer memories that allow for a sense of salience and pattern recognition (Benner, 1984a; Benner & Tanner, 1987; Dreyfus, 1979; Dreyfus & Dreyfus with Athanasiou, 1986). Norms, or even moral consensus, do not offer certitude, magical protection, or the capacity and ability to act, though they probably increase its likelihood:

> I think there's pretty much consensus on how people feel like it (death) ought to be, but you can't always actually actualize that. Like last night, that was one of the worst deaths I've ever seen. You have the other extreme in an emergency situation and you can't always create that situation. The consensus is that they want everybody to live and they're going to work really hard to make everybody live, but there is a pretty strong consensus that once they've decided that there's nothing more they can do that they would like

it to be as peaceful as possible. I think most people feel that way, but actualizing it is actually different. It's real scary.

This nurse puts her finger on the heart of the issue. No system of certain principles can be "applied," thereby taking the risk and uncertainty out of human relationships of care and responsibility, and this is even clearer in situations where one party is especially vulnerable. Skillful ethical comportment is based upon education about the principles as well as upon a dialogue over time and practice with patients' families and colleagues. This expertise is based on a better understanding gained over time in particular local, historical situations. This historical, perspectival dialogue is situated within the cultural-societal dialogue. We can never get beyond experience. We can only augment this acquisition of skillful ethical comportment by enhancing and enlarging the dialogue and narrative, and by expanding the moral imagination and consensus about what doing well means, and what that looks like in actual practice. Communities of scholars and practitioners can develop a nuanced conversation over time about what particular stories demonstrate, and about what knowledge, skill, and notions of good are evident or absent in the clinical stories.

Narratives of Disillusionment

Narratives of disillusionment are storylines of discovering the broken promises, the limits to others' knowledge, indeed, the limits to formal knowledge. They also cover encounters with limits to control, to understanding, and to the knowable. They are stories of times when rules, policies, and procedures do not match the situation. They are often filled with humor and self-discovery, and the stories of disillusionment have to do with confronting unavoidable suffering and death, because these are such central embodied concerns and the culture avoids and isolates these human events. Suffering and death, when addressed by the culture, are often presented as "problems" to be solved or as indicators of personal failure by the health care team or by patients and families (Benner, Janson-Bjerklie, Ferketich, & Becker, 1994; Callahan, 1993; Wros, 1994). The medical-technological cure model offers little cultural space, few metaphors, and no spiritual practices for facing suffering and death. And though the care of the dying is explored in nursing schools, nurses must learn firsthand from their practice how to be with the dying and about this cultural silence and avoidance. Narratives of disillusionment may include unresolved moral outrage, disengagement and disappointment or rage over helplessness in the face of suffering, ethical breaches, moral dilemmas, and conflict. Dana Marshall's narrative of disillusionment demonstrates a classic confrontation with the distance between theoretical and idealized versions of the practice and reality (Benner, 1974; Benner & Wrubel, 1989; Kramer, 1974).

"Being In Charge"
Dana Marshall, RN

I was first a Dental Hygienist for 3½ years, and then I went to nursing school. I received my RN and started working in a nursing home because my chosen field is gerontology. Because I chose to work the evening shift in order to continue my education, I was assigned to be charge nurse. Since I had to work evenings, I felt I had no choice. Besides, I rationalized to myself, I know the patients. They had been my dental hygiene patients. I was older and more mature than most newly graduated nurses, and the two LVNs that would be working with me had been RNs in the Philippines. Armed with my false sense of security, I made it through the first 1½ weeks without incident. The "honeymoon period," I like to call it.

We take our lunch breaks at different times to leave someone to cover the ward of 50 patients. On a good day, we have four to five staff; on a bad day, only three. This was a bad day. I was in the bathroom just finishing up when the nursing assistant called through the door: "I think Mr. D. just died." I hurried up and went into Mr. D's room. He was lying very peacefully in his bed. I hurried over to his chart to see if he was a DNR (do not resuscitate). While I was doing this I came to the realization that the LVN was at lunch, and I was the only licensed person on the floor, with only one nursing assistant to help me. I hate to admit it, but I was relieved when I saw the DNR order in his chart. We very respectfully cleaned him and prepared him in bed for his family to "view the body." We also called the Medical Officer on duty to pronounce the patient dead. All these thoughts were whirling round my head, my first dead patient, my first crisis, my first nursing job, maybe even my first nervous breakdown! Before the physician arrived, I got my stethoscope from my last school year (we do not wear them routinely), the one with the pink hoses that used to hold a clinging Alf for Peds two semesters ago. When I handed the stethoscope to the doctor, the diaphragm fell off. So much for professionalism. But that's okay, I found out that the physician in charge was a psychiatrist! I had to spell all of the big technical words for him when he wrote up the chart.

Against this backdrop of panic and false bravado, I also had a real problem, one that couldn't be solved by a DNR order in the chart, and rationalizations about leading a long, full life. In our ward, we also have a five-bed hospice unit. The philosophy of hospice is death with dignity, and comfort measures only. When I came on that day, both the head nurse and our ward physician explained that Mrs. S., a lady of about 60, had visited her daughter for a week, on pass from the hospital. She had leukemia and was receiving morphine for the pain. This made her very constipated and she returned from her visit with impacted bowels. The nurses had to remove the stool, and it had caused her rectum to bleed. Because of her platelet problem, the bleeding was uncontrolled, and I was informed that she would probably bleed to death on my shift. This was said in the gentlest of tones, but when I went into her bathroom, it looked like Charles Manson had been there. Apparently, she had sat down on the toilet, and that's when the bleeding had started. All of a sudden, "bleeding to death" didn't sound quite so gentle as the doctor had described it. I went back to the head nurse and asked her to redefine "bleeding to death" in more realistic terms. Would it be buckets? Should I get one? Would it be fast or slow? Should her family be there? Or would it be more humane to all them after she had died? These theoretical questions began to take on real proportions when I saw the blood on the bathroom floor. We put a diaper on her to contain the blood, and I called her family. I felt relieved that some things were done, and I repeated to myself the philosophy of hospice, as if I were reciting the Apostle's Creed or the Hippocratic Oath. It was apparent that this bleeding episode had really frightened Mrs. S., a former nurse herself. I tried to reassure her that we were doing everything possible to stop the bleeding. This was only partially true, because the doctor had told me that they had decided against a blood transfusion because of the advanced progression of her disease. "Comfort measures only" had been his last words when he left the ward that dark and stormy night. When her daughter arrived, I thought that I would get a little support for the "comfort measures only" philosophy of life. But to my chagrin, she was even more frightened and even less willing to let go of the little life her mother had left. She and I were about the same age, and I, too, had lost my mother, so I knew how she felt. This was clearly not a situation that fit any stereotype, and I was hard put to be objective about any decisions that I made.

Right about this time, the OD had been called in to pronounce Mr. D. Seizing the opportunity to unload my problems on someone else, even if he didn't know how to spell big medical words, I asked him to take a look at Mrs. S. and see what he thought. He spent a lot of time with both Mrs. S. and her daughter, just talking. Now I was glad he was a psychiatrist. He came back with a very concerned look on his face, a good sign. He called Hematology, and they decided that in spite of the comfort measures only order, they would do a blood transfusion. I was very relieved, because in this case, I just didn't feel that the patient or her family were ready to let go yet. This would give them a little more time to sort things out. I thought if I were going to err, as a new nurse, I would rather err on the side of a conservative decision, especially when the family seemed in favor of that decision. It was decided by the ward physician that Mrs. S. would get blood transfusions to carry her through the holidays, and then we would go back to comfort measures only. She died quite peacefully 2 months later and required no further blood transfusions. Her daughter and I became quite close, and I was able to share my experience of losing my mother. This helped her not to feel so alone in her loss.

I have thought about this often because it shaped my perceptions about death and dying. I still believe in the philosophy of death with dignity and letting go, when it is appropriate. But sometimes people aren't ready to let go just yet. As long as the measures don't create undue suffering, and prolong someone's agony, we as nurses can respect someone's wishes with a clear conscience. Each case is an individual one, and each person must decide what is best. Sometimes you just have to throw away the book.

This story has all the classic ingredients of disillusionment stories, but it also contains a strong storyline about facing death and suffering. It is the narrative of a beginner, filled with beginner's questions, but it is clear that the experience is transformative. The broken promises and failed expectations are legion and are met with irony and wit, the only strategies available in the heat of the situation. An expert nurse would have most likely played the psychiatrist's role of clarifying the patient's and family's wishes in the thick of the situation, but the beginner was astute in calling for help. Planned decisions are often changed when the reality of the decision sets in. This is one of the conundrums of advanced directives about heroic treatments. Principles do not accommodate timing and context well. There is an ethical obligation to the community of memory as well as to the dying. The limits of "the textbook" are encountered, and the nurse is called to be open to learn from the situation at hand. In this situation, Marshall apparently gets a level of involvement that works and decreases the isolation and loneliness of the daughter in facing her mother's death.

Narratives About Facing Death and Suffering

The above example is also a narrative about facing death and suffering. The experience helped Dana Marshall learn about timing, openness and clarity about the patient and family's wishes. Typically, these narratives of learning help one see different possibilities and concerns related to death and dying and suffering. They help the nurse confront his or her own fears of suffering and death. A major cultural theme and good is to avoid suffering (Taylor, 1989). However, in practice, unavoidable suffering is often exacerbated by separation and lack of adequate language, metaphors, rituals, practices, and meanings in a secular, suffering-and-death-avoidant culture. We avoid our sense of finitude by technological promises of continuous progress and technical solutions. Suffering is removed to the hospital room, where patient, families, and nurses are left to work out ways to communicate and comfort one another. Calm voices and smooth technical descriptions are inadequate to convey the reality to be confronted. The narratives are moments where language, touch, rituals, intimacy, presencing and courage, and new understandings or possibilities are experienced. For example, a new graduate describes being taught how to presence and how to cry by a more experienced nurse:

I had been talking to him (a dying patient). But she was talking to him and telling him everything that I was doing. She was carrying on a conversation with him. The last thing she said was: "It's okay. Just go ahead and let go. It's okay to die. I know that you are afraid." And he started crying and she was crying, too. And I was just standing there. And she turned around and told me that it was okay to cry, so I started crying . . . It was tough, but it felt really good to let it out finally, instead of doing it (crying) on my way home.

Nurses learn many moral and practical lessons about presencing, comfort, and courage in the face of death, but they also learn how to be with their own and others' anger over failed expectations and hope. These are powerful, hard-learned narratives that could instruct the larger community about facing death.

Liberation Narratives

Nursing is a women's profession that has undergone profound change within the last 20 years. Nursing practice now includes many instantaneous therapies that require judgment. What was once called "doctor's orders" should now be called medical guidelines and parameters, because the therapies require moment-by-moment adjustment according to patient responses. These clinical judgments are made in the context of outdated views about medical and nursing decision making (see Chapter 11). Consequently, many of the liberation narratives have to do with discovery and assertion of worth of clinical judgment that is based on their nursing experience.

Liberation narratives also depict nurses finding their voice. These narratives are concerned not only with the status inequity of sexism, but also with the marginality of the caregiver's voice in a highly technical, cure-oriented health care system. Nurses must discover for themselves the worth of their work and the importance of their voice for the patient's and family's recovery, for dignity in death, and for survival in a system where loss of attentiveness can cause death, even though attentiveness does not show up on the accounting ledgers, and is frequently undermined by cost-saving and dilution of nursing expertise. Narratives of liberation often contain narratives of disillusionment within them:

[*A patient was showing signs of shock due to as yet unconfirmed bleeding. The doctor wanted the nurse to get the patient up.*]
    He said: "I want to try it again." I said: "Why do you want to try it again? You just saw what happened." It was tough. It just rang in my head, what that one doctor had said when I had called when I had been unsure of an

order just rang in my head: "When a doctor gives you an order, you follow the order, and you do not ask any questions." I don't agree with that, but it rang in my head as I insisted that the patient be checked for bleeding. But I wasn't going to go through the same thing, and watch her brady down (heart rate fall) and have her fall on me and to push her with a drug that she didn't need because of his lack of recognition. But it did ring in the back of my head, "Don't question." [*And I thought*] No way, she's compromised. We then did prepare her for gastroscopy. She had a bleeding vessel which the doctor cauterized and she was okay.

This is the narrative of a new graduate learning to stand firm with her clinical assessment against the gradient of a hierarchical power relationship. This is no empty assertion for the purpose of gaining professional power and control. The force of the assertion comes from the moral press to do no harm and to obtain a good outcome for the patient. Her clear recognition of the patient's condition makes the assertion possible. Narratives of liberation are examined in Chapter 11 in relation to the current status of the doctor-nurse game (Stein, 1967).

Liberation narratives are not limited to physician-nurse interactions or status inequity issues. They include many stories about breaking free of biases and misunderstandings that limit caring practices, whatever the source of inhibition—timidity, fear of risk, fear of disclosing vulnerability, fear of intimacy, fear of visibility and responsibility, distraction, avoidance of suffering, avoidance of openness, the tyranny of bureaucratic demands, or the tyranny of rules and procedures. Liberation themes are as varied as the demands of the caring practice and the human fears that stand in the way of openness and connection, and the ethical demands of caring for the vulnerable.

THE FUNCTIONS OF NARRATIVE
AND COMMUNITY

The themes of the narratives presented here are the result of studying paradigm cases presented by nurses in classes, workshops, and in two research studies (Benner, 1982, 1984a; Benner, Tanner, & Chesla, 1992) over the past 15 years. Paradigm cases are narrative accounts of clinical situations that open up new areas of practice or teach the nurse something new about nursing practice. They are the stories that the nurse carries forward, not just in memory but as prereflective concerns that cause them to notice salient events and patterns as an instance of or a situation similar to the concrete narrative event. The embodied skills learned in the actual concrete event are taken up with emotional responses to the situation. The narrative memory of concrete events can evoke perceptual or sensory memories that enhance pattern recognition. For example, corrective narratives just make the world of the nurse a place where certain warnings stand out and must ever after be attended to, or are ignored with great deliberation ('I refuse to attend to that issue this time') or are overridden by great distraction and distress.

The thematic categories presented here tell something about the ethical concerns and ethical comportment of nurses. It would be a mistake, however, to give them a cognitive or "belief system" gloss. Nurses do not go looking in a deliberate fashion for "constitutive or sustaining narratives" or "learning narratives." The narratives are experientially given as a result of engagement in concrete situations. Nurses can tell stories from their practice about clinical situations that stand out as memorable, but they do not easily recall categories given to conjure up stories, and this seems to be the way narrative memory works . . . by actual story lines, rather than intellectual categories (Dreyfus & Dreyfus with Athanasiou, 1986).

Narrative memory and the telling and retelling of actual events in story form are signaled by concerns that order the story.[2] Some aspects of the situation are emphasized where others do not figure in at all. Without ethical concerns, it is difficult to tell a coherent story with a sensible beginning, middle, and end (see Chapters 7, 9). "Stories" without a point don't seem to be stories at all, but rather litanies of events or tasks. Furthermore, stories—as opposed to case studies or analytic reports—engage the person in a dialogue of learning with their own historical understanding and personal knowledge.

It is difficult to imagine a practice complete with notions of good embedded but without stories to convey the living-out and doing of the practice. It is also difficult to imagine a practice without a community of practitioners, because a practice (present or in memory, even scientific practice) is based on socially embedded knowledge. "The status of an observer who withdraws from the situation to observe implies an epistemological, but also a social break . . . leading to an implicit theory of practices that is linked to forgetfulness of the social conditions of scientific activity" (Bourdieu, 1990, p. 33).

Individuals make contributions to communities, but these contributions are never really the product of insular, disconnected individuals. The reception, production, transformation, and transmission of knowledge is social. Communities are not inherently good, as the Nazi Holocaust and the Jonestown mass suicide teach us. But they are the only place where human concerns can be instantiated and worked out for good or evil. The good that communities express and live out is dependent upon their cultural traditions, shared narratives, habits, practices, concerns, and experiential wisdom. A community offers the human possibility of dialogue and correction through multiple perspectives and memory of experiential learning from the past. Public moral space is created in community through dialogue and experience lodged in narratives.

THE NATURE AND FUNCTION OF A PRACTICE

Caring practices cannot be reduced to abstract concepts or psychological attitudes, but must be carried out by embodied caregivers and embedded in actual caring practices (see Chapter 2; Benner, 1990; Benner & Gordon, in press; Benner, Wrubel, Phillips, Chesla, & Tanner, 1994; MacIntyre, 1981). Ruddick (1989), Whitbeck (1983), MacIntyre (1981) and Taylor (1989) have defined a practice as characterized here. The following definition draws on all these authors:

> Practice is defined as a coherent, socially organized activity that has a no-
> tion of good and common meanings embedded in the practice, i.e., internal
> to the practice (MacIntyre, 1981). A practice is located within a tradition and
> is continually being worked out in history and through the ongoing devel-
> opment of the practice. A practice has a referential context of meanings, skills
> and equipment and has the capacity to be worked out in contexts that allow
> actualization of the notions of good embedded in the practice. A practice
> has the capacity for being worked out in novel or new situations. (Benner,
> 1990, p. 8)

A practice cannot be completely objectified or formalized because its complex social, practical, local, and historical bases make formalization in discrete objective elements impossible, both in terms of the sheer volume of words such formalism would require and in terms of radically altering the relational and concrete historical reality of the practice (Dreyfus 1979; 1991). This is why a practice requires narrative for constituting and sustaining it. Those expert in a practice can recognize strong instances of excellent or poor practice. Furthermore, the notions of good inherent in a practice are continually being extended and elaborated, in dialogue with the historical understanding of the practice.

The distinction I am making here is between traditionalism—a dead or ritualistic repetition of past conventions—and a living tradition that is continuing to be developed and worked out (Shils, 1981). MacIntyre (1981) notes that tic-tac-toe is not a practice in this sense, nor is the action of an isolated skill, such as hitting golf balls; however, the more socially organized game of golf is. In nursing, inserting an IV in a skills lab or in an isolated skill training session where only this task is done is not a practice; however, inserting an IV with concerns related to the care of a specific person with specific needs is a caring practice (Benner & Wrubel, 1989). Notice that a "caring attitude" or abstract sentiment is not sufficient to make the action a caring practice (Benner & Gordon, in press). The practice must be carried out in an excellent manner that is true to the notions of what constitutes good practice (Brown, 1986). Bellah, Madson, Sullivan, Swindler, and Tipton (1985) define practices of commitment, in contrast to mere means or technique, as follows:

> Practices are shared activities that are not undertaken as means to an end but are technically good in themselves (thus close to praxis in Aristotle's sense). A genuine community—whether a marriage, a university, or a whole society—is constituted by such practices. Genuine practices are almost always practices of commitment, since they involve activities that are ethically good. In the strict sense, "practices of separation" is a contradiction in terms, since such activities are undertaken in the interest of the self at the expense of commitments to others. (p. 335)

In the context of generous knowledgeable caring practices that are finely tuned by one's own sentient and skilled embodiment, the level of mutual respect and knowledge of the other will allow for more than mere rights and justice. The language of cost-benefit analysis and other forms of rational calculation will seem like impoverished "outside-in accounts" that miss the human connection and community and particular human concerns in the situation. It is in this sense that the ethics of rights and justice are always remedial (Sandel, 1982).

Since the Enlightenment we have assumed that theory liberates while tradition and practice enslaves (Taylor, 1985). However, the genesis of liberating theory is dependent on practice and practical know-how (Benner, 1985; 1990; Dreyfus, 1979; Dreyfus & Dreyfus with Athanasiou, 1986; Heidegger, 1962; Taylor, 1985c; 1989). A life well lived is required for developing new moral possibilities and stirring the moral imagination that may then be articulated as theory and further influence and refine practice.

The ethicist has no foundation for ethical judgment and wisdom that can be used in template fashion without considering community, history, personal and social concerns, and religious, cultural, and practice narratives. Here, as was evident in numerous other discourses with nurses, knowing the person is required for an effective assessment in formal terms. Practical moral reasoning and skilled ethical comportment ultimately determine our moral possibilities. Procedural ethics based upon rights and justice alone cannot answer all the hard questions about what constitutes care and how we ought to care, because a principle-based ethical discourse is not automatically translated into everyday ethical comportment, engaged ethical narratives, and genuine care. One can be well versed in ethical principles without noticing the actual qualitative distinctions and ethical concerns in actual practical situations.

The rational-technical quest for fairness and certainty through rational procedures offers little protection against the danger that old norms will remain unquestioned, even though the practice and cultural dialogue may have extended or altered the understanding of them. Normative ethics alone do not easily call attention to radical changes in the ethical context and landscape because the rational-technical model assumes that the notions of good are not in question. The point of scrutiny is limited to the means for achieving the established norm. In sum, normative ethics do not easily deal with identifying the salient ethical issues, the context, cultural diversity, and change, or with questions about choosing worthy norms (Taylor, 1991, 1993).

For example, the recent tendency to view the relationship of the health care provider and the patient as a buying and selling of goods, that is, health care bought and sold as a commodity by free autonomous agents in a free market, constricts the range of moral issues to stories of "bad" salespersons and patients either as helpless marks—subject to the whims of personal gain from profiteering practitioners—or as aggressive, informed consumers wary of what they are "buying." One can hold up ethical practices of the good salesperson, selling needed and worthwhile goods, but the responsibility for choosing wisely in the free marketplace is left to the economic free agent, the "consumer." Vulnerability or suffering ("compromised consumers") cannot be sensibly introduced into this practical moral equation. This is why managed competition introduces the ethical temptation of undertreatment whereas a fee-for-service approach creates the ethical temptation of overtreatment.

Nor can science modeled strictly on the physical sciences offer reliable ethical wisdom, because human significance terms are left out (Taylor, 1985b). To contribute to skilled ethical expertise, health care science must be conversant with the human terms of health and illness, as well as disease (Benner, 1994d; Kleinman, 1988). Ethics in health care must start with a practice-based understanding of what it is to be a person; what constitutes the relationships among the health care worker, patient, family, and community; and what constitutes care and responsibility toward one another (Benner, 1985; Benner & Wrubel, 1989; Leonard, 1989). The gap between theoretical and practical moral reasoning contains all the lived examples and narrative of what the ethical distinctions look, sound, and feel like when they are expressed in actual situations. Unlike normative approaches, the unfolding process changes or may even reconstitute the norms, because embodiment and being *in* the situation influence practical moral comportment. The first-person narrative accounts of first-person experience point to issues of relations between the embodied member and participant nurse as well as the patient, family, and other health care workers. Narratives exemplify positive notions about what is good and not just the problems or deficits, and this is so whether or not the person can state formally or explicitly the notions of good that are being exemplified

Narrative accounts of clinical situations where the nurse learned something new or felt good about his or her caring practice demonstrate moral discourse. Seeing the person as member and participant in a human community gives a more adequate account of caring for the vulnerable than utilitarian individualism, and challenges us to transform this ethical theory by enlarging it to account for the moral possibilities found in caring practices between persons who are interdependent, or unequally dependent, rather than autonomous (Benner, 1985; Benner & Wrubel, 1989; Zagarell, 1988). The dominant modern view of the person is oppositional (Whitbeck, 1983) or adversarial (May, 1988). In this view the person stands in competitive opposition to others so that self-interests, more often than not, compete with others' interests and are typically defined in isolation to the concerns and needs of others. Consequently, in the oppositional account, one has to assume that any "caring" or "giving" is at the expense of the self, or that it is based upon some overt or hidden need in the self that must be fulfilled. In this view, caring and relatedness are transformed into economic exchanges, social conventions, interpersonal skills, and control strategies. But a hidden motive of self-gratification is not the *only* explanation for caring and having people and things show up as meaningful, as illustrated in the moral discourse of these nurses. Indeed, self-gratification or even caring for the sake of caring do not qualify as care, because care necessarily focuses on the particular good of the one cared for, or else occurs in response to the other.

Fortunately, our ethical comportment often exceeds our formal ethical theories. The call is to shape our ethical theories by our most liberating and enlightened caring practices. And for this we need to increase our public story, telling our engaged actions and stories rather than our abstract theorizing. In the best of our caring practices we will find that people have learned ways to traverse the tension that is sometimes created between caring and curing and even economic exchanges, so that caring practices in local specific situations through knowing the person and community can guide our approach to cures and act as guides for shaping resource allocation questions. Much of our waste comes from the drive to break the tasks down and increase efficiency while diminishing the practitioners' ability to know their patients, and vice versa (Tanner et al., 1993).

We can work out precise formal rules and ethical theory, but our intellectual capacity to do this does not guarantee that we can transfer this knowledge into actual ethical comportment. We cannot get beyond experience, and we must not rely on our theories to distance us from skillful ethical comportment in concrete, specific relationships and local situations. The Platonic quest to get beyond the vagaries of experience was a misguided turn, a heroic quest to put us beyond habits, skills, practice, and experience (see Chapter 2). We can redeem the turn if we subject our theories to our unedited, concrete moral experience and acknowledge that skillful moral comportment calls us not to be beyond experience, but to be tempered and taught by it. The relationship, then, between ethical theory and skillful ethical comportment must be a dialogue between partners, each shaping and informing the other. Disengaged reason and rational calculation cannot replace engaged care as a moral source of wisdom (see Chapter 10). Increasingly, however, our communication is shaped by technical, analytic reporting of the "objective" facts and the measurable observations. Generalization and the search for commonality take the form of abstract principles or objectified accounts. But these forms, abstract principles, analytical reporting, and objectified generalizations do not evoke the caring relationships and clinical wisdom required in everyday ethical comportment. They cannot attend to qualitative distinctions, relational and contextual issues, or engaged care. Here we need to reintroduce narrative in our practice and in our discourse on ethical practice in order to preserve ethical distinctions and concerns. Polanyi (1958) noted that a clinician always knows more that he or she can tell. The clinician may also know more than she or he can practice. And this ethical tension requires an openness to learning from our practice, and the vision to design our large health care systems to support caring and attentiveness rather than indifference. Ethical expertise requires skill that must be experientially learned, but it also requires moral vision for ways of connecting with others and for designing our public systems so that care and equity are facilitated rather than impeded.

NOTES

1. Patricia Benner is indebted to Cynthia Stuhlmiller for the concept of sustaining narratives. Stuhlmiller found "sustaining narratives" in her dissertation research just as this work was being developed. See Stuhlmiller, C. (1991). *An interpretive study of appraisal and coping of rescue workers in an earthquake disaster: The Cypress collapse.* Unpublished doctoral dissertation, Uni-

versity of California, San Francisco. See also Stuhlmiller, C. (1994), "Narrative methodology in disaster studies, rescuers of Cypress." In P. Benner (Ed.) *Interpretive phenomenology: Embodiment, caring and ethics in health and illness* (pp. 323–349). Thousand Oaks, CA: Sage.

2. This was an insight given us early in our interpretive research sessions by Jane Rubin. See Chapter 7.

Chapter **10**

IMPLICATIONS OF THE PHENOMENOLOGY OF EXPERTISE FOR TEACHING AND LEARNING EVERYDAY SKILLFUL ETHICAL COMPORTMENT*

Hubert L. Dreyfus, Stuart E. Dreyfus, and Patricia Benner

A better understanding of the acquisition of everyday ethical expertise illuminates current debates in biomedical ethics and has implications for teaching everyday ethical comportment in health care. We have described the role of emotion in developing ethical sensitivity and perceptual acuity and in the discernment of qualitative distinctions central to clinical and ethical judgments at each stage of skill acquisition. We have also described clinical and ethical reasoning in transitions as central to clinical expertise (see Chapters 1, 7, and 9). Each of these aspects of acquiring everyday ethical expertise has implications for the current approaches in biomedical ethics and for teaching and learning to be an excellent practitioner.

A phenomenological understanding of skillful ethical comportment can augment the study of quandary ethics and illuminate both normative and casuistic methods. Our claim is that ethical theories and judgments are dependent upon background meanings, skills, habits, and practices and that approaches such as quandary ethics would not be possible unless people shared a background of common cultural meanings, i.e., expertise concerning everyday skillful ethical comportment.

---

*This chapter draws on the following published paper: Dreyfus, H. L., & Dreyfus, S. E. (1991). Towards a phenomenology of ethical expertise. *Human Studies,* 14:229–250.

Biomedical ethical theorists have focused on quandary ethics. Being an expert has meant being schooled in the formal moral principles and theories used to deal with ethical conflicts, dilemmas, and puzzles. Thus, expertise in quandary ethics is based upon applying ethical principles to breakdowns in everyday skilled ethical comportment, or, in the case of casuistry, expertise in delineating paradigm cases that support the extension of ethical principles to new situations (Jonsen & Toulmin, 1988). The focus on quandary or breakdown of ethical problem solving methodically excludes consideration of the good embedded in everyday skillful ethical comportment because only instances of breakdown are held up for scrutiny. Taken-for-granted references to what is good or appropriate, or what works smoothly in everyday coping, are overlooked.

One may well ask what counts as success or failure in ethics. It turns out that in ethics what counts as expert performance is doing what those who already are accepted as ethical experts do and approve. Aristotle tells us: "What is best is not evident except to the good man" (V1.12). This is circular but not viciously so.

Learning exhibits the same circularity. To become an expert in any area of expertise, one has to be able to respond to the same types of situations as do those who are already expert. For example, to play master level chess, one has to see the same board positions as masters do. This basic ability is what one calls having talent in a given domain. In addition, the learner must experience what society considers the appropriate satisfaction or regret at the outcome of his response. To become an expert nurse one should feel concern, not indifference, about the patient's and family's plight. To acquire ethical expertise, then, one must have the talent to respond to those ethical situations to which ethical experts respond and one must have the sensibility to experience the socially appropriate sense of satisfaction or regret at the outcome of one's action.[1]

Ethical mastery is just one kind of expertise. We are all experts at many tasks, and our everyday coping skills usually function smoothly and transparently so as to free us to be aware of other aspects of our lives where we are not so skillful. However, in a field where caring practices (recognition and respect for the other as other, mutual realization, nurture, and protection of vulnerability) are central, it is difficult, if not impossible, to have encounters that do not encompass both clinical and ethical expertise (see Chapters 1 and 7). John Dewey introduced the distinction between *knowing-how* and *knowing-that* to call attention to just such thoughtless mastery of the everyday:

> We may . . . be said to *know how* by means of our habits. . . . We walk and read aloud, we get off and on street cars, we dress and undress, and do a thousand useful acts without thinking of them. We know something,

namely, how to do them. . . . [I]f we choose to call [this] knowledge . . . then other things also called knowledge, knowledge *of* and *about* things, knowledge *that* things are thus and so, knowledge that involves reflection and conscious appreciation, remains of a different sort . . . (Dewey, 1922, pp. 177–178)

We should try to impress on ourselves what a huge amount of our lives—working, getting around, talking, eating, driving, and responding to the needs of others—manifests *know-how*, and what a small part is spent in the deliberate, effortful, subject/object mode which requires *knowing-that*. Yet deliberate action, and its extreme form, deliberation, are the ways of acting we tend to notice, and thus are the only ones that have been studied in detail by philosophers.

Our hypothesis is that if one returned to the phenomenon and tried to give a description of ethical expertise, one might find phenomenology has a great deal to contribute to contemporary debate, particularly since the focus of discussion has shifted from interest in meta-ethical issues to a debate between those who demand a detached critical morality based on principles that tells us what is *right* and those who defend an ethics based on involvement in a tradition that defines what is *good*. This new confrontation between Kant and Hegel, between *Moralität* (principles) and *Sittlichkeit* (customs and practices), has produced two camps which can be identified with Jürgen Habermas and John Rawls on the one hand, and Bernard Williams and Charles Taylor on the other. The same polarity appears in feminism, where the Kohlberg scale, which defines the highest stage of moral maturity as the ability to stand outside the situation and justify one's actions in terms of universal moral principles, is attacked by Carol Gilligan (1982) in the name of an intuitive response to the concrete situation.

What one chooses to investigate as the relevant phenomena will prejudice from the start where one stands on these important issues. If one adopts the usual phenomenological approach, one will focus on the rationality of moral *judgments*. Edmund Husserl proceeded in just this way. Likewise, on the first page of his classic text, *The Moral Judgment of the Child*, Jean Piaget explicitly restricts ethics to judgments. He states at the start that "It is moral judgment that we propose to investigate, not moral behavior" (Piaget, 1935, p. *vii*). "Logic is the morality of thought just as morality is the logic of action," and in the end concludes, "Pure reason (is) the arbiter both of theoretical reflection and daily practice." (Piaget, 1935, p. 404)

This is still the approach of Maurice Mandelbaum (1955) in his book, *The Phenomenology of Moral Experience*, a more recent but unsuccessful attempt to introduce phenomenology into current ethical debate.

The phenomenological approach's . . . essential methodological conviction is that a solution to any of the problems of ethics must be educed from, and verified by, a careful and direct examination of individual moral judgments. (p. 31)

But Mandelbaum does not seem to realize that he has already made a fateful exclusionary move. He claims that: "Such an approach . . . aims to discover the generic characteristics of *all* moral experience" (Mandelbaum, 1955, p. 36, our italics).

Why equate moral experience with judgment, rather than with ethical comportment? Mandelbaum's answer to this question is, we think, symptomatic of the intellectualist prejudice embodied in this approach. He first gives a perceptive nod to spontaneous ethical comportment:

I sense the embarrassment of a person, and turn the conversation aside; I see a child in danger and catch hold of its hand; I hear a crash and become alert to help. (Mandelbaum, 1955, p. 48)

He then notes:

Actions such as these (of which our daily lives are in no small measure composed) do not . . . seem to spring from the self: in such cases I am reacting directly and spontaneously to what confronts me. . . . [I]t is appropriate to speak of "reactions" and "responses," for in them no sense of initiative or feeling of responsibility is present. . . . [W]e can only say that we acted as we did because the situation extorted that action from us. (Mandelbaum, 1955, pp. 48–49)

Mandelbaum next contrasts this unthinking and egoless[2] response to the situation with deliberate action in which one experiences the casual power of the "I."

In "willed" action, on the other hand, the source of action is the self. I act in a specific manner because I wish, or will, to do so. . . . the "I" is experienced as being responsible for willed action. (Mandelbaum, 1955, p. 48)

He continues:

To give a phenomenological account of this sense of responsibility is not difficult. It is grounded in the fact that every willed action aims at and espouses an envisioned goal. When we envision a goal which transcends what is immediately given, and when we set ourselves to realizing that goal, we feel the action to be *ours*. (Mandelbaum, 1955, p. 48)

And focusing on willed or deliberate action and its goal, we arrive again at rationality.

In willed actions . . . we can give *a reason*: we acted as we did because we aimed to achieve a particular goal. [W]hen asked to explain our action, we feel no hesitation in attributing it to the value of the goal which we aimed to achieve. (Mandelbaum, 1955, p. 49)

Thus the phenomenology of moral experience comes to focus on judgment and justification. Granted that one aspect of the moral life, and most of moral philosophy, has been concerned with choice, responsibility, and justification, we should, nonetheless, take seriously what Mandelbaum sees and immediately dismisses, viz., that most of our everyday ethical comportment consists in unreflective, egoless responses to the current interpersonal situation. But this unreflective, egoless coping is a perceptual skill that must first be learned in a community tradition. These habits and skills are both received, created, and developed in dialogue with others and are amenable to correction, even though they cannot be completely formalized (spelled out completely and comply with the demands of criterial reasoning). Why not begin on the level of this spontaneous coping?

Several methodological precautions must be borne in mind in attempting a phenomenology of the ethical life.

1. We should begin by describing our everyday ongoing ethical coping.
2. We should determine under which conditions deliberation and choice appear and under what conditions are attunement and responsiveness to the other central.
3. We should beware of making the typical philosophical mistake of reading the structure of deliberation and choice back into our account of everyday ethical comportment.

In nursing, the ethical comportment, which we presume a nursing student has already acquired, is modified by the new ethical demands of nursing practice. This is different than the clinical skills that the nurse must learn *de novo*; e.g., no background experiential learning prepares the nurse to titrate vasopressor drugs to maintain a patient's blood pressure. The distinctions between learning a new clinical skill and augmenting ethical and interpersonal skills show up particularly in the first three stages of the model (from novice through competency) but converge in expertise. Novice nursing students have no experience of the medical and nursing technical situations in which they are expected to perform, thus they are taught objective attributes and formal theories about diseases. However, they do come to their practice with interpersonal skills and ethical concerns which are further developed and modified. Communication theories are taught to help the students be more open, less judgmental, but as one new graduate explained in trying to account for his ability in working with the family of a dying infant, his everyday skillful ethical comportment was essential (see Chapter 3):

Int: How did you know how to bring this father along? Did you ask people?
Nurse: No. How did I know? I don't know. They don't teach you that. . . . In my undergraduate psychology program we tried specifically to teach people how to do active listening, how to empathize, how to do all these things, and some people were just good at it and others were just out to lunch, no matter what theory they read or what happened in the practice sessions.

This new graduate was asked about how he had learned to be so attuned and skillful in dealing with a father whose baby was dying. He answered that he had learned in part from nursing school, but that he had prior work experience and personal experience that prepared him for this occasion. Thus, those skills such as ethical comportment and communication skills that are modified or extended, rather than learned from the ground up, may proceed unevenly, with some situations close enough to prior learning to afford expert performance.

Learning to relate the theories to practice depends on prior skills, practices, habits, and meanings. Growing up in a culture teaches one the common background meanings, habits, practices, and skills necessary for ethical comportment. For example, in this individualistic culture children first learn respect, reciprocity, and relational skills in myriads of nonreflective practices and skills. When children are old enough to understand, they are taught rules for sharing and turn-taking. The effectiveness of this rule-based instruction will depend upon how closely the child's experiential learning matches the rules. With expertise, these rudimentary skills for respecting others develop complexity and flexibility, as the imitation and rule-based learning are experienced in many contexts and social situations. The expert becomes skillful in everyday ethical comportment, living out the meanings of respectful relating to others.

When *adults* learn a practice such as nursing, teaching, law, or medicine, they are again inducted into skillful ethical comportment, taught by imitation and questioning, skills, habits, practices, and theories about what is considered skillful ethical comportment in the field. This presupposes the background understanding acquired as a child. Nurses talk about gaining skill in achieving the right kind and level of involvement as they expand their skillful ethical comportment to meet the demands of nursing.[3] However, skillful ethical comportment as a nurse calls for a different kind and level of involvement than was required as a child, student, worker, friend, or family member. The skills of connection and involvement must be modified to meet the demands of caring for strangers in extreme circumstances that range from birth to death. The nurse must learn skillful ethical comportment that protects the vulnerability in complex clinical situations, in health promotion, and in crises.

Recognizing vulnerability, developing interventions to deal with it and managing one's own feelings are all involved in modifying skillful ethical comportment as a nurse. If the nurse overidentifies with the patient/family he or she will be too flooded with painful emotions to be able to perform effectively. On the other hand, rigid defenses that numb the pain can make the nurse oblivious to the patient's/family's suffering and prevent effective caring practices. The rule-governed behavior typical of the novice is limited and inflexible. As noted in Chapter 9, being given rules to guide performance does not guarantee that one will recognize when the rules are relevant. And since the rules dictate what novices notice, they may not notice situations not covered or pointed up by the rules.

In nursing, developing skillful ethical comportment must compete with the demands of gaining technical, medical and nursing expertise. The newly graduated nurse is an advanced beginner and is confronted with a complex clinical world with many tasks and weighty responsibilities. Focusing on basic skills and organizing the task world is a priority, and "psychosocial" skills are exercised deliberately and worked in with effort, rather than being smooth, flexible, and nonreflective. The advances in psychosocial skills learned in nursing school may deteriorate to a novice level in high demand situations. For example, in the excerpt below a new graduate reflects on her hard-won advances in skillful ethical comportment. She notices the situational components that make a difference in approach to the possibilities of the situation.

> My organizational skills are really bad. I'm playing catch-up. The psychosocial gets put in the backdrop. The more technical things that would take a more experienced nurse less time will take me half an hour to do, because I'm more conscious of everything that could happen. I am always making sure that what I am doing is the right way . . . The first month practicing alone, I hardly ever used psychosocial skills, just the basic questions of: "How are you doing? Are you in pain? Do you know where you are?" . . . I am getting better with talking to the patient and being a little more sociable, because . . . we forget that they're human, and we just treat them like bodies. [*Later in this interview she describes working with her second patient with a gastrointestinal bleed as an advance in her psychosocial skills.*] I started lavaging with iced normal saline, and at the same time, I was asking my patient: "Are you O.K.? Are you comfortable?" . . . I didn't forget about her, in all my anxiety, that she was bleeding. She wasn't bleeding as profusely as my other patient was, and this bleeding occurred in this middle of the shift rather than at the end . . . But what was good about this patient is that I didn't forget that she was a patient, and I was talking to her, and it made me feel good because I was so scared.

This description is very different from ones given by expert nurses who typically fill in who the person is and what the particular concerns are, as opposed to the advanced beginner's effort just to talk to the patient with general reassuring phrases and questions.

As the nurse develops competency, agency is increasingly focused on organization and planning. Successful plans induce euphoria, and mistakes are felt in the pit of the stomach (see Chapter 4). In the chess and nursing cases, we find a common pattern: detached planning, conscious assessment of elements that are salient with respect to the plan, and an analytical rule-guided choice of action, followed by an emotionally involved experience of the outcome. The experience is emotional because choosing a plan, goal, or perspective is no simple matter for the competent performer. Nobody gives him any rules for how to choose a perspective, so he has to make up various rules, which he then adopts or discards in various situations depending on how they work out. This procedure is frustrating, however, since each rule works on some occasions and fails on others, and no set of objective features and aspects correlates strongly with these successes and failures. Nonetheless, the choice is unavoidable. Familiar situations begin to be accompanied by emotions such as hope, fear, etc., but the competent performer strives to suppress these feelings during his detached choice of perspective.

Nurses remember clinical situations that stand out because the nurse made a difference, felt good about his or her practice, learned something new, or experienced breakdown or conflict. In narrative accounts of nursing practice we find discourse about errors and false caring, such as inappropriate "taking over" or controlling, instead of enhancing the person's/family's sense of possibility. These distinctions about "getting it better and worse" are at the heart of skillful ethical comportment. The practitioner must find out directly what the good feels like and looks like in many particular situations. And this discourse is nurtured and continued in caring for and about others. This is illustrated in a nurse's dialogue with herself:

I thought this was going to be a great assignment because the patient was young, could talk, and even get out of bed. But he was depressed. [And I still continued] "How are you doing. We had a teacher here before that had a transplant." And he said: "Well, he did all right for a while then, didn't he?" I responded: "Yeah, he did really well." And he did for 10–12 years. He went back and taught. But I could tell that he was winding down away from me, like pulling back. I think to myself: "O.K., calm down, this person isn't going to talk to you." So that was kind of a negative experience. I think I overstepped my boundaries by probably talking too much . . . He's had so many different nurses that he doesn't need to keep getting close to each one that comes in and talks to him. He has his primary nurses and he can be close to them . . . He didn't want to interact with me because he doesn't have that much energy to bond with me. Which is fine . . . You really have to be sensitive to their needs, and I usually am, but I was being more sensitive to my needs, I think. At that particular time, I wanted a fun assignment. I had taken care of unconscious people for so long.

This nurse demonstrates the reflection on practice that enables her to learn the skill of involvement, the right level and kind, given the patient's needs. One can imagine that this dialogue will be extended in future situations modifying her skillful ethical comportment so that it is appropriate to nursing practice. Such skill requires active experiential learning.

As noted in Chapter 5, the hallmark of proficient ethical comportment in nursing is the ability to get beyond the technical demands of the task world and regain skillful involvement in the patient's world that is neither too distant nor too close. The following nurse describes her ability to change her mode of care when the situation has moved from the possibility of saving a life to the situation of the patient dying:

> I've been on the unit for 2 years now, and I'd say that within the last year or so, I stopped doing so much of the uniform looking to see when everything looks perfect, and looking more at the person first instead of all the equipment. That has kind of been a real good thing for me, although it's been a lot harder because now I'm getting more involved . . . We work with so much equipment. When you're oriented to an ICU that's what you're oriented to. You are oriented to the person also, but the numbers, the flow sheet, all the monitors, the lines, the dressings, what you have to do on your shift—I mean this is just a body in the bed with all these dressings and numbers . . . [Now if a patient is dying] I get more involved with the families. I don't really worry about taking their blood pressure or maybe checking their labs. I'm more interested in talking to the family and seeing how they're dealing with what's going on in the situation.

Although it may seem obvious to an outsider that one would change perspective and approach once a patient has no more medical options, recognizing this change in the situation and the ability to respond to the new situation is not easy, and indeed, not possible, if one is still caught up with mastering the task world. Moreover, once they notice the family issues, nurses still have to learn how to respond to the family.

As soon as the competent performer stops reflecting on problematic situations as a detached observer, and stops looking for principles to guide his actions, the gripping, holistic experiences from the competent stage become the basis of the next advance in skill.

Having experienced many emotion-laden situations, chosen plans in each, and obtained vivid, emotional demonstrations of the adequacy or inadequacy of the plan, the performer involved in the world of the skill "notices" or "is struck by" a certain plan, goal, or perspective. No longer is the spell of involvement broken by detached conscious planning.

Since there are generally far fewer "ways of seeing" than "ways of acting" after understanding without conscious effort what is going on, the proficient performer will still have to think about what to do. During this thinking, elements that present themselves as salient are assessed and combined by rule and maxim to produce decisions.

In the following excerpt, the proficient nurse recognizes that the patient is in pain, and that the interns are not sufficiently experienced with the situation to respond appropriately. She recognizes the problematic situation and, using her knowledge of the patient's cultural background, plus rules of thumb, decides what to do:

> So I finally interrupted them [the interns] and said: "When can I give her some pain medication? When are you going to do this [remove chest tube]? She really needs it." They responded: "Oh, she doesn't need any pain medication." It really irritated me. They were both young, probably younger than me, and probably had never pulled out a chest tube. They probably had no idea that it hurt. [And I thought] it was like, why don't you realize this is a person laying in this bed? You shouldn't be standing beside her bed and describing in graphic detail what you're going to do to pull this chest tube out, much less, not give her any pain medicine. This [Samoan] lady was very stoic. You had to anticipate her pain. That's a culturally based thing: In a Samoan culture, she would never have said that she needed something for pain anyway. Finally, I got them to tell me when they were going to do it so I gave her the pain medication.

She overrides the physicians' resistance, uses a pre-established order for pain, and times the administration of pain medication. Implicit in her description is the well-known maxim that it is easier to anticipate and prevent pain than to try to alleviate severe pain.

The proficient performer, immersed in the world of skillful activity, *sees* what needs to be done, but must *decide* how to do it. With enough experience with a variety of situations, all seen from the same perspective but requiring different tactical decisions, the proficient performer gradually breaks this class of situations into subclasses, each of which share the same decision, single action, or tactic. This allows an immediate intuitive response to each situation.

In nursing, we encounter expert skillful ethical comportment that responds immediately to the demands and takes into account the context of the situation. For example, a nurse describes choosing the right time to talk about decisions around heroic medical care:

> We prepare people for living as well as dying . . . This man is 86 years old and he could die. But it didn't feel right to talk to him or his anxious family

about code status. In the light of the fact that his health is declining—he's 86 years old; at some point that does need to be discussed between him and his family. But I didn't feel that it was appropriate with the time I spent with him, as nervous as he was. The last thing I would need to say to him is: "Have you ever thought about heroic measures?" . . . At this point he is not even close to a situation really where he needs to decide. There's really still no reason to think that he shouldn't be able to go home and continue on with an 86-year-old life at this point.

This discussion occurred in the context of other examples where nurses expressed strong values for fully informing patients and families about heroic measures and living wills. However, as we probed the question with this nurse, the possibility didn't even come up in her caring for this 86-year-old man and his family, since such a conversation would be misinterpreted given their anxiety.

DELIBERATION

We have shown so far that everyday intuitive ethical expertise, which Aristotle saw was formed by the sort of daily practice that produces good character, has, from Aristotle himself to Mandelbaum been passed over by philosophers, or, if recognized, distorted by reading back into it the mental content found in deliberation. It would be a mistake, however, to become so carried away with the wonder of spontaneous coping as to deny an important place to deliberative judgment. Getting deliberations right is half of what phenomenology has to contribute to the study of ethical expertise. One should not conclude from the pervasiveness of egoless, situation-governed comportment that thought is always disruptive and inferior.

More specifically, expert deliberation is not inferior to intuition, but neither is it a self-sufficient mental activity that can dispense with intuition. It is *based upon* intuition. The intellectualist account of self-sufficient cognition fails to distinguish the *involved* deliberation of an intuitive expert facing a familiar but problematic situation from the detached deliberation of an expert facing a *novel* situation in which he has no intuition and so, like a beginner, must resort to abstract principles.

A chess master confronted with a chess problem, constructed precisely so as not to resemble a position that would show up in a normal game, is reduced to using detached analysis. Likewise, an ethical expert when confronted with a quandary case may have to fall back on ethical principles. But since *principles* are unable to produce expert behavior, it should be no surprise if falling back on them produces inferior responses. The resulting decisions are necessarily crude, since they have not been refined by the experience of the results of a variety of intuitive responses to emotion-laden situations and the learning that comes from subsequent satisfaction and regret. In familiar but problematic situations, therefore, rather than standing back and applying abstract principles, the expert deliberates about the appropriateness of his *intuitions*. Common as this form of deliberation is, little has been written about such buttressing of intuitive understanding, probably because detached, principle-based deliberation is often incorrectly seen as the only alternative to intuition.

Let us turn again to the phenomenon. Sometimes, but not often, an intuitive decision maker finds himself torn between two equally compelling decisions. Presumably this occurs when the current situation lies near the boundary between two discernable types of situations, each with its own associated action. Occasionally one can compromise between these actions, but often they are incompatible. Only a modified understanding of the current situation can break the tie, so the decision maker will delay if possible and seek more information. If a decision maker can afford the time, the decision will be put off until something is learned that leaves only one action intuitively compelling. As Dewey (1960) puts it:

> [T]he only way out [of perplexity] is through examination, inquiry, turning things over in [the] mind till something presents itself, perhaps after prolonged mental fermentation, to which [the good man] can directly react. (p. 131)

Even when an intuitive decision seems obvious, it may not be the best. Dewey (1960) cautions:

> [An expert] is set in his ways, and his immediate appreciations travel in the grooves laid down by his unconsciously formed habits. Hence the spontaneous "intuitions" of value have to be entertained subject to correction, to confirmation and revision, by personal observation of consequences and cross-questioning of their quality and scope. (p. 132)

Aware that his current clear perception may well be the result of a chain of perspectives with one or more questionable links, and so might harbor the dangers of tunnel vision, the wise intuitive decision maker will attempt to dislodge his current understanding. He will do so by attempting to re-experience the chain of events that led him to see things the way he does, and at each stage he will intentionally focus upon elements not originally seen as important to see if there is an alternative intuitive interpretation. If current understanding cannot be dislodged in this way, the wise decision-maker will enter into dialogue with those who have reached different conclusions. Each will recount a narrative that leads to seeing the current situation in his way and so as demanding his response. Each will try to see things the other's way. This may result in one or the other changing his mind and therefore concluding in final agreement. But, since various experts have different past experiences, there is no reason why they should finally agree.

RELEVANCE OF SKILLFUL ETHICAL COMPORTMENT FOR CONSIDERING THE PARTICULAR AND THE GENERAL

The phenomenology of expertise allows us to sharpen up and take sides in an important contemporary debate. The debate centers on the ethical implications of Lawrence Kohlberg's (1981, 1984) cognitivist model of moral development. Kohlberg holds that the development of the capacity for moral judgment follows an invariant pattern. He distinguishes three levels: A Preconventional Level, on which the agent tries to satisfy his needs and avoid punishment; a Conventional Level, during the first stage of which the agent conforms to stereotypical images of majority behavior, and at the second stage, follows fixed rules and seeks to retain the given social order; and a Postconventional and Principled Level. The highest stage of this highest level is characterized as follows:

> Regarding what is right, Stage 6 is guided by universal ethical principles . . . These are not merely values that are recognized, but are also principles used to generate particular decisions. (Kohlberg, 1981, p. 412)

Jürgen Habermas (1992) has taken up Kohlberg's findings and modified them on the basis of his own discourse ethics, adding a seventh stage— acting upon universal procedural principles that make possible arriving at rational agreement through dialogue.

Charles Taylor has remarked that for Habermas, "'Moral' defines a certain kind of reasoning, which in some unexplained way has in principle priority" (Taylor, 1989, p. 88). Kohlberg's developmental stages are supposed to explain the priority; they serve to give empirical support to Habermas's claim that detached moral reasoning develops out of and is superior to ethical intuition. As Habermas explains: "The stages of moral judgment form a hierarchy in that the cognitive structures of a higher stage dialectically 'sublate' those of the lower one" (Habermas, 1992, p. 162).

Habermas sees Kohlberg's work as evidence that moral consciousness begins with involved ethical comportment, but that the highest stages of moral consciousness require the willingness and the ability to "consider moral questions from the hypothetical and disinterested perspective" (Habermas, 1982, p. 253). Thus, according to Habermas, Kohlberg's research lends empirical support to his modified, but still recognizable, Kantian view that the highest level of moral maturity consists of judging actions according to abstract, universal principles. He tells us that "The normative reference point of the developmental path that Kohlberg analyzes empirically is a principled morality in which we can recognize the main features of discourse ethics" (Habermas, 1992, p. 150).

It follows for Habermas that our Western European morality of abstract justice is developmentally superior to the ethics of any culture lacking universal principles. Furthermore, when the Kohlberg developmental scale is tested in empirical studies of the moral judgments of young men and women, it turns out that men are generally morally more mature than women.

In her book, *In a Different Voice*, Carol Gilligan (1982) contests this second result, claiming that the data on which it is based incorporate a male bias. She rests her objection on her analyses of responses to a moral dilemma used in Kohlberg's studies. She explains as follows:

> The dilemma . . . was one in the series devised by Kohlberg to measure moral development in adolescence by presenting a conflict between moral norms and exploring the logic of its resolution. . . . [A] man named Heinz considers whether or not to steal a drug which he cannot afford to buy, in order to save the life of his wife. . . . [T]he description of the dilemma . . . is followed by the question, "Should Heinz steal the drug?" (Gilligan, 1982, p. 27)

Kohlberg found that morally mature men, i.e., those who have reached stage 6, tended to answer that Heinz should steal the drug because the right to life is more basic than the right to private property. Women, however, seemed unable to deal with the dilemma in a mature, logical way. We quote from Gilligan's analysis of a typical case:

> Seeing in the dilemma not a math problem . . . but a narrative of relationships that extends over time, Amy envisions the wife's continuing need for her husband and the husband's continuing concern for his wife and seeks to respond to the druggist's need in a way that would sustain rather than sever connection . . . Seen in this light, her understanding of morality as arising from the *recognition* of relationship, her *belief* in communication as the mode of conflict resolution, and her *conviction* that the solution to the dilemma will follow from its compelling *representation* seem far from naive or *cognitively* immature. (Gilligan, 1982, pp. 27–30)[4]

The first point to note in responding to these interesting observations is that many women are "unable to verbalize or explain the rationale"

(Gilligan, 1982, p. 49) for their moral responses; they stay involved in the situation and trust their intuition. Many men, on the other hand, when faced with a moral problem, attempt to step back and articulate their principles as a way of deciding what to do. Yet as we have seen, principles can never capture the know-how an expert acquires by dealing with, and seeing the outcome of, a large number of concrete situations. Thus, when faced with a dilemma, the expert does not seek principles, but, rather, reflects on and tries to sharpen his or her spontaneous intuitions by getting more information until one decision emerges as obvious. Gilligan finds the same phenomenon in her subjects' deliberations:

> The proclivity of women to reconstruct hypothetical dilemmas in terms of the real, *to request or to supply missing information* about the nature of the people and the places where they live, shifts their judgment away from the hierarchical ordering of principles and the formal procedures of decision making. (Gilligan, 1982, pp. 100–101, our italics).

Gilligan, however, undermines what is radical and fascinating in her discoveries when she seeks her subjects' *solutions to problems*, and tries to help them articulate the *principles* underlying these solutions. "Amy's moral *judgment* is *grounded* in the belief that, 'if somebody has something that would keep somebody alive, then it's not right not to give it to them,'" she tells us (Gilligan, 1982, p. 28; our italics). Yet, if the phenomenology of skillful coping we have presented is right, principles and theories assist the novice in learning a new skill, and, in the case of skillful ethical comportment, serve to modify earlier skills so they are appropriate for the demands of the new practice. No principles or theory "ground" an expert ethical response, any more than in chess there is a theory or rule that explains a master-level move.

As we would expect, Gilligan's intuitive subjects respond to philosophical questions concerning the principles justifying their reactions with tautologies and banalities, e.g., that they try to act in such a way as to make the world a better place in which to live. They might as well say that their highest moral principle is "do something good." If Gilligan had not tried to get her intuitive subjects to formulate their principles for dealing with problems, but had rather investigated how frequently they *had* problems and how they deliberated about their spontaneous ethical comportment when they did, she might well have found evidence that moral maturity results in having fewer problems, and, when problems do arise, being able to act without detaching oneself from the concrete situation, thereby retaining one's ethical intuitions.

The second, and most important, point to consider is that Gilligan correctly detects in Amy's responses to the Heinz dilemma an entirely different approach to the ethical life than acting on universal principles. This is the different voice she is concerned to hear and to elaborate in her book. In answering her critics, she makes clear that it is not the central point of her work that these two voices are gendered.

> The title of my book was deliberate. It reads, "in a *different* voice," not "in a *woman's* voice." . . . I caution the reader that "this association is not absolute, and the contrasts between male and female voices are presented here to highlight a distinction between two modes of thought . . . rather than to represent a generalization about either sex." (Gilligan, 1986, p. 327)

She calls the two voices "the justice and care perspectives." Under one description to be good is to be *principled*; on the other, it is to be *unprincipled*, i.e., without principles.

Although Gilligan does not make the point, it should be obvious to philosophers that we inherit the justice tradition from the Greeks, especially Socrates and Plato. It presupposes that two situations can be the same in the relevant moral respects, and requires principles which treat the same type of situation in the same way. The principle of universalizability thus becomes, with Kant, definitive of the moral. All of us feel the pull of this philosophical position when we seek to be fair, and when we are called upon to justify what we do as right, rather than merely what one happens to do in our society. Moreover, we seek universal principles guaranteeing justice and fairness as the basis of our social and political decisions.

The other voice carries the early Christian message that, as Saint Paul put it, "the law is fulfilled," so that henceforth to each situation we should respond with love. Proponents of this view sense that no two situations, and no two people, are ever exactly alike. Even a single individual is constantly changing, for, as one acquires experience, one's responses become constantly more refined. Thus there is no final answer as to what the appropriate response in a particular situation should be. Since two abstractly identical situations will elicit different responses, caring comportment will look like injustice to the philosopher but will look like compassion or mercy to the Christian. We feel the pull of these Christian caring practices when we respond intuitively to the needs of those around us.

It is important to be clear, however, as Gilligan is not, that the care perspective does not entail any particular way of acting—for example, that one should promote intimate human relationships. The Christian command to love one's neighbor does not dictate how that love should be expressed. Caring in its purest form is not ordinary loving; it is doing spontaneously whatever the situation demands. As we have seen, even if two situations were identical in every respect, two ethical experts with different histories would not necessarily respond in the same way. Each person must simply respond as well as he or she can to each unique situation with nothing but experience-based intuition as a guide. Heidegger captures this ethical skill in his notion of *authentic care* as a response to the *unique*, as opposed to the *general*, situation (Heidegger, 1962, p. 346).

Responding to the general situation occurs when one follows ethical maxims and gives the standard acceptable response. This would correspond to the last stage of Kohlberg's Conventional Level. For Kohlberg and Habermas, on the next level the learner seeks principled justification. On our model, however, reaching the Postconventional Level would amount to acting with authentic care. When an individual becomes a master of his culture's practices or a professional practice within it, he or she no longer tries to do what *one* normally does, but rather responds out of a fund of experience in the culture and in the specialized practice. This requires having enough experience to give up following the rules and maxims dictating what *anyone* should do, and, instead, acting upon the intuition that results from a life in which talent and sensibility have allowed learning from the experience of satisfaction and regret in similar situations. Authentic caring in this sense is common to Paulian *agape* and Aristotelian *phronesis*.

This gets us back to the debate over which is more mature: acting upon rational judgments of rightness, or intuitively doing what the culture deems good. On the one hand, we have Kohlberg's stage 6 and Habermas' stage 7, both of which define moral maturity in terms of the ability to detach oneself from the concrete ethical situation and to act on abstract, universal, moral principles. On the other hand, we have John Murphy and Gilligan who, following W. B. Perry, view the "transition to maturity as a shift from 'the moral environment to the ethical, from the formal to the existential'" (Perry, 1968, p. 205). According to this view, the mature subject accepts "contextual relativism" (Murphy and Gilligan, 1980, p. 79). Murphy and Gilligan (1980) state the issue as follows:

> There are . . . people who are fully formal in their logical thinking and fully principled in their moral judgments; and yet . . . are not fully mature in their moral understanding. Conversely, those people whose thinking becomes more relativistic in the sense of being more open to the contextual properties of moral judgments and moral dilemmas frequently fail to be scored at the highest stages of Kohlberg's sequence. Instead, the relativizing of their thinking over time is construed as regression or moral equivocation, rather than as a developmental advance (p. 80)[5]

Habermas recognizes that "the controversy [raised by Gilligan] has drawn attention to problems which, in the language of the philosophical tradition, pertain to the relation of *morality* to ethical life (*Sittlichkeit*)"

(Habermas, 1992, p. 223). He, of course, continues to contend that rational morality is developmentally superior to *Sittlichkeit*.

If one thinks of morality exclusively in terms of *judgments* which are generated by *principles*, ethics looks like a form of practical reason, and the ability to stand back from the situation so as to insure reciprocity and universality becomes a sign of maturity. But if being good means being able to learn from experience and use what one has learned so as to respond more appropriately to the demands of others in the concrete situation, the highest form of ethical comportment consists in being able to stay involved and to refine one's intuitions.

It looks like we should follow Murphy and Gilligan in recognizing that at the Postconventional Level the learner accepts his intuitive responses, thus reaching a stage of maturity that leaves behind the rules of conventional morality for a contextualization.

None of the above is meant to deny that an ethical quandary could occur so unlike any previous situation that no one would have an expert intuitive response to it. Then, no amount of involved deliberation would serve to sharpen the expert's intuitions. In the face of such a total breakdown, and in that case alone, the ethical expert would have to turn to detached reflection. But the need to appeal to principles in quandary cases does not support the claim that ethical comportment normally involves implicit validity claims, nor that grasping rational principles of morality is the *telos* of ethical practice. We need to distinguish such breakdown cases from the cases of everyday intuitive ethical comportment and deliberation *internal* to our *Sittlichkeit*. If we fail to distinguish these two sort of cases and read the breakdown case back into the normal one, then ethical comportment looks like an incipient form of practical reason and ethical expertise is "rationally reconstructed" as a cognitive capacity which shows the same development as other cognitive capacities.

But there is no evidence that intuitive ethical expertise can be *replaced* by rational principles. Even if the principles of justice show the sort of equilibrium and reversibility that cognitivists like Piaget hold are characteristic of cognitive maturity, and situated ethical comportment lacks reversibility and universality, this does not show that acting on abstract, universal moral principles is developmentally superior to an intuitive contextual response. The cognitivist move looks plausible only because the tradition has overlooked intuitive deliberation and has read the structure of detached deliberation back into normal ethical comportment.

Thus when one measures Gilligan's two types of morality—her two voices—against a phenomenology of expertise, the traditional western and male belief in the maturity and superiority of critical detachment is reversed. The highest form of ethical comportment is seen to consist in being able to stay involved and to refine one's intuitions. If, in the name of a cognitivist account of development, one puts ethics and morality on one single developmental scale, the claims of justice, in which one needs to judge that two situations are equivalent so as to be able to apply one's universal principles, looks like regression to a competent understanding of the ethical domain, while the caring response to the unique situation stands out as practical wisdom.[6] If so, the phenomenology of skill and expertise would not be just an academic corrective to Husserl, Piaget, and Habermas. It would be a step toward righting a wrong done to involvement, intuition, and care that traditional philosophy, by passing over skillful coping, has maintained for 2500 years.

IMPLICATIONS OF THE PHENOMENOLOGY OF EXPERTISE FOR HEALTH CARE ETHICS

Skillful comportment is more complicated than any theoretical account. For example, a theoretical discourse about rights and justice is deprived for two reasons. First, the formal theory cannot point out all the embodied skilled know-how that is encountered in practice and, second, a formal procedural ethics cannot account for the qualitative distinctions and complexities encountered in living it out. Formal accounts of rights and justice alone cannot depict the know-how and lived meanings of being in the right relationship to concrete specific others in ways that protect their vulnerability while nurturing their strengths and sense of possibility. Where caring practices offer generosity and love, a discourse on rights and justice may cause the situation to deteriorate (Sandel, 1982). In the context of generous, knowledgeable, caring practices, finely tuned by one's own embodiment, the level of mutual respect and knowledge of the other will allow for more than mere rights and justice. The language of cost-benefit analysis and other forms of rational calculation will seem like an impoverished outside-in account that misses the particular human concerns of the situation. Of course, in situations of oppression and corruption, the ethics of rights and justice will improve the situation offering liberation and empowerment.

Our intellectual capacity to work out precise formal rules and moral theories for deliberation and justification does not guarantee that we will have the communities of practice, moral courage, habits, skills, and practices to live out and extend these theories in our everyday lives. First, we have to have the vision and courage to trust our intuitive responses. The phenomenology of the development of expertise predicts that skillful ethical comportment will deteriorate to a competent level if we apply norms and principles to complex practical situations where we have the potential for skillful recognition of patterns and intuitive responses. Strategies of adjudication and the search for certitude through the application of norms and principles, though comforting, do not produce expert skillful ethical comportment.

Second, a phenomenology of acquiring expertise illustrates that we must have the courage to face the limits of our predictive theoretical knowledge. Clinical situations are open-ended, changing, and ambiguous. Ambiguity resides not only in the knowledge of disease and treatment, but also in understanding the concerns of the patients and families. Skillful ethical comportment in a caring practice must include not only clinical knowledge about disease and cure but also knowledge of patient/family concerns— what they are trying to conserve and live out. Health care practitioners must have the moral courage to face up to the limits of existing knowledge and continue to act as prudently as possible given these limits. After the fact, when the situation becomes clearer, and it becomes evident that they have erred in their practices and judgment, they must have the courage to learn from the failure and not rationalize it away; otherwise they will not improve their performance.

Experts cannot get beyond experience, and formal theories cannot provide certitude or prevent error; that is, theory cannot get us beyond skillful ethical comportment in concrete, specific, local situations. The Platonic quest to get to the general in order to get beyond the vagaries of experience was a misguided turn, a heroic quest to transcend our habits, skills, practice. It has failed. We can redeem this mistake if we subject our theories to concrete ethical experience and acknowledge that skillful ethical comportment calls us not to be beyond experience but tempered and taught by it. The relationship, then, between moral theory and skillful ethical comportment must be a dialogue between respected partners, each shaping and informing the other. Theory is shaped by practice, and in turn may influence practice.

Examination of the process of acquisition of a new skill, such as assessing clinical signs and symptoms (see Chapter 3), shows that beginners make judgments using strict rules and features, but that with talent and a great deal of involved experience the beginner develops into an expert who sees intuitively what to do without applying rules and making judgments at all (Benner, 1984a; Dreyfus & Dreyfus with Athanasiou, 1986). The intellectualist tradition has given an accurate description of the beginner and of the expert facing an *unfamiliar* situation, but normally an expert does not *solve problems*. He does not *reason*. He does not even act deliberately. Rather, he spontaneously does what has normally worked and, naturally, it normally works.

To sum up, we can distinguish four different contexts in which ethical considerations come up for phenomenological analysis: comportment, communication, education, and justification.

1. *Comportment.* We have so far been discussing ethical action, and how one learns to produce and improve expert performance. Our question has been: How does one develop the ability to respond appropriately to ethical situations? We have seen that what is needed is involved activity plus the ability to learn from one's successes and mistakes. This experience produces learning without the learner needing conscious reflection, indeed, without his or her needing to remember anything, as long as emotionally involved experiences serve to modify future intuitive behavior.

2. *Communication.* This is a short name for the complex process of forming a community around shared experiences and responses. Such a community is formed by sharing exemplars which focus shared practices and make manifest that they are shared. Exemplars take up the past history of the group, show what the group is committed to, and thus serve to orient beginners and pass on wisdom to those who already have some understanding of the domain.

3. *Education.* Learning new skills can be facilitated by pointing out prototypical aspects to advanced beginners, and whole paradigmatic situations to those who already have experience. Thus the learner is led to pick out relevant aspects and to see the situation as those already in the community see it.

4. *Justification.* When an expert ethical response must be explained and defended, there is nothing the expert can do which captures his or her expertise but tell a story which leads other experts to see the situation in such a way that the action performed is seen to be appropriate. If some further justification is demanded by outsiders and nonexperts, the expert can appeal to principles, but it will always turn out that such principles will not generate an expert response in other situations, and so are not really reasons underlying the decision. Thus, there can be no genuine justification; only rationalization.

The best one can do is interpret one's response to a *specific* situation as a response to a specific *type* of situation for which a response is already accepted. One assumes that the case in question is similar enough to the typical case or strong instance to count as the same situation and therefore to require the same response as has already been found to be appropriate. Such "justification," while better than an appeal to principles, can never fully capture the expert's expertise, since what is basic but cannot be rationally explained is the reason the expert takes the current situation as sufficiently similar to the typical case to count as the same type.

The implications of our view are that ethical experts are those who have profited from many concrete experiences to move beyond a less nuanced competent level based on formal principles. Detachment is generally not desirable, and an outside-in perspective does not preserve wisdom.

NOTES

1. Without a shared ethical sensibility to what is laudable and what condemnable, one would go on doing what the experts in the community found inappropriate, develop bad habits, and become what Aristotle calls an unjust person.

2. "Egoless," as we are using the term, means free of mental content. It does not imply selflessness or self-sacrifice and the like.

3. This study did not include beginning nursing students; therefore, we can only provide retrospective accounts from recently graduated nurses. Examining "novice" skillful ethical comportment in nursing awaits future studies.

4. The cognitivist vocabulary we have italicized should warn us that, in spite of her critique, Gilligan may well have uncritically taken over the cognitivist assumptions underlying Kohlberg's work.

5. Again, note the cognitivist vocabulary: thinking, judgment, dilemmas.

6. If one accepts the view of expertise presented here, one must accept the superiority of the involved, caring self. But our skill model does not support Gilligan's Piagetian claim that the *development* of the self requires crises. Skill learning, and that would seem to be *any* skill learning, requires learning from *mistakes* but not necessarily from *crises*. A crisis would occur when one had to alter one's criterion for what counted as success. Aristotle surely thought that in his culture, the men, at least, could develop character without going through crises. The idea of the necessity of moral crises for development goes with an intellectualist view of theory change that may well be true for science but which has nothing to do with selves. This is not to deny that in our pluralistic culture, and especially for those who are given contradictory and distorting roles to play, crises may be necessary. It may well be that women are led into traps concerning success and need crises to get out of them. Thus Gilligan may well be right that crises *in fact* play a crucial role in modern Western women's moral development, even if they are not *necessary*.

Chapter 11

THE NURSE–PHYSICIAN RELATIONSHIP: NEGOTIATING CLINICAL KNOWLEDGE*

The importance of positive nurse–physician relationships has been widely acknowledged (Baggs, 1989; Baggs & Schmitt, 1988; Eubanks, 1991; Fagin, 1992; Mechanic & Aiken, 1982; Prescott & Bowen, 1985). There is increasing evidence that positive relationships between physicians and nurses contribute to improved patient outcomes. A study conducted in the mid-70s produced some evidence that interdisciplinary collaboration and high levels of collegiality resulted in positive patient outcomes (Schmitt & Williams, 1985). More recently, a widely cited study by Knaus, Draper, Wagner, and Zimmerman (1986) examined treatment and outcome in intensive care units at 13 tertiary care hospitals. Variations among hospitals in effectiveness were attributed, in part, to the degree of interaction and communication between physicians and nurses. In a demonstration project sponsored by the American Association of Critical Care Nurses (Mitchell, Armstrong, Simpson, & Lentz, 1989), high nurse-physician collaboration was identified as one of four major factors related to positive clinical outcomes (i.e., low mortality ratio, absence of new complications, and high patient satisfaction).

Stein (1967), in a now classic article, described the "doctor-nurse" game, in which physicians and nurses interacted in ways to avoid open conflict at all costs. The nurse could make recommendations, but could do so only indirectly, to avoid the appearance of making recommendations; the physician, in asking for a suggestion from the nurse, could do so only without

---

*Substantial contributions to the interpretation of text and to drafting this chapter were made by Sheila Kodadek, Martha Haylor, and Peggy Wros of Oregon Health Sciences University.

appearing to. The game served to preserve the dominance of medicine over nursing and the higher status afforded the physician. Recently, Stein and his associates (Stein, Watts, & Howell, 1990) asserted that interactions between nurses and physicians are now characterized, in large measure, by different but equally valued contributions to decision making. This view is contrary to much of the nursing literature of the 80s, suggesting that relationships between physicians and nurses are far from peaceful, and that a pattern of physician dominance and nurse subordination continues to prevail (for example, Prescott, Dennis, & Jacox, 1987; Spoth & Konewko, 1987; Weiss, 1982).

In a national survey conducted between 1980 and 1984, a majority of both nurses and physicians reported that their relationships were satisfactory (Prescott & Bowen, 1985). Interestingly though, the reports of what constituted a satisfactory relationship differed for nurses and physicians. The nurses emphasized mutual respect and trust, while physicians cited how well the nurse communicates with the physician, her willingness to help, and her competence. To receive a rating of satisfactory, the relationship apparently did not require a high degree of collaboration. When disagreements between physicians and nurses occurred, resolution was handled through competition (assertiveness and uncooperativeness) or accommodation (unassertiveness and cooperativeness), rather than through collaboration and joint problem-solving. Both nurses and physicians commonly viewed the process of joint decision making as being comprised of nurses' providing input to physician decision makers.

This pattern of physician dominance and nurse subordinance has a long history (Campbell-Heider & Pollock, 1987; Darbyshire, 1987; Keddy, Jones-Gillis, Jacobs, Burton, & Rogers, 1986; Lovell, 1981). Feminist analyses suggest that the pattern is purposeful and institutionalized, reflecting the dominant power and gender relationships within society (Ashley, 1976; 1980; Reverby, 1987); relationships which have resulted in the elimination of the predominantly female lay movements of disease prevention (Ehrenreich & English, 1973).

Data from our study suggest that relationships between nurses and physicians are far from ideally collaborative and that issues of status inequity, gender bias, and power imbalance are commonplace. While we do not want to ignore these issues, we are hopeful, like Stein and his associates, that change is possible given the influx of men into nursing, women into medicine, and feminist thought into the discourse of both practices. While acknowledging the central role of status inequity and power imbalance in shaping troubled nurse-physician relationships, we offer an interpretation of the genesis of the problem that turns on a different set of interdisciplinary issues: the blurring of boundaries between medicine and nursing, and the eclipse of both clinical knowledge and knowing the pa-

tient by formal scientific knowledge. We will also show that skillful negotiation between nurses and physicians is a practical skill gained through
experience; its development roughly parallels the skill acquisition model
and the developing sense of agency described in earlier chapters.

To introduce the central issues in the nurse-physician relationship, we
have selected one exemplar which is typical of numerous accounts in our
study. This exemplar illustrates particularly well the negotiation of clinical knowledge and the role of experience in shaping interdisciplinary communication patterns.

The patient was an elderly woman who had had an abdominal aortic
aneurysm repair and was being cared for by an inexperienced nurse. A
more experienced nurse who is telling the story recognized, "by the flurry
of activity" in the room, that things were not going well. The new nurse
was busy managing intravenous therapies, as the patient's blood pressure
was very labile and required continuous monitoring and adjustment of a
nipride drip. The patient also required large amounts of fluid and was in
metabolic acidosis. The clinical understanding of the situation by the house
staff and the new nurse was that the patient was "taking her time to warm"
after this major surgery, and would be expected to do fine after she
"warmed up." The more experienced nurse provides this account of how
the story unfolded:

Nurse: I went by the room and I looked at the patient and she was very cold
and clammy and you could see, looking at her vital signs, that she was still
hypothermic. I had a sense of what was going on. There were two things that
I noticed right off. One, that her abdomen was very large and very firm, and
the other thing was that her knees were mottled and I said, "She has a dead
bowel." And they [the house staff] said, "She doesn't have a dead bowel." So
backing off a little bit I said, "Would we consider an ischemic bowel?" They
asked why I thought that and I said "You can't maintain her blood pressure.
We're playing nipride/fluid, nipride/fluid. She's acidotic as all-get-out. She's
hypothermic and tachycardic. Her abdomen is taut and firm." They really just
thought that she was just not having a smooth recovery from her operation. I
went on with them: "This nipride game has got to stop. This is ridiculous. As
soon as you put it on, she drops her pressure. She's cold, she's clamped. She
needs to be warmed, she needs fluid." So they started to come around a tad,
then they hung lactated Ringers. I said, "Wait a minute, she's got a lactic acidosis, the last thing you need to do is throw more lactic acid into her with the
Ringers." "Oh yeah, get some saline."

We finally paged the senior resident who was unavailable, he was in the
operating room, but the attending was there, so he just came up and he still
felt that the patient was just not recovering smoothly, that in another few hours,
if we get the patient warm and clear the lactic acidosis, they would all of a
sudden turn the corner and be fine. And he left the hospital, out of beeper range
for some time.

Finally, one of the surgical attendings who was in the house over the week-end came up to the unit and she said "What's going on with this patient?" She'd been following the patient through the computer . . . the blood gases. And she looked at the patient and said "Dead bowel," and I said "Yeah, I've been try-ing to tell them for three hours." . . . They finally began to believe that this pa-tient had a problem with dead bowel, but now the attending cannot be reached. Finally, the senior surgical resident comes out of the OR and he sees it, but everyone's going to wait. I said "You don't have time to wait for this attend-ing. Someone's just going to have to make a decision and do it. The senior resi-dent has the ability to operate." I said, "This woman is going to die."

Int: You really felt that sense of urgency.

Nurse: Yes, the patient was starting to get less tachycardic. The blood pressure was starting to slowly drop off. And we had fluid wide open. So I thought someone should go talk to the family, to let them know how sick she was but also to discuss no code, because this woman was going to die. And the resi-dent said "Keep your pants on. What are you getting all in a wad for?" and this is like 3 hours later. And I said, "Excuse me. I'm going to get the emer-gency cart." And he said, "You're crazy." I went to get it. As I brought it to the door, she arrested. And we went through a round of drugs, and of course at this point now they realize that there's nothing we can do, so they let the woman die. I really still didn't believe that they believed it was dead bowel, but unfor-tunately on autopsy, they proved it was dead bowel. And it's one of those situ-ations, the physicians are in the room, they had the ability to look at the same things that I saw, I mean maybe in their eyes I'm just a nurse, but they had someone even telling them what the problem was. And not just saying "I think it's dead bowel" but "I think it's dead bowel because she's tachycardic, she can't maintain her blood pressure, she's spiking up and down with the pressures, she's cold, she's clammy, her temp's down, her belly's up, knees are mottled, she's got metabolic acidosis that won't quit." I could show them exactly what it was. They still either couldn't see it, didn't believe they were seeing it, or maybe hoped that that wasn't what it was.

Int: Did they talk to you afterwards?

Nurse: No. They were very . . . when I said to them, "What did the post show?" they said, very quietly, "Dead bowel." The poor nurse taking care of the patient was devastated. She had been trying to manage this all morning and not having the experience, you know. She's kind of going along with what they're doing, which is fine. Very frustrating situation. . . . She was like "What else could we have done?" And I thought, "We even had the attending in the room" and I probably wasn't as strong with the attending as with the interns. I did point it out to him. I did present my ideas to him, not as strongly, but he's someone who should have the experience and should have the knowledge and shouldn't need to be hit over the head with a bat. I mean an intern that's never seen it, you have to tell them point blank what it is and why it is. But in the case of this attending, with his many years of experience, I thought being subtle was the way to go.

Evident in this narrative is the nurse's frustration and sense of failure at not getting the action needed for this patient to survive. There is no gaming quality to her interactions with the physician, at least as she recounts them. Rather, there is a skillful appraisal of a rapidly changing situation, and an honest and straightforward effort to help the physicians see the situation as she did. Her clinical knowledge is at the heart of her assessment; even though she did not know this patient, she recognized a clinical picture that was ominous. She reported, on questioning, that she had seen patients with "dead bowel" enough so that she could recognize the problem when she saw it. She also discussed having considered other explanations for the woman's deteriorating condition, including the physician's hypothesis of slow warming, as well as an arterial bleed and, finally, superior mesenteric artery occlusion resulting in necrosis; this consideration, or deliberative rationality, helped bolster her own confidence about her appraisal and her ability to make the case with the physicians. Even when the resident began to concede that her assessment might be correct, he did not have the same sense of urgency that this nurse did. She later described her recognition of this rapid, downward trajectory, knowing that a cardiac arrest was imminent. Also apparent in the text is the nurse's consideration of how to best present the case to the physicians: that she thought "subtle was the way to go" with the attending who was more experienced and, she presumed, able to respond to her communications about the patient's deteriorating state.

Obviously, in rapidly changing situations such as this, errors in judgment will be made. But without a sense of mutual collegiality and respect among care providers, and a setting in which discussion and debate about the meaningful clinical picture and the appropriate medical responses are possible, errors like this are far more likely. Another disturbing aspect of this account, and many others like it, is that there was no formal mechanism for case review, in which the judgments and the actions of the nurses and physicians could be discussed and used as a resource for further clinical learning. The discussion was closed down with the tacit recognition that an error had been made.

The narrative also illustrates the role of experience in negotiating clinical knowledge. The advanced beginner nurse initially assigned to take care of this patient lacked the recognitional abilities evident in the the expert nurse's account, and she clearly relied on the judgment of others, essentially "delegating up" decision making. The inexperienced residents also lacked the ability to see important aspects of the clinical situation; moreover, with no practical understanding of this patient's likely trajectory, they missed the sense of urgency apparent to the experienced nurse. The more experienced nurse, on the other hand, understood the complexities of communication patterns, believing that the more experienced attending would be able to read her signals, and respond appropriately. Her sense of responsibility in this situation is characteristic of the expert practice described in Chapter 6.

This exemplar of breakdowns in physician-nurse collaboration is like countless others provided by experienced nurses in this study. In this chapter, we will explore what were found to be the central themes related to this breakdown in nurse-physician collaboration:

1. the blurring of disciplinary boundaries between nursing and medicine, in which nursing has assumed much more responsibility for medical decision making without the corollary explicit recognition of this contribution;

2. the eclipse of clinical knowledge by formal scientific knowledge;

3. the role of experience in clinical judgments and interdisciplinary communication patterns; and

4. the covering over of concerns about illness and suffering.

We also offer an analysis of interdisciplinary collaboration which presents it as a clinical skill, developed through experience and hard-won transformations in understanding.

BLURRING OF DISCIPLINARY BOUNDARIES

The practice of nursing in intensive care units has markedly changed the ways in which physicians make medical judgments. Therapies are instantaneous, most often administered intravenously, and require astute, instantaneous clinical judgment by the clinician at the bedside. The style of physician orders has changed from precise mandates to guidelines or parameters; often these "orders" instruct the nurse to keep the patient within certain physiological parameters (e.g., "Keep serum potassium between 4 and 5") and within certain therapeutic dosage ranges of medication. The judgment of when to alert the physician to changes in the patient's status may be guided to a limited extent by "orders" (e.g., "call if BP< 90"), but because not all contingencies can be anticipated in the "order" writing, nurses must often decide when to alert the physician. No nurse questions the physicians' legally and socially mandated prerogative and responsibility to make medical decisions. But the responsibility of the nurse is to make all the moment-by-moment clinical judgments, such as recognizing that the patient is not within the set guidelines (e.g., serum potassium may be low) or that the patient no longer seems to be responding well to the ordered treatment regimen and then deciding how to keep the patient within the set guidelines, given the possible drugs identified in the order.

The language used to describe these guidelines, i.e., "physicians' orders," covers over the significant responsibility nurses have in medical decision-making and maintains the traditional unidirectional line of authority from physician to nurse. In addition to the obvious responsibilities of nurses in managing instantaneous therapies and alerting the physician of changes in the patient's status, there are many more subtle ways in which experienced nurses inform and influence medical judgments.

In the following excerpt, nurses are describing the way they interpret and present clinical data to physicians. In this particular case, they are describing what's needed to differentiate hypotension from hypovolemia in preterm infants.

Nurse 1:   I think if your blood pressure is low and you go to him and tell him "the pressure is falling," he's going to want to know other things. Like, how much is the kid peeing, what's his specific gravity, what's his skin color, what's his skin turgor, is his fontanelle sunken?

Nurse 2:   You have to have made the diagnosis yourself . . . because that's how you present your case . . .

Nurse 1:   Either you want him to go up on the Dopamine or you want him to give the kid some blood . . . We don't have autonomy to turn up the drip, even if we're sure that's what he needs. We still have to get an order for it, which you do when you make your case. It is one of the hardest decisions for anybody to make and if you give volume when the kid is hypotensive you end up in worse trouble than you were before and if you don't give volume when they need it, the same thing is also true. How you present the information is important. Whether you say "Do you want to turn up the dopamine?" or "We're this far behind on cells," you can make a difference in what they decide to do next. I don't like to have to be the one who is essentially making this decision. But you're in that position from time to time, especially in the middle of the night when it's an inexperienced physician on.

Here, the nurses are describing their responsibility for diagnosis, differentiating between hypotension and hypovolemia. The way in which nurses present data may determine what actions the physicians take, particularly with inexperienced physicians. Some nurses describe this as a deliberate strategy, to get what they believe the patient needs. In many other situations, it shows up as nurses' responding to the physician based on their reading of his understanding. When the nurse makes the case to the physician, she expects a certain response. When the expected response is not forthcoming, she may shift to a different approach to make the case. It is interesting to note in this excerpt that nurses are not counting on physician skill in decision-making. Rather, their emphasis is on the skill that they as nurses acquire in what they refer to as "making the case." It is clear in this and other excerpts that nurses see it as their responsibility to present the information to the physician in such a way that he or she will make the correct medical judgment.

The assumption of responsibility in medical judgments is born of experience. Advanced beginners unquestioningly rely on the experience and judgment of other nurses and physicians for even the moment-to-moment decisions. There is little evidence in their narratives of a sense of agency and responsibility for making many medical decisions; they never seriously doubt the judgments of physicians. Expert practice, on the other hand is characterized by the tacit acceptance of responsibility for much of medical decision making—to recognize when a physician needs to be alerted to changes in patient status, *and* to have already worked out an expected response, *and* to present the information in such a way that the physician responds in the anticipated way. Nurses refer to this skill as "making the case." They see it as their responsibility to persuade the physician to pay attention and to respond in certain ways, and they feel that they have failed when they are unsuccessful. In all circumstances reported by nurses in this study, "making a case" was not about power, nor about conforming to the rules of a game in order to minimize conflict. Instead, it was viewed as a necessary part of their practice to get what they felt the patient needed:

Nurse 1: It's sad when you have to manipulate them like that. Why can't you just tell the truth? "You're supposed to do this. Why should I have to tell you this; you should know it."

Nurse 2: Especially if it's a resident. Sometimes you know that you know more in this particular situation, how to deal with this certain patient. From my own experience, though, just going up to somebody and challenging him and putting him on the defensive doesn't get you what you want. And you end up fighting with each other and you're just against a brick wall. And he's not going to move because he's the physician. You can have screaming battles at the bedside and you can be right, and the attending can come in the next morning: "Why didn't you call me?" Which is exactly what I thought should happen, but the resident wouldn't do it.

Nurse 3: But you're being right didn't save the patient.

Nurse 2: Exactly. And you've been sitting on a bombshell for 12 hours.

This new sense of responsibility is hard-won. Many of the expert nurses recounted narratives which transformed their practice, such as the exemplar which follows:

The incident that happened with me involved a vascular patient, an elderly lady who had vascular bilateral femoral-popliteal bypass in her groin and her blood pressure was, on her first full postop day, 190/110 and that's just too high. Anybody else would have been on nipride to keep it down. Otherwise it would blow her graft. And I was working with a new orientee at the time and I remember being very concerned about this lady's blood pressure and her being fairly refractory to any of the oral agents that they were using on her. They tried all kinds of things like nitropaste and she was still sitting at 170/100 and the third-year resident came by [this really causes me chest pain when I think about it now] and I said, "This lady's blood pressure is this and we can't get it down; what would you like us to use to get it down further?" He says, "That's OK," chewing his gum. And I said, "Well, as a rule, vascular patients are not allowed to have a blood pressure higher than this," and he said "We'll go with that." I said, "Her blood pressure's usually x/x and now its 180/120," and he said "Well, we should give her something for pain." And I should have fought harder. I should have gone up [*meaning "go up the ladder" to the next resident*] because a few moments later, I was helping another nurse with a patient and the orientee says, "C., come here" and I go "I'll be there in a minute," and she says "It can't wait." So I go whipping around the corner and she's blown her graft. She's got arterial blood pumping from her groin into the bed with a thigh this big around, and I just killed myself over that; if I had fought it harder, maybe that wouldn't have happened. We start doing all the appropriate things, dipping her head down, calling over to the OR, calling the physicians who are not coming and this physician in question did not respond to the stat pages . . . So since then, when I'm fairly convinced about something, then I'll fight for it.

This excerpt illustrates several issues which emerge repeatedly in our data. First, although the nurse has clear clinical data pointing to a potentially serious problem, she is unable to persuade an inexperienced resident that immediate attention is needed. His seemingly cavalier attitude (he says, chewing his gum, "OK") is also not uncommon. Second, the nurse's learning in this situation is painful, and her practice is transformed by her experience; never again, she insists, will she avoid going to bat when she's so certain that she is correct. Her narrative reveals an enormous sense of responsibility for a clinical situation gone awry, although she had objectively done all that is presumably required of the nurse in reporting to the physician signs of complications.

Experienced nurses also cue physicians to what is important from the tremendous amount of data available to them. In the following excerpt, a group of nurses is discussing the importance of this practice:

Nurse 1: Doesn't the doctor look at the baby every day?
Nurse 2: They don't check every . . .
Nurse 3: (laughter) They don't. What they do is they . . .
Nurse 2: Take a glance and that's it.
Nurse 3: That's right. Or they just look at the flow sheet and they may go through the steps of an exam, but they may not. I mean, they may not do it that in-depth if they're not clued in that there is a problem here.
Nurse 2: And, usually, some of them really rely on what the nurses tell them, because usually it is only through the pushing of the nurses that something gets done.

The importance of cuing the physician to salient data shows up most clearly in circumstances of breakdown. In the following excerpt, a competent level nurse describes a situation in which she learned the importance of this aspect of nursing practice:

This is a traumatic one I'll never forget. I was on nights and I was really green and I had received this patient who had surgery that day. I don't remember what the surgery was, but he had a glucose of around 400. He was admitted about noon and he had that elevated glucose on admission and there were several notations on his 24-hour flow sheets that he had a high glucose and that he was a diet-controlled diabetic. So I assumed since that was his admission, it had been documented and we even had a doctor come in that evening and look at it before he went to bed. So I assumed that they had seen that and decided that because he was a diet-controlled diabetic that it would resolve itself. Anyway, this one doctor could be very harsh and the next morning when he went on rounds he just nailed me. He nailed me hard, and he yelled at me. He goes. "What level do you think you'd report it?" and on and on and . . . I was just devastated. But the assumption I made was that they had already assessed it and made their decision because it had been recorded at least four times since noon and this was midnight. And that was a bad assumption. . . . Now, I never assume, because millions of times I go "Well, did you happen to see . . . ?" even though they had just looked at the 24-hour flow sheet, what was documented. "Did you happen to see or did you note that his urine output is low?" I always say that. Now I'm very good at it. I mean, I never assume. Even if they get irritated because they feel that I am encroaching on their decision and giving mine . . . And, you know, they have 20 million things on their mind. They come wandering in; they see about five different sheets and they haven't been with the patient and haven't seen this progression and they're not as acutely aware of what's going on with this patient as we are, so I think that they need a little reminder. I make sure that my preceptees know to present the data and the majority of them are saying "It's right there and he just looked at it but that does not make a difference. I think all they look at sometimes is the blood pressure. They see they're alive and ticking, so they're healthy."

Physicians may develop some expectations about the kind of information that they receive from nurses. In this case, there was a tacit assumption that the nurse had distilled the relevant information from the flow sheet and pointed it out to the physician. The nurse also describes why this kind of practice is so important. The nurse is there with the patient for hours a day; they know the minute-by-minute changes and they know what is salient for this patient. Of course, not every physician seeks or attends to this kind of input from nurses, setting up more possibilities for conflict and for inappropriate medical judgments.

ECLIPSE OF CLINICAL KNOWLEDGE
BY FORMAL SCIENTIFIC KNOWLEDGE

All practice disciplines suffer from the obscurity of practical or clinical knowledge in an era in which formal scientific knowledge and rational technical decision making are the only legitimate forms of knowledge (Benner, 1984a; Dreyfus & Dreyfus with Athanasiou, 1986; Schon, 1983). Clinical knowledge shows up as recognition of familiar patterns, an understanding of changes in human responses over time, and the ability to make qualitative and perceptual distinctions that augment or go beyond the "objective" evidence or hard laboratory data. Clinical knowledge encompasses a particular patient's responses in relation to the general expectations for similar patients; it includes both detailed knowledge of a particular patient's patterns of responses (Jenks, 1993; Jenny & Logan, 1992; MacLeod, 1993; Tanner et al., 1993) and in-depth, often tacit, understanding of how particular groups of patients typically react. Both physicians and nurses alike would probably favor the use of objective clinical evidence that a patient's condition is changing; both would also favor practices based on sound scientific theory and research (Prescott et al., 1987). But expert practitioners in both disciplines must rely on advanced clinical knowledge as the skilled know-how that makes recognition of subtle changes possible (Benner, 1983; 1984a; Schon, 1983) and that allows for nuanced interpretations of "objective" evidence. All clinicians must deal with historical understanding of a particular patient.

The expert nurse is able to recognize what is salient in particular situations because of her advanced clinical knowledge and because she knows the patient. Nurses who spend hours a day with the patient learn how the patient typically responds to therapies, how he usually communicates, and what his likes and dislikes are. They know the appearance of patients' wounds, the sound of their chest, the degree of movement and strength in their extremities, the kind of eye contact they usually make, and the way they respond to their family's presence. When there are subtle changes in the patient, the nurse who knows the patient recognizes the changes. In the following excerpt, two nurses talk about the beginning awareness that something is wrong with a patient and how this awareness depends on knowing the patient.

Nurse 1:   It's so gradual, sometimes, and you're getting the feeling that something's up because you've just spent the last 3 months with this kid and you know him inside out, and if you try and describe it in words or do it in physical symptoms . . .

Nurse 2:   . . . It sounds dumb . . .

Nurse 1: And they come and look . . . "The kid looks fine, he's pink, his color is good."

Nurse 2: . . . "Labs look fine."

Nurse 1: . . . Yeah, his fluid status is fine but . . . it's like being a parent. You know your children and you know what they do day after day after day, you know when they're coming down with a cold, you know if it's teething, you know that something's up.

Here the nurses express the frustration of trying to put into words their indeterminate clinical knowledge of the patient. Because they know the patient well, they're able to detect subtle changes in his condition. These changes don't add up to an objectively clinically significant picture yet, but they often serve as a warning of more dramatic changes to follow. In the case of infants, children, and critically ill adults, this lead time can be life-saving.

Knowing the patient is a vital aspect of interpreting early warnings and of managing instantaneous therapies. The nurse's capacity for knowing a patient contributes in significant yet invisible ways to medical diagnosis and management. The following excerpt clearly illustrates the importance of knowing how a patient typically responds to medical therapy.

Nurse: This person had a failing myocardium, labile blood pressure and his pressure—he went into episodes of SVT vs. just a sinus tach. He had a fixed sinus tach, almost like a fixed cardiac output syndrome, where his cardiac output was only maintained by a heart rate of 120 or greater, because he just had such a lousy myocardium. He started to drop his pressure and he went into an episode of flash pulmonary edema. And the trauma team was managing him and they're planning along with medicine and cardiology. And this is after I had been taking care of him about 3 or 4 weeks. And they were saying, "We want to start him back on Dopamine." He was on Dobutamine at the time and I said, "No, he needs both drugs." "No, we want to start him on the Dopamine." I was fighting and fighting, saying, "He needs both drugs." And I lost that fight momentarily. So we put him on the Dopamine and took him off the Dobutamine. He did much worse. He had more ectopy. He had chest pain. I mean, of course he did. We all knew what he was going to do.

Int: So how did you know that he needed both drugs?

Nurse: Dobutamine, he had intravascular volume to support blood pressure. His heart—he had a flabby heart. The Dobutamine would just give him inotropic support. Whereas the Dopamine is just going to flog his heart out and increase his myocardial work and his myocardial oxygen consumption and would kind of aggravate the situation. They were taking away the drug that was supporting him and putting him on a drug that I thought was going to hurt him. I thought he needed both. To have both those drugs in moderation would help him. And we ended up doing that the next day.

Int: When you say "moderation," what do you mean?

Nurse: I mean, give him the Dobutamine—moderate, like maybe 5 mics of Dobutamine which was what he liked. Keep the Dopamine in between 3 and 6 because he is very sensitive to Dopamine. I mean, I knew from before that if you
try to drop his Dopamine from 2 to 1, he would bottom out his pressure and
you know, 2 mics is a renal dose; it shouldn't do anything with him, but it did.
He was so catecholamine-dependent by that time. I just had a sense of, look, I
had seen him try just the Dobutamine, I had seen him try just the Dopamine
and I thought, I think he needs both. It was just a gut feeling; "Let's try this—
we haven't tried this and there is nothing wrong with both drugs."

On questioning, the nurse goes on to relate more specifics about this
particular patient's experience with Dopamine and Dobutamine. She has
in-depth knowledge of this patient's response to the drugs, and of how he
differs from what might be anticipated. A wise physician would use this
nurse's expert grasp of the patient's particular response in working out the
next treatment plan. Because physicians aren't with patients day in and
day out, monitoring their response to treatment, there is no way they can
have the kind of grasp that an expert nurse has by virtue of having managed the moment-to-moment administration of drugs to a particular patient over days or weeks.

Interestingly, this way of knowing a patient can serve to maintain the
status inequity between nurses and physicians, even while granting a
source of informal power to the nurse. Campbell-Heider and Pollock (1987)
point to the contrast between

> the physician's contacts with hospitalized patients, which are characterized
> by brief, highly structured, almost ceremonial interactions, and those of the
> nurse, who may spend hours in direct, unstructured contact with patients,
> from casual conversation to assisting with the most intimate bodily func-
> tions. The nurse's closeness to the patient and the physician's remoteness
> are pervasive features of the ideology of social relations within hospitals,
> in which status is proportional to separation from patients. In such settings,
> physicians become dependent on nurses, and often believe that nurses with-
> hold from them important information (Stein, 1967), or that nurses will
> "pollute" their relationships with patients. (p. 422)

Differences in the extent to which nurses and physicians know their
patients is a very common source of conflict. The nurses in these intensive
care units worked with the patients for long periods of time. They knew
the patients' typical pattern of responses and had learned to adjust their
practices accordingly—e.g., titrating drugs, changing positions, managing
airways, etc. based on the patient's response (Tanner et al., 1993). Teams
of physicians, particularly in teaching hospitals, often know neither the
patient nor their ways of responding. Enlightened interactions between

nurses and physicians were characterized by a recognition on the part of the physician of the nurse's knowledge of the patient, which was sought out in developing or modifying a treatment plan.

Of course, clinical know-how is not limited only to experienced nurses. Experienced physicians rely on such perceptual and recognitional skills in the diagnosis and management of disease. The following excerpt illustrates the nurses' recognition and appreciation of this clinical wisdom in a physician, and the way in which the physician draws on and uses nurses' skilled observations of the patient.

Nurse: We have one doctor who to me is—I'm always amazed—but he can come in and spend 15 or 20 minutes with a baby who's on, say, 22,23,24% oxygen, and after he's spent that time with the baby he either takes the hood off or he doesn't and he says, "This baby is going to do fine." And the baby does fine.

Int: How does he know?

Nurse: Lots of experience. He doesn't articulate it any better than the rest of us do. He's got a vast wealth of experiential knowledge that he hasn't entirely put together in a form that can be used by other people. But just ways the baby responds to stimuli, to its environment, just to things, to its IV, just the whole number of things that seem to provide him with enough information that the rest of us wouldn't even begin to attempt.

Int: It's interesting, it does require the 20 minutes with the baby.

Nurse: Oh yeah! He asks questions about the baby, "Well, how does the baby do when you do this, and how does it do when you do that?" I mean it's not hocus-pocus.

Int: He's gathering information.

Nurse: He's gathering information but, you know, the way he puts it together isn't always readily apparent. But he's one of the ones that asks us often when we're primary, "Do you think the baby wants to go up on the feedings? Is he hungry? Is the baby satisfied? Do you think the baby wants the oxygen, or does he seem to be trying to get rid of it?" I mean, half the time they're there with the cannula off. So you begin to get a sense of paying attention to what it is that the baby's trying to tell you and can't tell you.

The nurse describes well the often ineffable nature of clinical knowledge—"He's no more articulate about it than we are." This excerpt also illustrates a skillful negotiation of clinical knowledge between an experienced physician and nurses who are sufficiently experienced to have made relevant observations. The more typical descriptions of interactions between physicians and nurses were those in which nurses struggled to get a physician to pay attention to exactly the kind of clinical data described in this excerpt. When claims for final authority supersede the need for skillful negotiation of clinical knowledge, then both disciplines and the patient are likely to lose.

THE ROLE OF EXPERIENCE

Most advocates of collaboration between physicians and nurses, and many of the critics of the extant nurse-physician relationship, seem to assume that there is an ideal kind of relationship. This assumption, of course, requires that all physicians and nurses are equally competent and equally knowledgeable about a particular patient's situation; clearly, however, a renowned attending physician and a clinical nurse specialist with years of experience do not function in the same way as a resident or a new graduate nurse. It is ludicrous to assume, for example, that the physician is always in the most knowledgeable position when, for example, the physician is a relatively inexperienced resident working with an experienced and well-educated clinical nurse specialist. It is also ludicrous for a physician to assume that all nurses are equally skilled in recognizing salient aspects of a situation and in recommending appropriate treatment. It is, of course, difficult for the new resident, unfamiliar with any of the nurses on the unit, to sort out the nurses who can be trusted for reasonable advice. As nurses in this discussion point out:

> It really makes me nervous when I see interns and residents asking inexperienced nurses for the same kind of input and they haven't got it to give. They do tend to look at all nurses as being the same. It is hard for them because they are here for 1 month and there are 100 and some of us. There is no way they're going to know who knows what they're doing and who doesn't. So you really get it from both ends. You have some intern trying to teach you your business and you just want to punch his lights out. Then you have another one who's going to a new grad saying, "What do you think I should do about this?"

In our data, we found that the classic nurse-doctor game was far more likely to occur between the inexperienced resident and the expert nurse. The more enlightened and liberated exchanges occurred between expert nurse clinicians and clinically expert attending physicians. With clinical expertise, the dialogue is a lively discussion of qualitative distinctions situated by the concerns of the particular patient. The exchange does not deteriorate into a confused power play with the decision resting on rank, but rather the decision is weighted by the clinical issues at hand.

Physicians may develop some expectations about the kind and quality of information they receive from nurses. An expert nurse provides clinical data to the physician, ordering it according to relevance, salience, and the interrelatedness of the facts. Moreover, the expert nurse knows by the physician's response whether she or he has "heard" the clinical story with the correct weighting and significance. If the nurse is surprised by the physician's response, he or she can ask directly why the physician is not worried about the same thing that he or she is worried about.

In the following excerpt, a breakdown occurs because expected communication patterns were not followed. A beginning nurse, working nights, is assigned to the care of a man dying of AIDS with multiple system problems including DIC, ARDS, septicemia, a pneumothorax, bladder infection and renal failure. He was bucking the ventilator, so had been pavulonized. The family had wanted everything done.

It was a lack of knowledge on my part. When I got his blood gas back, even though it looked similar to the previous ones, I should have noted that this man was in metabolic acidosis. As the night went on, I felt really uncomfortable with him. Just looking at him, saying this man just looks like he's going to die any moment now. You know, his heart was taching at 150s. His blood pressure was OK. He was breathing real fast in the 28–30s, and I guess they had done gases before that and they had said that was fine, satisfactory. Well, I was uncomfortable. So by 5:00 AM I had done gases and I called and told the doctor that I was really uncomfortable, that this man didn't look good. I gave him the gases and I gave him my assessment. And he didn't want anything done about it. His neuro status, he was getting a little more lethargic, his blood pressure was dropping, his urinary output was real low, his gases were not looking so good. I guess they were the same. The 7:00 crew came on and the nurse who had come on had taken care of this patient now for a couple days, so she knew him too. And he was being dialyzed and she pointed out, "Yes, he's in metabolic acidosis. He should have been dialyzed a lot sooner than he's going to be." You know dialysis, usually they come at 6:00. He should have been dialyzed a lot earlier.

But I gave the little scenario to the doctor, two of them, and they didn't do anything about it . . . the head nurse [*who later counseled the nurse about this incident*] said that the doctor had felt that I hadn't given him enough information when I had called and I had stressed something different . . . than the metabolic acidosis. So he didn't catch it.

The physician received a report from an inexperienced nurse, and being accustomed to a nurse's report shaped by the subtleties of sequencing and which points out saliences, he missed the relevant points. The inexperienced nurse does not know how or when to present the most salient clinical facts to the physician because he or she has not yet learned to weigh the clinical issues. Thus, an inexperienced nurse's report to the physician will most often be factual with almost equal weight given to all the "facts." The inexperienced nurse, unsure of her own clinical knowledge, and feeling dependent on the authority of the physician, doesn't recognize when the report has been misunderstood. In the above example, the inexperienced nurse was unable to read from the physician's response that he had not picked up on the abnormal blood gas report; instead, she doubted her own judgment that something should have been done, and so didn't push the issue. This breakdown in expected communication patterns resulted in the patient not receiving timely treatment.

Inexperience on the part of the physician also contributes significantly to conflicts between disciplines. Nurses in the study repeatedly discussed situations in which their own clinical knowledge was overlooked or ignored by inexperienced physicians who wanted to claim superior status by virtue of greater education and presumed social mandate.

> I think one thing they don't realize is that I've been in the NICU for 10 years and I'm there for at least 40 hours a week. They come once a year for 6–10 stints, 3 years in a row. When I was in graduate school, I spent 17 weeks with a resident during my internship, making calls with the doctors, so I also know some of that aspect. And so, then to have them tell me in so many words that I don't know what I'm talking about can sometimes make me irate.

In the following clinical episode, the frustration of the nurse in working with inexperienced physicians is apparent:

> I was taking care of a 39-year-old Samoan lady who had a renal transplant, then rejected it, and then got a huge necrotizing fasciitis in her wound. She was on the ventilator and developed pneumos [*pneumothoraxes*] and had chest tubes. The residents came in one afternoon and wanted to pull the chest tubes on one side and proceeded to get ready to do it without any warning, didn't allow me to give her any pain medicine. And then, because it was early July, I don't remember exactly, they were teaching. They were doing it because there were new residents there, they were describing it in the most graphic terms. They might as well have said they were going to pull the garden hose out of this lady's chest, because that's what it sounded like. It made *me* squeamish, and I've seen hundreds of tubes pulled out. So I finally interrupted them and said, "When can I give her some pain medication? When are you going to do this; she really needs it." "Oh, she doesn't need any pain medication." It really irritated me; they were both young, probably younger than me and probably never had a chest tube pulled out. They probably had no idea that it hurt, and it was like, why don't you realize this is a *person* laying in this bed. You shouldn't be standing beside her bed and describing in graphic detail what you're going to do to pull this chest tube out, much less not give her any pain medicine. This lady was very stoic. You had to anticipate her pain. In a Samoan culture, that's a culturally based thing, so she never would have said if she needed something anyway. This was a lady who was getting 300 micrograms of fentanyl for every dressing change. So she needed a lot of pain medication. And she would lay there and not say a word. Some patients will stiffen up; she wouldn't even do that. Finally, I got them to tell me when they were going to do it, so I gave her the pain medication. Then I proceeded to get ready to do her dressing change

after they pulled the chest tube, and they were going to do it with no sterile gloves, no nothing. And she had this huge wound. And true, it wasn't clean per se; it wasn't like it was sterile, but I felt like pulling gloves out of a box on the other side of the room. She had very resistant Pseudomonas in her lungs that could have contaminated those gloves. At least they could have used sterile gloves. The difference between clean and sterile in that room might have been significant.

The nurse wasn't successful in getting young residents to stop talking in the room. She gave pain medication, without "asking their permission." When asked how she convinced them that they needed to use sterile gloves the nurse responded . . .

"I think I said, `What size gloves do you need so you can do [it right]?'"

In this situation, the nurse knew the patient, knew her usual response to pain, and knew what was needed to try to control the pain. She showed a grasp of the patient's situation that was overlooked and ignored by the medical staff. Because of the power afforded even beginning residents, they could decide to proceed to do the painful procedure despite the advice of the nurse who knew this patient and knew what she needed. The nurse also understood the risks involved in contaminating an open wound of this person who already had compromised immune function. Through an indirect approach ("What size gloves would you like?") the nurse was able to assure the patient some protection from further contamination. In these circumstances, the nurse covers over her well-founded rationale for suggesting an appropriate course of action. To expound on the reason for her suggestions may call too much attention to the fact that she's making a suggestion. However, this covering over may contribute to the continuing perception of physicians that nurses have little role in decisionmaking, and little scientific basis for their suggestions. In this situation, the doctor-nurse game continues, due, in part, to the extreme breakdown caused by the physicians' inexperience.

The inexperienced physician who has been socialized in medical school to believe that she or he is the "captain of the ship" and must have the leadership authority cannot tell when he or she is being harassed by trivial suggestions or when she or he is missing the boat, overlooking important details, or paying too much attention to the abstract, general science and not enough to this particular patient's responses. Munday (1990), in her response to Stein et al. (1990), expresses well the dilemma of the new physician trying to assert the authority of the role based upon formal education:

As a young female physician, perhaps I am more sensitive to this issue of hierarchy. Some nurses resent receiving orders from a younger colleague and offer resistance at every turn. I am tired of defending literally every order I write. Question me when it is warranted, show me my mistakes when I have made them but give me credit for my years of college, medical school, and postgraduate and residency training. Also, remember in the eye of the patient and my colleagues, I am ultimately responsible for your actions as well as my own. In return, I will value your ideas and listen when you have a grievance. I will view you as an ally. (p. 201)

No doubt fledgling physicians and nurses receive more than their share of advice. Once credibility is lost in the clinical situation, it is hard to regain it. But the way out is not to insist on authority based on education and credentials alone, but rather to be a clinical learner open to the issues in the particular situation. Physician and nurse allies are needed in order for fledglings from both disciplines to learn from experience. The grim truth is that there is no *real* delegation of responsibility in a patient's death, or when a terrible clinical mistake is made. No professional can morally or legally shrug off the human responsibility to use their knowledge to the best of their ability in the situation. The worth and dignity of the work require that the nurse and physician draw on their own and other's clinical wisdom, expertise and science when a patient's life is at stake, regardless of the social conflict that may ensue.

COVERING OVER THE HUMAN SIDE OF DISEASE, SUFFERING, PAIN, FEAR, AND CONFLICT

As Stein et al. (1990) and response letters indicate it is a mistake to assign all the caring and compassion function to nurses and all the instrumental functions of cure to physicians. The current commodification of health care serves to diminish the relationship between providers and clients to a mere economic exchange. The healing function of all health care workers breaks down without care and compassion. There is no cure without care. But the culturally and socially mandated healing roles of nurses and physicians are, in fact, different. Nurses are culturally expected to attend to alleviation of vulnerability and to coaching patients toward recovery of social and physical integrity. Patients seek help from nurses in practicing their "medical questions" and in framing their complaints prior to asking physicians. Nurses are socially and culturally more approachable than physicians.

In this project, for example, we found that nurses frequently assumed the role of translator for families once the physician left the scene. They coached family questions in the presence of the medical team, and/or interpreted into medical terms the family's concerns:

> A lot of the attending physicians have a kind of abrupt manner. "Well, this is the way it is and I think you should do this," and the families say "Well, OK, you're the doctor and I won't question your judgment." But they do have questions, and I ask them, "Are you wondering about anything?" A lot of the time, they do not know the questions to ask. So when the families come in, it's very important to discuss what is going on. And what these tubes are, and these lines, and it's OK to touch them. By having the family get close to the patient physically, then they start asking more and more questions. . . . When the doctor is around, I'll say, Oh excuse me, they have questions here. And if they can't ask it . . . then you facilitate that. "Well, are you referring to this?" They'll say, "Yes, this is what I'm talking about." Getting them to communicate is the hard thing to do. But then they feel like they are participating and they care, too, which is important.

This social and cultural distinction usually works well as long as the healing role does not drop out of either profession and as long as the communication between nurses and physicians works.

Physicians and medical students alike are willing to grant decision-making authority to nurses in certain aspects of care: psychosocial aspects of care, discharge planning, assessing what a patient can or can't do physically, dealing with the family, and evaluating a patient's abilities to perform life functions (Prescott et al., 1987; Webster, 1985). Prescott et al. (1987) reported that there was a general lack of value accorded to decisions within the domain of nursing. One physician reflected a view, apparently echoed by others, that "in something like how to feed or manage a depressed patient, if I don't think it makes a difference, I think it is important to let a nurse choose, to give her respect in the management" (p. 59). The view is that nurses have decision-making authority over aspects of care that don't matter.

Nursing judgment, in the view of these physicians, then relates to the impact of the illness and treatment on the patient's daily life, his psychological state, and his personal values. Pfifferling (1981) referred to medicine's selective inattention to these aspects of illness, or the redefining of patients' complaints only into biophysical derangements, as "medicocentrism." Of medicocentrism, Barnard (1988) writes:

> This tendency to view the world of health care through the providers' eyes is not surprising. Medicine and its allied disciplines in the humanities and social sciences have long been afflicted with this disturbance of vision. For most of medicine's modern history, physicians have distrusted patients' views of their own experience. The scientific physician's goal has been to replace the patient's subjective language of distress with data from the labo-

ratory; to translate idiosyncratic or culture-bound expressions of discomfort into the supposedly universal categories of biomedicine. (pp. 89–90)

Given this understanding of the assumptions underlying medical practice and the physician's interpretation of what constitutes the domain of nursing practice, it is not surprising that nurses find themselves at odds with physicians when there is conflict between the medical plan of care and the nursing plan of care. Nurses can do what they wish, as long as it does not cross the boundaries of or interfere with medical practice.

Both professions suffer to some degree from medicocentrism and from the Cartesian suspicion that seeks to determine the "validity" of the patient's complaint. Are the complaints related to "real" pathology? If they are not "real," then the respect and attention to the suffering may be withheld or relegated to psychiatrists or alternative health care practitioners (Benner & Wrubel, 1989; Cassel, 1989; Lock & Gordon, 1988; Lowenberg, 1989).

THE SKILL OF NEGOTIATION

Negotiation between physicians and nurses is a skill acquired through experience. From nurses' accounts, negotiation clearly rests on: (1) having a strong clinical grasp and the judgment that this situation needs to be attended to; (2) knowing the physician and having developed a relationship of trust; and (3) skill in making the case.

Clinical Grasp

Nurses learn through experience, often in difficult circumstances of extreme breakdown, that they should trust their clinical sense and be more aggressive in negotiating with the physician for a different management plan. They also learn from experience what situations require immediate attention, which can wait, how long they can wait, and what the risks are of either pursuing physician intervention or not. Here is a conversation among a group of nurses about weighing the pros and cons of pushing through the line of authority to get medical action.

Nurse 1: You're always confronting people, whether it be other nurses or physicians even. It seems like that's acceptable here. You certainly get the people who say, "Do it because I told you to do it." The hierarchy of the authority line here is certainly more open to communication than in some other areas. Once again, you get to the situation where if you question a physician why they're doing that, they always have the out of saying "Because I'm writing the orders, and you follow the orders." That's the way the old structure was, and it's going to be a long time before it changes.

Nurse 2: But if you do that, and you get that kind of response, you always have the opportunity to ask your colleague or your charge nurse, "Is this important enough that I should carry it any further? Or is this something that I should just do?"

Nurse 1: Do you have enough energy to pursue it? I think it is self-motivated.

Nurse 3: I always think you pick your battles, though. And if you're argumentative and you're resistive to everything, what's the point?

Choosing one's battles is an important judgment on the part of nurses. They must balance the immediate risk to the patient, and the possibilities they have for being successful in making the case. There are also long-term risks; if not for this particular patient, then for the nurse's relationship with the physician and her credibility when future issues surface.

Sometimes it is obvious to the nurse that when the risk for the patient of doing what the physician wants is not great, and the likelihood of successfully making a case is not good, it is better not to pursue it further. The nurse in the following excerpt describes her disagreement with the physician that a newborn needed bili lights. Her assessment of the physician was that his primary concern wasn't about the baby, but rather that it was a "power thing:"

Nurse 1: This physician felt [that the bili lights could not be turned off since the bili's not below 5.] I left the bili lights on because it wasn't worth fighting about.

Nurse 2: It does depend on what the issue is. You know if they [the physicians] are just being a stinker.

Nurse 1: Yeah, you know. In that case, it didn't matter with me, it wasn't any big deal that the bili lights were left on; it clinically isn't going to affect the baby tremendously in any way other than he has to wear little eye patches and pretend he's laying in Mazatlan, but there are other situations where the impact will be much greater.

Nurse 2: It takes judgment, though, and time to figure out what argument is worth fighting for and what argument isn't worth fighting over in the long run.

Knowing the Physician

Negotiating with a physician also rests on a firm relationship between the nurse and physician, in which communication patterns have been established, there is at least tacit recognition of one another's abilities, and there is a sense of mutual trust and respect. In teaching hospitals, where physician turnover is rapid, particularly among first- and second-year residents, the possibilities for developing this kind of relationship are limited. In these circumstances, nurses express great frustration when they have to prove themselves competent before physicians will take their recommendations seriously. While they don't necessarily expect that the physicians will just do what they suggest, they do wish for a serious discussion in which their clinical understanding of the particular situation can be explored, and different treatment options examined.

In contrast, when experienced nurses and attending physicians have worked together for extended periods of time, negotiating clinical knowledge is not such a challenge. The following excerpt is particularly rich in its illustration of nursing judgment in indeterminate clinical situations. The nurse is describing a premature baby who began to show early signs of deterioration. She describes how she recognized the signs, and how she attempted, unsuccessfully, to get medical attention for the infant. Finally, a more experienced nurse knew exactly how to make the case with this physician. Here's how the story unfolds:

Nurse 1: I had a baby who was about 26 or 27 weeks, who had been doing well for about 2 weeks. He had open ductus. The difference between the way he looked at 9:00 and the way he looked at 11:00 was very dramatic. I was at that point really concerned about what was going to happen next. There are a lot of complications with patent ductus. It is not just in itself, but the fact that it causes a lot of other things. I was really concerned that the baby was starting to show symptoms of all of them.

Int: Just for 2 hours?

Nurse 1: Yes, you look at this kid because you know this kid and you know what he looked like 2 hours ago. It is a dramatic difference to you, but it's hard to describe that to someone in words. There are clusters of things that go wrong . . . The kid is more lethargic, paler, his stomach is bigger, he's not tolerating his feedings, his chem strip might be a little strange. The baby's urine output goes down, they sound like they're more in failure. At this time I think I had been in the unit 2 or 3 years. I was really starting to feel like I knew what was going on but I wasn't as good at throwing my weight in a situation like that. And I talked to a woman I knew who has more experience and I said, "Look at this kid" and I told her my story and she goes "OK." Rounds started shortly after that and she walks up to the attending and very quietly sidles up and says, "You know, Carol's really worried about this kid." She told him the story, and said "Reminds me about this kid we had 3 weeks ago," and he said "Oh." Everything stops, he gets out the stethoscope and listens to the kid, examines the kid and he says, "Call the surgeons." It's that kind of thing where we knew what had to be done. There was no time to be waiting around. He is the only one that can make that decision. It was a case that we had presented to other physicians who should have made the case, but didn't. We are able in just two sentences to make that case to the attending because he knew exactly what we were talking about. . . . And this physician relies at least half the time on anecdotal medicine. So that was one thing. The other thing was that this particular nurse knew what she was doing. He knew that she knew what she was doing and she also practiced a lot of anecdotal medicine. So between the two of them she knew what button to push.

Here the nurse was contrasting a scientific rational approach to "anecdotal medicine." While in many instances, nurses may be criticized for this practice, in this situation it may have been the only approach that would have worked with this attending physician. By providing an exemplar from their shared practice, the nurse helped the physician to immediately grasp the current situation in the same way that the nurse did. Stein and associates (1990) have suggested that using anecdotes is a way of avoiding direct suggestions in order to maintain the rules of the game. In this situation, it appears that the use of an anecdote was a deliberate effort to provide a frame of reference for the physician.

Skill in Making a Case

Expert nurses take on as their responsibility the task of making a case—for example, persuading the physician that a change in therapy is needed. In actual practice, this is not framed in a quest for more power, or to usurp the physician's legally and socially mandated role to provide medical diagnoses and treatment, but rather in terms of getting adequate attention paid to patients' responses to treatment and adequate changes made in therapies that are not working well for the patient. Making a case can be a particularly difficult task in situations that call for indeterminate clinical knowledge, where the quest for certainty in medical decisions cannot be attained through objective medical data, and where the judgment call is based on knowing the particular patient's responses to therapy rather than on abstract scientific facts about the properties of the drug. Nurses frequently talk about avoiding open conflict that may deteriorate into power plays and interfere with making clear and accurate judgments about patient needs.

There are circumstances, of course, where the physician recognizes the nurse's expertise, and the nurse can say, simply and directly, "I believe that this patient needs something different medically." But there are many other circumstances in which the nurse must find other ways to capture the physician's attention or in some way alter his or her perception of the situation. Expert nurses recognize this as an important part of their practice and feel that they have failed the patient when they are unsuccessful in making a case.

A variety of approaches for making a case have been described in the literature (Damrosch, Sullivan, & Haldeman, 1987) and appear in our data. The first approach is coaching the physician by asking questions. For example:

> Sometimes you are saying "Explain your reasoning behind this to me" without saying "This is a dumb order," which is tempting to say sometimes.

The question prompts a perceptive physician to reconsider his or her choice, and it may also provide information to the experienced nurse about whether she or he should pursue the problem further, picking this as a battle, or going up the ladder. The second approach involves coaching the physician by pointing out facts that contradict or contraindicate a chosen plan, or that will lead to an obvious plan of treatment; for example:

> When I came in on Saturday night, they weren't giving enough osmotic diuretics. This is not a nursing judgment call, but it's certainly something that a nurse who would take care of these patients would know, that the serum osmolarity is only 280 and you can bump it up to 310 or 320. And you can't say "I'm going to give 25 more grams of Manitol" but you can certainly tell the physician "the CO_2 is 19 and his osmolarity is only 280, maybe we should do something else here."

The third approach is to frequently remind the physician of the continuing changes in the patient condition. For example, one nurse referred to this practice as "nudging:"

> And it's that kind of nudging that you do all day long every day, if you have the experience to do it. And it's just that exact situation that I think is the difference between people who have the experience and know exactly what you need to do and how you need to nudge it and who you need to nudge, and people who say "She told me that in this case you know you give the manitol and we're giving it." And you're going to go back 3 or 4 or 5 times until you get the answer you want.

When all else fails in persuading the primary physician that the patient needs a change in medical therapy or in altering his or her perception of the situation, nurses may resort to going up the ladder—in teaching hospitals from the first year resident, to the senior resident to the attending; in private hospitals, from the attending to the chief of the service or director of the unit. Expert nurses again see this practice as part of their responsibility; one nurse explains:

> If you don't get a good answer, you're expected to do that. Sometimes the intern or the junior, whoever you jump over, gets a little upset. But if it's serious enough, I'll go to the top."

Another nurse expresses a common view when discussing her decision to go up the ladder:

> "It's a balance—just not wanting to step on toes, yet wanting to be sure that the patient gets the adequate treatment. It's something that you kind of get a feel for. It's like "I can wait" or "I can't wait" or "If I step on toes, I'm sorry but my goal is the care of this patient and it needs to be addressed. And if your toes get stepped on, too bad."

As described by nurses in our study, finding ways to negotiate with the physician does not rest on a context-free set of strategies, but rather on a deep understanding of the clinical situation, the physician's likely response, and the physician's usual pattern of responses; moreover, the skillful negotiation requires reading the physician's demeanor and responses, and modifying the approach accordingly, all in an effort to help the physician share the same perspective, and enter into a discussion of the best treatment options.

SUMMARY AND CONCLUSIONS

A central focus of the narrative accounts by experienced nurses, particularly those practicing at the proficient and expert levels, was negotiating patient care decisions with physicians. Experienced nurses feel enormous responsibility for what might ordinarily be viewed as medical practice; when nurses have a strong clinical sense that a patient is not responding to treatment as expected, they view it as their personal responsibility to persuade the physician to change the treatment plan. Often their clinical sense is based on knowing the particular patient's usual pattern of responses and a tacit understanding of the usual course for patients like this, rather than solely on scientifically based predictions or on objective clinical evidence. Just as these clinical judgments are based on situated understanding, so is skillful negotiation with physicians. Breakdowns in expected communication patterns occur when either the nurse or physician is inexperienced and unskilled in soliciting and/or reading the other's response.

Many writers have attributed the continued problems in physician-nurse collaboration to a failure in our educational systems. They argue that improved education of both medical and nursing students would promote mutual understanding of the practices of medicine and nursing and thereby enhance possibilities for collaboration (Darbyshire, 1987; Mechanic & Aiken, 1982; Webster, 1985). Webster (1985), in an extensive field study of 60 medical students, found that the vast majority seemed to assume that, "in practice, nursing is essentially a lower level of the practice of medicine or entirely dependent on the physician's instigation and supervision, rather than a separate role characterized by variable degrees of overlap or intersection with the physician's role." (p. 316). Webster also noted that "even when both medical students and nurses were at the patient's bedside, they often carried out activities in a parallel fashion without acknowledging each other's presence" (p. 315). Darbyshire (1987) commented: "This is a sobering thought: that the extent of our ability to work together has risen to the level of parallel play exhibited by toddlers" (p. 34).

More recently, reports on medical and nursing education reform emphasize interdisciplinary education (NLN, 1993; Pew Health Professions Commission, 1991) as central to improved health care. It is clear that early significant interactions between nursing and medical students are important for laying down patterns of interdisciplinary collaboration. Recognition of the role of clinical knowledge and knowing the patient in both medical and nursing care decisions is central to developing meaningful collaborative educational experiences. Opportunities should be provided for both medical and nursing students to participate in patient care conferences, where the contributions of nurses and physicians to medical decision making is explicit, and where areas of ambiguity, conflict, or disagreement are surfaced and explored. Both medical and nursing education could benefit from greater clarity about the relationship between the two disciplines in patient care—nursing responsibility in monitoring patient responses to therapy and managing changes in therapy, in helping patients and families cope with changes necessitated by illness, and in serving as advocate and interpreter for patients and their families.

Over a decade ago, Mechanic and Aiken (1982) recommended a number of changes in practice settings to support interdisciplinary collaboration, recommendations echoed more recently by Fagin (1992), and dramatically supported in our data. Specifically, they suggested that:

1.   nurses should have greater authority to act on matters "within their spheres of competence" such as modifying medications when indicated, including dosage and mode of administration, changing special diets, and contributing to decisions regarding time and place of hospital discharge; and

2.   greater attention should be paid to clearly differentiating nurses by experience and education, so that those more competent in handling complex judgments are clearly identified" (Mechanic & Aiken, 1982, p. 749). Wandel and Pike (1991) recently reported the outcomes of a unit dedicated to the development of positive collaborative relationships, in which physicians and nurses develop mutual trust and respect, an appreciation for the interdependence of the two practices, and an alliance between the two disciplines that enhances patient care.

Chapter 12

IMPLICATIONS FOR BASIC NURSING EDUCATION

Our work on this project has inevitably led to lively discussions about its implications for our day-to-day practice as teachers of nursing. Although we did not study educational practices per se, we believe that this study has profound implications for the education of our basic nursing students. First, the understanding of professional practice advanced by this work challenges some of the very basic assumptions which undergird our educational practices. Through our discussions, we have explicated some of these assumptions and reevaluated them in light of our new understandings of nursing practice. The effect has been a transformation in our thinking about nursing education and educational practices. Second, our work with narratives for this study has opened up new possibilities for their use in undergraduate education. And finally, our study of the new graduate group helped us identify clinical learning issues which seem to be underattended in basic educational programs, and which require some further exploration and adjustment.

ASSUMPTIONS CHALLENGED BY THIS STUDY

The Relationship Between Theory and Practice

In our traditional approaches to nursing education, we have assumed that practice is the instrumental application of research-based theory to the solution of patient care problems. The direction between theory and practice is predominately one-way—theory guides practice. The students are taught theory in the classroom; then clinical experiences are sought which help them apply this theory to the care of their patients (sometimes with great difficulty, since available practice situations seldom correspond directly with what is taught in "theory" classes).

Our research has pointed out that the relationship between theory and practice is far more complex than the traditional assumptions and educational practices suggest (see Chapter 2). Theory is extremely important for guiding the beginning clinician to the right region—for example, to know *that* he or she should evaluate a patient for fluid in the lungs or crepitus. Theory is also important for helping nurses learn to expect certain kinds of responses when addressing illness, suffering, and comfort issues—for example, that a grieving family may show a range of emotions, from rage to complete denial. Such theory, however, by definition an abstraction, falls short of the mark in describing the particular situation and in guiding even the beginning clinician's response. Practice is also guided by attention to individual patient and family responses, how clinical problems are manifested in particular patients, and the human concerns of illness and suffering, by understanding particular patients' and families' issues, concerns, and ways of coping.

This correspondence view of the nature of clinical practice obscures several significant aspects of clinical learning. Clearly students do need experience in applying theory to practice, recognizing the limitations of theory in predicting particular patients' responses or specifying nursing actions. What is less apparent from this view are the limits of formalism— the possibility that theoretical language can ever adequately describe the concrete manifestations and qualitative distinctions that are central to clinical understanding.

The limits of abstract theory were evident in all levels of practice, and nursing students can be prepared to experience the support and the gaps in support that theory will supply their practice. In beginning practice, advanced beginners instruct us that the central dilemma is in recognizing the concrete manifestations of syndromes and conditions that they have learned in the abstract. Competent nurses experience the crisis of recognizing that formal and abstract knowledge provides precious little guidance in working out a plan or agenda for the immediate care of a particular patient. Proficient nurses evidence a decline in their reliance on the calculative rationality, and begin to take up the situation more intuitively than as a problem to be solved with selected abstract knowledge. With openness and willingness to learn from continued experience, experts practice intuitively rather than through rational calculation in both their understanding and management of the patient's situation. Students need experience to help fill out theory and to learn to make qualitative distinctions. They need experience working side by side with an experienced nurse who can point out saliences, nuances, and qualitative distinctions.

What is also obscured by this view is learning the clinical practice for which there is no formal theory, what has been defined by the Dreyfuses (Chapter 2) as the tact of nursing, or as existential skill, or as skillful ethical comportment (9). Narrative accounts from nurses at all levels of practice point to learning issues that can be resolved only through learning from practice, rather than through filling out or applying formal theory in practice. The knowledge of nursing practice includes large domains of knowledge that have traditionally been in the private, rather than public, discourse, worked out in the practice, but not well articulated either within or outside the discipline. These domains include knowledge of caring practices, personhood, world, care of the body and embodied skills during recovery, comfort, safety, and health promotion practices. Much of this knowledge is relational and contextual. Students need experience in practice to articulate this knowledge in the public world, while attending to and preserving the relational and contextual nature of the knowledge.

Nurses in this study have an elaborate discourse on the right kind and level of involvement with patients and families. They tell stories of being overinvolved, or overidentified, so that the ability to offer alternative perspectives, or even offer support as an interested "other" are lost. From these nurses' perspective, this is clearly getting it "wrong." Examples of leaping in, taking over, and making the patient and family excessively dependent were retrospectively considered misguided. Situations where nurses felt good about their skill of involvement were told in terms of being in tune with the patient's or family's needs and wishes, recognizing early warning signs of harm or danger, facilitating the next step in recovery, understanding and coaching, and being able in some situations to just be present in silence and tears. There is no way to learn the skill of involvement without experientially learning when help is helpful, intrusive, or disruptive. Similar kinds of learning issues include coping with human suffering and death or personal anxieties about doing harm; negotiating clinical knowledge with other disciplines; and developing the skill of staying open to a clinical situation, without being overwhelmed or closing down prematurely. These are all existential caring and coping skills.

In our educational settings we have long taught the power of critical thinking, judgment, distancing, and disengaged reasoning. We have all but ignored the centrality of emotional engagement to learning, thinking and being with others. There are traditional reasons, even prudent reasons, for this emphasis on disengaged critical reasoning and silence on relational skills and engaged reasoning. It is easier to teach critical thinking, disengagement, and judgment than it is to teach openness, being with, dwelling, engagement, and discerning qualitative distinctions. Adjudication and arguing about what is right are heady intellectual activities. Furthermore, we depend on the primacy of trust, involvement, and openness in our most basic and primary relationships. We expect our students to come with these qualities from their families of origin and life experience. And as educators, we explain that we cannot "teach" these things. But our reasons for emphasizing critical powers also have to do with our instrumental and information-giving view of what it means to "teach."

The skills of involvement, when taught, are taught as corrective "boundary work." The hazards of overinvolvement, hyper-responsibility, and overidentification are likely to be emphasized, while an embarrassed silence may develop around incidents where a helping relationship with patients and families was positive and even healing. We intuitively know that we mustn't burden students with the expectation that they always enter their nurse-patient relationships in this way. We defend and protect our students from unrealistic expectations. Instinctively, we know that since the skill of involvement has to do with our ways of being in the world, we cannot and must not ask another to *be* a certain way, or enter relationships in certain ways. Human involvement is not an area that can be legislated or "behaviorally controlled."

But this does not mean that we are bound to educational silence and embarrassment about advancing involvement skills. We can tell our stories and listen to others' stories about being in relationship to others. We can treat our existential skills of relating as sacred and respect them as ways of being while entering into narratives of learning and dialogue about them. What we are suggesting is that there are skills of involvement, relational ethics, and even caring practices for teachers too (Phillips & Benner, 1994).

We do not need to instrumentalize all our educational efforts, nor do we need to make the oppositional swing to pure expressivism, subjectivity, or emotivism. By focusing on caring practices and relationships with our students and patients, we can teach ourselves and our students to articulate narratives of learning how to be attuned to others. We can make the qualitative distinction between using rituals and routines to open up safe caring spaces with patients and using standardized strategies that create a false justice of treating everyone the same. In our practice and our concrete relationships, we can identify qualitative distinctions between caring, coercing, controlling, and being sentimental. We can increase the safety and capacity for being open and having the moral courage to learn from our mistakes.

The Nature of Clinical Judgment

As pointed out in Chapter 1, the prevailing conception of clinical judgment in nursing is the diagnosis-treatment model, which relies on explicit identification of patients' deficits and deliberation on and selection of treatment options most likely to eliminate these deficits. It is assumed in this view that disengaged reasoning is always more reliable than practical, engaged reasoning.

We have found in our work that disengaged, analytic thinking, that is, standing back from a situation, is a useful strategy for the beginner who is flooded with anxiety or emotion. Our work also shows that, with experience, nurses become more involved, rather than more detached; they grasp the meaning of the situation directly, rather than through analytic thinking. Knowing the patient, his usual patterns of responses, and knowing him as a person in embodied, direct ways are prominent aspects of nurses' clinical judgments. Detached analytic reasoning is needed in cases of breakdown, where direct apprehension doesn't occur, or when the nurse notices that vague, uneasy feeling of not having the right clinical grasp.

The technical-rational model of professional practice holds that practice is the instrumental application of research-based knowledge and scientific theory to the problems in practice. Clinical learning, on this view, is supported by creating opportunities for the direct application of theory to practice. The translation of this conception of professional practice and clinical learning to the design of undergraduate educational experiences has resulted in two dominant practices in nursing education:

1.   the use of total patient care experiences, in which the student is responsible for planning and implementing care for one or two patients, and where the patients are chosen, to the extent possible, for the application of classroom learning to their care; and

2.   extensive reliance on nursing care planning, in the form of the academic care plan, to help students learn application of theoretical knowledge to a particular patient situation.

The care plan is additionally used to support the development of clinical judgment skill, both in planning for and anticipating likely events in patient care, and in thinking analytically about clinical problems and their resolution.

The underlying conception of clinical practice and clinical learning has its place in the undergraduate nursing curriculum as do these two dominant educational practices. But our expanded understanding of clinical judgment suggests that the range of clinical learning experiences for our undergraduate students must be greatly augmented beyond the dominant practices. Clearly both of these practices contribute to students' developing skill in recognizing relevant theory and its applicability to a particular clinical situation; they encourage students to prepare for their clinical learning experiences by helping them set up expectations of what they will encounter, and by guiding conscious, deliberative, and theoretically based planning for possible events. But their utility, perhaps, ends there. (To our knowledge, there have been no studies of the effectiveness of total patient care experiences or academic nursing care plans in helping students learn even these fundamental aspects of clinical thinking.)

Moreover, there may be unintended consequences of overuse of either or both of these approaches. Reliance on total patient care for the majority of clinical experiences may provide students with some diversity in patients, particularly if the patients are chosen to provide students with the opportunity to apply the theoretical learning of the week. It may also serve to reinforce a strong value in nursing for care of the whole patient, a value that many fear would be lost if we had students do only certain components of care. Until recently, total patient care also mirrored the "real" practice of nursing under a primary nursing model; of course, this is no longer true, in light of the changes in acute care nursing practice buttressed by "restructuring" and allocation of nursing care to unlicensed assistive personnel. But, clinical learning experiences which focus solely on the provision of total patient care reduce the opportunities for other kinds of learning experiences—for example, seeing many patients within a particular patient population, and learning qualitative distinctions among the clinical manifestations of their disease; or having in-depth experience with one patient population or even one patient over time, which provides for other kinds of clinical knowledge development.

Reliance on the nursing care plan as an instructional device assumes that it helps the students in analytic thinking. Moreover, at one time we assumed that writing nursing care plans helped students learn to personalize care. The ready availability of standardized care plans, which busy students often tend to adopt wholesale, mitigates against any possibility of individualized care. Moreover, the frequent requirement that care plans be completed before care is actually provided, and sometimes before the patient is actually seen, as a means of preparing for practice, convey the implicit message that the most important knowledge for patient care decisions is that which can be applied to the practice from textbooks, more than that which can be learned from the patient, his story, and his particular manifestations of the condition. In addition, such practice overemphasizes planning and anticipation, perhaps limiting the possibility of being open to a clinical situation as it unfolds. Our information management and classification strategies of listing nursing diagnoses and nursing interventions must not be misconstrued as thinking in action (i.e., engaged clinical reasoning in transitions) or knowing and relating to patients and families.

While we would not expect basic students to become proficient or expert at engaged practical reasoning as new entrants to the practice, we do believe it is possible to begin to cultivate these skills, even within the context of the basic baccalaureate program. Specific suggestions for restructuring some aspects of undergraduate nursing education are offered at the end of this chapter.

The Separation of Thought from Emotion

In our traditional approaches to education, we have carried on with the Cartesian tradition of separating mind from body, and separating the objective, observable and measurable from the subjective, inner experience. By the nearly universal adoption of the behavioral model of education in nursing, we have directed our teaching only toward those outcomes which could be expressed behaviorally and measured objectively. We have gone to great extremes to write outcomes for programs and courses and sometimes even for weekly or daily behaviors. In these outcomes we carefully separate the cognitive from the affective from the psychomotor, but acknowledge that each are important only as long as we can formalize and "objectify" all that we intend to teach. Although this model has recently come under harsh criticism (Bevis & Watson, 1989; Diekelmann, 1993; National League for Nursing [NLN], 1988, 1989, 1990, 1991), the cognitive aspects of nursing practice continue to receive great emphasis. For example, occupying a central position in the nursing educational reform movement is the teaching of critical thinking (see NLN, 1993; NLN, 1992). There is little doubt that this is an important educational aim, but caution is also clearly warranted as we go about defining what we mean by critical thinking, deciding how we can measure the attainment of this outcome and considering learning activities that support its development.

The burgeoning literature on critical thinking continues the rational tradition in which anything other than logical thought processes, especially emotion, is suspect. That emotion and thought are mutually constituted is not a view recognized in most models of critical thinking. As Walters has pointed out,

> Conventional critical thinking mainstreamed in college and university curricula claims to be a technique that schools students in the rational justification of beliefs by providing a set of rules with which to analyze propositional arguments. The method it defends is best described as analytic reductionism . . . [In the professional literature] most educators, psycholo-

gists and philosophers who champion the critical thinking method as a top educational priority do so because they identify it, either implicitly or explicitly with rational thinking. (1990, pp. 451–452)

In nursing, with a few notable exceptions (e.g., Bevis & Watson, 1989; Ford & Profetto-McGrath, 1994) critical thinking has been equated with clinical judgment. The concern is not that critical thinking is an unimportant skill, because even in its most narrow definition of analytic reductionism, it is. Rather, the concern is that both the behavioral model and the current emphasis on critical thinking, with their attendant assumptions, overlook and in some ways cover over the possibility of embodied knowing, the role of emotion in skilled judgment, the skill of involvement, and the role of narrative in understanding a patient's experiences.

Expectations for Professional Role Acquisition

Often, the set given nurses in undergraduate education is that they graduate as full-fledged, independent, autonomous practitioners. In our educational practices we strive to have students adopt a responsible, self-reliant, professional stance. The assumption that nurses are fully ready to practice by the time they finish nursing education probably reflects the difficulty within the culture and the discipline in recognizing expertise acquired through experience in practice. The reluctance to admit that nurses don't graduate as fully skilled professionals, but rather as advanced beginners who require many years of experience to fill out their skills and become expert, also upholds a myth which is accepted in many health care institutions: that nurses of any skill or educational level are roughly equal in their abilities to fulfill staffing needs.

Although it is important to help students adopt a professional nursing role, this might be counterbalanced by also teaching the distinctions in the practice that exist in nurses who are new to a practice versus nurses who have practiced for one, two or more years and have acquired considerable experience and clinical knowledge in the practice. By acknowledging the distinctions in the nature of the clinical perception and agency in new graduates and nurses who have worked for even one year, educators legitimize the learning that is anticipated and necessary in the course of continued practice. Indeed, it sanctions and makes visible clinical knowledge. This acknowledgment orients students to the reality that clinical judgment and expertise develop gradually throughout one's practice career. This orientation might contribute to their openness to continued learning, and might relieve them of unnecessary guilt about their need to learn, and to rely on the expertise of others early in their careers.

THE ROLE OF NARRATIVE

Interpretation of narrative, as we have used it in our work, and as we are proposing as an educational innovation, draws on a long tradition of interpretive phenomenology (Benner, 1994b; Benner & Wrubel, 1989; Dreyfus, 1979; Leonard, 1994; Phillips & Benner, in press), an interpretive approach for studying embodiment, world and caring practices through the study of text, which can be narratives of every day life.

Interpretive phenomenology offers perspective on the nature of being human, and a method of interpretation that uncovers human concerns and practices (Benner, 1984a; Benner & Wrubel, 1989; Dreyfus; 1979; Dreyfus, 1991; Heidegger, 1962; Packer & Addison, 1989; Wrubel, 1985). It seeks to gain a different understanding and relationship to common taken-for-granted meanings habits, practices, skills and concerns central to being and dwelling in a world. Instead of the Cartesian epistemological assumptions about a private subject cognitively representing an objective world, interpretive phenomenology questions how the person's world, practices, habits, skills and concerns determine what is perceived and what can be talked about (Dreyfus, 1991; Guignon, 1985; Heidegger, 1962; Merleau-Ponty, 1958). Five common aspects of being that are explored in phenomenology are: 1) Situation. This includes an understanding of how the person is situated, both historically and currently. Questions related to the situation are whether the situation is understood as one of smooth social functioning or whether it is a situation of breakdown, novelty or confusion. 2) Embodiment. This includes an understanding of embodied knowing that encompasses skillful comportment and perceptual and emotional responses. Embodied understandings of the situation are explored as in highly skilled, taken-for-granted responses or bodily responses such as an early recognition of impending patient crisis as a result of perceptual acuity and pattern recognition, or anticipatory nausea experienced by a patient approaching a chemotherapy situation. 3) Temporality. The experience of lived time is the way one is projected into the future, and understands oneself from the past. Temporality is more than a linear succession of moments, it includes the qualitative, lived experience of time or timelessness. 4) Concerns. Concerns are the way the person is oriented meaningfully in the situation. Concerns will dictate what will show up as salient, and therefore what will be noticed in the situation. They constitute what matters to the person. 5) Common meanings. These are taken-for-granted linguistic and cultural meanings that create what is noticed, what are possible issues, what are possible agreements and disagreements between people. For example, a classroom situation is predicated on certain taken-for-granted meanings about what it is to be a teacher and a student. Even the disagreements about what it is to be a teacher and a student depend upon a taken-for-granted understandings that allow meaningful distinctions and disagreements to occur. (Benner 1994b, p. 104)

Examination of all these aspects of being is important in grasping and learning from a clinical experience, and thus reflection of practice via narratives logically draws on interpretive phenomenology.

We are proposing at least three ways in which narrative could become a significant aspect of undergraduate nursing education. First, assignments that help students learn the skills of gathering and interpreting clinical ethnographies or illness narratives can enhance students' powers of understanding others' worlds. Second, experiences in which students tell stories from their own practice can increase their skills in (a) recognizing patient and family concerns, (b) communicating with patients, (c) reflecting on ethical comportment and engaged clinical reasoning, and (d) articulating experiential learning and clinical knowledge development. Third, faculty stories from their own teaching practice can enhance faculty participation in pedagogical knowledge development and in building a narrative of community teaching practices. Each of these potentially transformative uses of narrative is detailed here.

Interpretation of Illness Narratives

Stories of lived experience with illness provide new insights for the clinician in the meaning of the illness for the patient, ways of coping with suffering and loss, and ways in which nursing and medical care can be more responsive to patients' understanding of their disease and experience with illness.

Interpretation of the lived experience is central to nursing practice as we have described in this volume. Students need opportunities to develop skill both in soliciting from patients stories of their illness, and in interpreting these narratives. Experience is required in hearing stories of others, exploring concerns and background meanings, arguing alternative interpretations, and reflecting back to the storyteller interpretations and questions that elicit significant, but perhaps forgotten, parts of the story.

Learning to enter the worlds of others through literature (poetry, biographies, drama, ethnographies, and novels) can increase the power of understanding and the capacity to articulate that understanding to others. For health care practitioners, reading narrative accounts of illness and recovery can augment explanations of disease and pathology with the human experience of living with illness, loss, recovery, and care. This background in developing interpretive skills and narrative understanding prepares the student to actively listen to first-hand accounts of illness experiences, informal models of illness and recovery and self-described relationships to illness (Benner, 1994b; Kleinman, 1988).

As a means to explore ways of helping students acquire these interpretive skills, we recently developed a course for beginning nursing students. The course titled "Living with Chronic Illness" was structured to focus on patients' narrative accounts of their experiences with chronic illness. We chose three conditions that we thought would be representative of some of the issues of living with a chronic condition—COPD, HIV disease and Alzheimer's.

Each of the three conditions was taken up by the class for a 3-week period. During the first of the 3 weeks, at least one patient, and in the case of Alzheimer's, three families, talked about their experiences of living with the condition. Prior to the discussion with the patient or family, students were given some basic reading—usually research about living with the condition and a brief, fairly simple reading outlining the pathology of the disease and its treatment. They were given a set of questions to guide their thinking and writing in preparation for hearing from the patient. The questions asked them to reflect on their own personal experiences, on what they knew theoretically about the condition, and what they expected to hear from the patient or family.

The patients and/or their families were asked to talk about significant events they could remember in living with their illness. We suggested that they recall the time surrounding the diagnosis, any hospitalizations, responses from family or friends, or particular times when their illness was especially challenging. We asked that they tell us stories.

After the patients' presentation, students were again asked to address the following in their writing: (a) reflections on what they had heard from the patients, describing and interpreting a particular instance reported by the patient, identifying the problems and central concerns, and suggesting in broad terms the nursing responsibilities and practices that might be responsive to these concerns; (b) how they felt in response to the patient; (c) their general expectations about the kind of nursing roles that experts might describe; and (d) one or more questions about facts, principles, or theory that would be needed to provide care to the specific patient who presented in class.

The second of the 3 weeks, we reviewed the students' reflections about the patients' experiences, spending a significant portion of the time interpreting the patients' stories. Expert clinicians also presented exemplars and paradigm cases from their practice and responded to students' questions about nursing practices in caring for these particular patients.

The third of the 3 weeks was devoted to discussion of the students' reflections, questions, and concerns. Prior to this class, they were encouraged to find ways to answer pressing questions that could be answered through textbooks or discussions with faculty and peers. They were also asked to write about their reflections on the clinician's accounts of particular situations.

The narrative accounts provided by patients have been both moving and profound. Many patients commented that they shared important aspects of their illness with the class that they had never discussed with their care provider. One account was particularly memorable for the students and was recalled several times during their subsequent practice as students. The patient was a young man in his mid-twenties, recently diagnosed with HIV disease. The students had asked him about things that he found helpful from health care providers, and this is the story he told:

> I was sure I had AIDS. I mean I've been gay, pretty active when I lived in San Francisco. I had this cough, fevers, weight loss, now I was really having trouble breathing. So I went to [*a small, rural hospital*] and was admitted, and was sure I'd be treated like the scum of the earth. A nurse came into my room to admit me. Everyone had been pretty brusque, you know, kind of efficient, just-the-facts kind of thing. She sat down to fill out some admission form, looked up at me, just kind of reached out and took my hand, and said "It's going to be OK. I know this is scary." [*Voice cracking*] Now that was helpful.

Students' interpretations of this account at the time focused on the act of touching, and how important that was for connecting to patients. ("The simple act of touching," as some referred to it.) Later they understood how overwhelming the stigma of this disease was for this young man, fearing both the disease and how people in this conservative community would respond to him, feeling perhaps already distanced and alienated because of his lifestyle and HIV status.

There was varying participation by students in the writing exercises. At least initially, some students found the exercises to be just another assignment to get through, and responded to the questions without participating in deep reflection about them. Others, however, wrote quite seriously. An experienced LPN returning for a degree used the writing as a way to explore involvement, reflecting on her experiences and hearing in clinicians' accounts their working out involvement. It was clear that one course in a whole curriculum that emphasized understanding lived experience was simply not sufficient. Although the students gained some skill in interpretation, more opportunities for follow-through in actual clinical learning would be necessary.

The strengths of the course were: (1) the experience provided in interviewing and actual interpretation; (2) the opportunity to experience emotional connection or involvement, and to reflect on and discuss that level of involvement; and (3) the possibility of exploring all relevant aspects of nursing care (including, for example, pathophysiology, pharmacology, other medical sciences, and family responses) through the interpretation of patients' experiences, and through raising questions about the scientific/ theoretical knowledge, as well as the human understandings needed to provide care.

Narrative Accounts of Clinical Practice

Seminar and classroom presentation of narrative accounts of clinical practice enables the clinical learner to hear his or her own voice and concerns in clinical situations. Articulating one's newly gained understanding in dialogue with others serves to extend experiential learning and make it available for others to contribute, alter, and extend that understanding. Teaching students to interpret, and to give language to what they are learning, creates an ongoing dialogue with practical situations, human relationships, and ethical comportment:

> Public storytelling among practitioners allows for noticing distinctions and clinical learning. The forming of the story, where it begins, how it develops, what concerns shape the story and how the story ends as well as the dialogue and perceptions of the storyteller present meaningful accounts of practical engaged reasoning. The narrative reveals what is significant and relevant to say about situations and events in the practice. The storyteller can be surprised by the way the story is formed and unfolds because the lived experience can take over the account in its immediacy. To tell one's story is also to hear one's story. Oral storytelling is more immediate than formal procedural or analytical accounts usually presented in formal documents or case presentations by professionals. The structure of the story, the chronology, asides, and the remembered dialogue can reveal assumptions, and taken-for-granted meanings of which the storyteller is only dimly aware. In presenting the paths chosen, one can reflect on the paths and options that were not taken, even the ones that did not occur to the person at the time. Thus, storytellers, hearing their own stories, can learn and experience consciousness raising and critical reflection. The listener can enrich and augment what is heard and understood by the storytelling. (Benner, 1994c, pp. 110–111)

As noted by Rubin (see Chapter 7) stories are organized by concerns, even though the storyteller does not know or may not even be able to clearly articulate these concerns. Telling stories in first-person language reveals and fosters a sense of agency. Telling a story reveals one's own stance and encourages the practitioner to clarify one's own responsibility for working toward the patient's good. The absence of a story seems to indicate a poorly developed sense of agency and connection to the situation. It signals alienation, disengagement, indifference, or *anomie* (Benner & Wrubel, 1989). Narratives are essential to conveying knowledge about the skill of involvement (getting the right level and kind of involvement with the situation and with the person, family, and community) because relational skills always involve particular other(s) and particular situations and are context-dependent. Stories reveal personal knowledge (Polanyi, 1958). Biases and exclusions are encountered so that new possibilities and constraints are discovered. Narratives can reveal openness or closedness to the other.

Oral and written first-person stories allow nurses to learn from their successes and failures. A collection of narratives of learning can form a body of both private and public student literature that can extend engaged learning about one's own agency and self-understanding as a practitioner. Narratives allow for internal dialogue, as well as continued dialogue with patients, families, communities, and coworkers.

Explanation does not always signal understanding. That is, knowing reasons and causes does not mean that one will understand the clinical and ethical implications, nor that one will become involved and respond (Benner, 1994a). Being placed in a situation with the best preparation for discerning qualitative distinctions about involvement, caring, suffering, hope, recovery, and loss does not ensure that the learner will engage in a dialogue that will enhance experiential learning. The goal of education is to enhance dialogues fostered by the notions of good internal to the practice, the clinical and ethical demands of the situation, and one's own skills of seeing and responding to the situation. One can learn techniques and abstract knowledge, but to be a practitioner requires a helping relationship with particular persons, families, and communities. Ethical learning and skillful ethical comportment are based upon a continued dialogue with doing better and doing worse in specific situations. It is the domain of professional education to ensure that dialogue is taken up in actual practice with actual situations in ways that augment and extend the notion of good internal to the practice (MacIntyre, 1981). Abstract rigorous knowledge about science, technology, and ethical principles are essential for guiding and extending practice, but they cannot ensure that one will recognize in practice when these norms might be relevant, nor can they guarantee that the technological ideal can be actualized.

Storytelling is central to developing our self-understanding and the understanding of the good and the goods in life that we care about preserving. A story is not a purely subjective construction, although one can only tell about what one sees and knows. In telling stories of practice, the storyteller constitutes and is constituted by the story. To be given a story is to be a member-participant. To narrate is to participate in narratives that allow one to understand what is worth talking about, where the story ought to begin, what it ought to be about, and where it ought to end. The storyteller reports thoughts, feelings, and experiential knowledge of an event.

The practice of storytelling requires a climate of trust and disciplined attention to learning from experience, rather than focusing on grading academic performance. Since experiential learning always entails correcting, extending, or adding nuances to one's pre-understandings, the focus is on learning and change, rather than achievement. In clinical practice, the goal is to avoid as many mistakes as possible, and the ethical demand is that one learn from one's own and others' mistakes.

Storytelling requires a "learning space," as Palmer (1966, p. 69) describes it, with at least 3 different dimensions: openness, boundaries, and an air of hospitality. Teachers participate with students in creating space, removing impediments to learning, and avoiding the tendency to clutter both consciousness and classroom. As Palmer (1966) points out, one way in which we create obstacles to learning is out of fear of appearing ignorant. We prepare long detailed lectures, "parsing out concepts without end, unwinding the interminable and irrelevant illustrations" (p. 71). Boundaries are also required because without them a learning space is "not a structure for learning, but an invitation to confusion and chaos" (p. 72). Hospitality means "receiving each other, our struggles, our newborn ideas with openness and care" (p. 74).

Creating a learning space requires a countenance on the part of the teacher that shows openness to clinical learning and a willingness to listen to and hear the students' interpretation of the clinical situation. It is essential that we as teachers see ourselves in practice as clinical learners who are open to clinical situations. It is important that we demonstrate our own learning and talk about the ways in which experience taught us who we are as nurses, how to cope with illness and suffering, and how to develop the skill of involvement. In the classroom, this means that as teachers we talk about lived experiences in nursing and present particular clinical situations that were a source of learning through narratives where learning shows up as the situation unfolds. In the clinical setting, this means showing students their own natural curiosity about particular clinical situations and seeking to understand, with our students, particular patients' lived experiences with illness.

Narratives of Teaching

Just as narratives of practice are central to clinical knowledge development and building a community of understanding among clinicians, so too can storytelling build knowledge and community among teachers. In our busy academic lives, we seldom have the opportunity to tell stories from our teaching practice. As Shulman describes:

We close the classroom door and experience pedagogical solitude, whereas in our life as scholars we are members of active communities: communities of conversation, communities of evaluation, communities in which we gather with others in our invisible colleges to exchange our findings, our methods and our excuses. I believe that the reason teaching is not valued in the academy is because the way we treat teaching removes it from the community of scholars. (1993, p. 6)

Of course, we all talk with one another about all sorts of things related to teaching. We argue endlessly in curriculum meetings about the selection and sequencing of content. Those of us involved in research on teaching may have conversations about the implications of our latest study, or about some new pedagogy that we're interested in exploring. We may even exchange amusing anecdotes about students' faux pas, or complain about the failure of our students to adequately prepare for class. These kinds of conversations rarely push us to seriously consider how we teach in the classroom, in clinical settings, or in our interactions with students.

As Diekelmann (1992) is finding in her studies of teaching practices, narratives reveal human meanings and concerns, moral issues, and the practical know-how embedded in concrete teaching episodes. Edgerton (1993), Hutchings (1993a; 1993b), and others suggest that dialogue about particular teaching incidents may contribute to a richer understanding of teaching and is, in fact, a kind of scholarship of teaching (Boyer, 1990). Teachers know much more than they can ever say about teaching. The precepts offered by any pedagogical theory inevitably fall short in prescribing teaching practices, since the theory must be filled out, refined, or challenged by the particular teacher, with particular students and particular subject matter. This kind of practical, pedagogical knowledge development can occur through discussion and interpretation of narrative accounts of particular teaching incidents.

EDUCATIONAL STRATEGIES AND INNOVATIONS

This study has led us to a deeper understanding and appreciation of the centrality of experiential learning for the development of truly expert practice. We believe that a project of undergraduate nursing education is to lay the groundwork for nursing students to enter their practice with an orientation to learning from practice. We have already identified the transformative and constitutive power of narrative in educational practices. In addition, we here outline some additional aspects of undergraduate education that might shift to help the learner take a more open stance in adopting this practice that is morally directed, practically and experientially grounded, intuitive, historical, contextual, and supported by a community of practice and understanding.

Teaching Clinical Judgment

1. For rank beginners, we recommend continued effort directed toward helping students learn to do rule-based activities and *apply theoretical knowledge*, where the major clinical judgment is recognizing which rules may be relevant, identifying which signs and symptoms should be watched for, and listing possible nursing actions that may be appropriate given a patient's medical problems.

Having students do a simple prep sheet ahead of clinical practice may help them focus their attention on relevant theoretical understandings. The emphasis on preparation, rather than care planning, conveys its real purpose: to help students identify what is relevant, and to ensure at least minimal preparation for clinical practice. The overall goal is to teach clinical forethought.

2. Also early in the program, we recommend continued emphasis on *analytic clinical thinking*, including planning for decision making and considering what information will be relevant in particular situations. In actual clinical situations, analytic clinical thinking is promoted by providing help in recognizing aspects (rather than context-free features) of the situation, noticing relevant and ignoring irrelevant information, generating possible explanations for clinical data, collecting additional data to test out explanations, and so on. Here, students need the guidance of a clinical coach to have relevant aspects pointed out to them and to begin to compare and contrast among clinical situations. Both total patient care experiences and opportunities to see many patients with similar concerns or problems support the development of this analytic thinking.

Questioning students in a way that opens them up to the clinical situation, rather than shutting down or creating a one-way dialogue from the textbook to the clinical situation, is critical for developing skill. Also important are experiences where students are provided a safe environment for thinking aloud (see Corcoran & Tanner [1988] and Corcoran, Narayan, & Moreland [1988]), in which they can reveal to themselves and the teacher, where their knowledge may be limited or lacking, and where the clarity of their thinking breaks down.

3. As the student advances in analytic thinking, emphasis should turn to *learning about individualizing care*. Again, clinical learning opportunities need to be provided for the students to have experience in (a) knowing the

patient, with articulated understanding of the patient's pattern of responses and ways of being in the world; (b) interpreting the patient's concerns through narrative accounts of illness experiences; (c) shaping nursing actions through understanding the patient's concerns and ways of coping; and (d) recognizing how this patient is similar/dissimilar to others in the patient population (e.g., by health problems, culture, etc.)

Learning experiences that allow students to work closely alongside more experienced nurses are warranted. Close preceptorship and modeling can help students advance their perceptual and care skills. Close work with a more experienced nurse is the *only* way that students can learn embodied nursing skills. Only by seeing the nurse model these behaviors and by trying to imitate the skill can learners begin to appreciate and acquire the technical skills of comforting and being-with that are embodied. For example, learning to turn terminal cancer patients so that additional pain is not inflicted, or to swaddle a baby during a procedure so that a child can self-comfort or maintain a reasonable level of calm, can only be demonstrated. The requirement that students have close contact with one or two nurses may argue against the common practice of having 7–10 student nurses on the same unit during one particular shift. That load of students may overwhelm staff nurses engaged in practice and make them less willing to pull a student in the room, model a skill, or point out a change in a patient condition. More sparse assignments of students to units and clear identification of nurses that students might follow, observe, and work with in developing their skill would be optimal for learning from direct modeling.

4. Students should also be guided in *clinical knowledge development*. Specifically, they need help in recognizing the practical manifestations of textbook signs and symptoms, learning graded qualitative distinctions, and seeing and recognizing qualitative changes in a particular patient's condition, as well as learning qualitative distinctions among a range of possible manifestations, common meanings, and experiences. Opportunities to see many patients from a particular group, with the skilled guidance of a clinical coach, should be provided. For example, students could participate in clinical rounds with an expert nurse clinician who could point out commonalities and graded qualitative distinctions in patients' symptoms and life experience with similar disease processes.

5. Students need the opportunity to *develop habitual practices and skills in reflection on practice* in ways that stay true to the clinical issues at hand. Nurse educators have traditionally emphasized evaluation—either overall self-evaluation of clinical performance, or outcomes of patient care. Both of these are important activities, but must be examined in light of the overall aim of developing the habit of critical reflection on practice.

First, let us try to be clear about what we mean by reflection on practice. There is a burgeoning literature in many practice disciplines about developing reflective practice, perhaps spawned in part by the influential works of Schon (1983; 1987). (See, for example, reviews in Clift, Houston, & Pugach, 1990, for examples in education, and for examples in nursing, Clarke, 1986; Powell, 1989; Saylor, 1990.) Many writers have emphasized a kind of reflection in practice. As Schon (1983) has characterized it:

> If common sense recognizes knowing-in-action, it also recognizes that we sometimes think about what we are doing. Phrases like "thinking on your feet," "keeping your wits about you" suggest not only that we can think about doing but that we can think about doing something while doing it . . . Much reflection-in-action hinges on the experience of surprise. When intuitive, spontaneous performance yields nothing more than the results expected for it, then we tend not to think about it. But when intuitive performance leads to surprises, pleasing and promising or unwanted, we may respond by reflecting-in-action . . . Such reflection tends to focus interactively on the outcomes of the action, the action itself, and the intuitive knowing implicit in the action. (pp. 55–56)

We have characterized this sort of thinking in action as deliberative rationality, clearly an important part of the practice of nurses (See Dreyfus & Dreyfus with Athanasiou, 1986).

The kind of reflection we are referring to is recollective, occurring after the situation has passed. Such reflection may be prompted by something in the situation that troubles us, and we may focus on what we did or did not do that the situation may have warranted. We most often try to link a patient's responses or other outcome to what we did or did not do. We try to be "mindful of whether the action in the . . . situation was appropriate (good, right, best under the circumstances) . . ." (van Manen, 1991, p. 116). Through reconsideration and discussion of concrete whole experiences, we reach new understanding of the meaning of the experience. We may uncover taken-for-granted assumptions about the meaning of particular practices, or habitual ways of being. Such reflection heightens our sensitivity and capacity for appropriate responses in subsequent experiences. Reflection in the sense we mean it is not objective, detached, standing away from the situation. The particular experience is separated by time, not necessarily by engagement.

Both self-evaluation and evaluation of patient outcomes are important aspects of or results of reflection on practice. But they must be done in ways that support the development of the habit and skills of reflection. They must focus on:

1. concrete, particular experiences or specific interactions;

2. experiences where both immediate and long-term consequences can be seen and where there may be a possibility to link the nursing action with the patient response; and

3. the clinical learning possible in the situation, including learning from errors in judgment and lack of knowledge.

Students also need to develop habits and skills for reflection outside of these somewhat traditional and formal expectations. This requires the skill in noticing and attending to problematic situations in practice, seeing when things may go awry, paying attention to those gnawing feelings that things didn't go quite as expected, and sorting out relevant dimensions of those events.

Teaching Nursing as a Moral Practice

We have argued that nursing practice is a form of engaged moral reasoning and that expert nurses enter the care of particular patients with a fundamental sense of what is good and right. Many of the suggestions we have made for teaching engaged reasoning in action or clinical judgment also address this additional concern that nurses learn moral agency. For example, learning the importance of knowing a patient's pattern of response, his habits and practices, and how he is situated in his world all contribute to the nurse's moral sensitivity. Additional educational approaches that specifically focus on supporting the moral groundedness of the nurse-learner can also be suggested.

Undergraduate nursing students may benefit by learning ethical principles and reasoning based on ethical theories, especially if the limits of this practice are taught at the same time. Principles might be taught alongside practicalist and relational ethics. This may become important because in most situations where moral decisions are explicitly discussed, many in the room, including perhaps the person with most power in swaying the decision about action, may rely on traditional ethical principles. Nurses who have been educated in not only the principles, but their limitations, are better able to defend their judgments and to argue effectively in favor of a particular team response to a patient situation which has set up a moral concern or dilemma.

When studying the narratives of practice of others, the moral dimensions should be given attention and emphasis that parallels the emphasis placed on the practical learning that narratives set up for engaged care of the person. Particularly for nursing students who are anxious about the care of the body and the specialized knowledge they must acquire to accomplish that care, shifting their focus to larger questions of what is good and right in a clinical situation is difficult. Reflection through narrative study of their own practice and the practice of others helps students to approach a case with multiple levels of concern and begins to strike a balance in care of the body and care of the embodied person-in-context.

The socially constructed and embedded nature of the moral basis of practice can be addressed in undergraduate education. In an age when ethical sensitivity is commonly translated as moral relativism (Taylor, 1992) it seems essential that students begin to understand in their basic education the responsibility of attending to and embracing the moral concerns of the discipline. It seems imperative that nursing be taught as a *practice*, which has a different structure and set of concerns than other career choices (e.g., being a laboratory or X-ray technician) and that the goods internal to the practice differ from the goods internal to other practices (e.g., law). These discussions are most logically placed in courses on "leadership" or "professional development" where the notions of a profession are discussed alongside the notions of a practice.

Teaching a Socially Embedded Practice

Much of our cultural and disciplinary self-conception orients students away from entering the practice in a way that acknowledges that the knowledge for practice is worked out and largely maintained within the daily practices of nurses caring for patients, families, and communities. A true acknowledgment of the socially embedded nature of nursing knowledge and practice heightens the importance of attending to a) skills in communicating both one's grasp and one's confusion about a clinical situation; b) skills in striking the right balance between relying on the clinical knowledge of others and taking the ever-present risk of relying on one's developing ability in reading and managing a patient condition; and c) the developmental cycle of nurses in relation to knowledge for practice that includes sampling and learning, maintaining, and finally extending clinical knowledge in the course of their practice.

Clinical supervision groups in undergraduate education might focus explicitly on developing skills in communicating in a concise but intelligible fashion what one does and does not understand about a clinical encounter. For this to work effectively, the group must have a tone that is supportive of learning, that accepts rather than blames the student for misjudgments, and that establishes an ethic of group responsibility for the clinical outcome. In this atmosphere, students can begin to learn the collegiality that is required in a discipline where the knowledge for practice is shared. It also may represent a shift—from the individual competitiveness that characterizes some academic environments, to group support and shared responsibility for furthering the abilities of the learner and the care of the patient. Establishing this ethic of group responsibility helps nursing students to learn how nurses work together for the betterment of the patient overall. Of course, this effort to teach students to communicate their knowledge and their blindness does not overcome the problem of secondary ignorance, but it does begin to establish a stance of openness about one's abilities and need for further skill development.

A more complex endeavor is fostering the appropriate balance of acting independently in situations where one is marginally prepared, and relying heavily on the knowledge and judgement of others. In a discipline where the young practitioner is always operating at the edge of knowledge and capabilities, explicit attention should be given to the skill of negotiating clinical assignments where only partial independence is possible. Early in their education, students can be coached in how to work interdependently with staff nurses on the units on which they train, and to turn to those staff for advice and guidance instead of relying solely on the advice of their nursing instructor. Clear negotiations with clinical units about the role of staff in training students must be completed before introducing students to units with these learning expectations, particularly if this represents a shift in practices, away from the direct and fairly exclusive consultation of students with nursing instructors.

Finally, students can be helped to see that no nurse is a fully autonomous practitioner; that experience and seasoning in the practice of nursing brings with it a different but not diminishing quality of embeddedness and reliance on others. Students can be taught that social embeddedness of knowledge is a good, not a state to be overcome or outgrown. They can additionally be helped to see that throughout their professional careers, the likely trajectory in their situatedness with the community of other nurses is from a position of high dependence and learning to a mutually supportive position as a peer with other experts in the practice.

SUMMARY

In the name of self-mastery, autonomy, and self-esteem, as educators we structure learning for success as early and as often as possible, and this is good. Wherever the educator can instruct so that the student need not learn by failure, this is best for the student—not to mention the patient! But no clinical encounter is without its edges of learning and mystery. And we must also take our students to the edges of understanding and point up the risky areas in our caring and clinical practice where we do not know the answers, where there is no time to do adequate library research. It is here that we must teach the best possible engaged reasoning and openness to learn from questions, unknowns, mistakes, shortcomings, misperceptions, contingencies, and imperfections, etcetera. This is after all, what it means to learn from experience. There is a kernel of "failure" in all experiential learning if the focus is on perfect performance and achievement. But if the focus is on the moral courage to learn from our limited, temporally and relationally constrained encounters, experiential learning becomes an adventure requiring courage and openness rather than bravado and the cultivation of fragile false egos. For every clinical assignment there is the possibility of learning from success and learning from the unknown and failures. As educators we must be open, and teach our students to be open, to both kinds of clinical learning.

Our zeal to teach for certainty, science, and disengaged criterial reasoning creates an eclipse of clinical knowledge, clinical inquiry, and clinical knowledge development. Where possible, exactitude and certainty are good. But where certainty is not possible, it is dangerous and damaging to offer illusions about the possibility for certainty. This is an academic formula for creating closed minds. Even our teaching strategies designed for objective grading create a false sense of certainty that makes us focus on areas of learning where we can be objective, and de-emphasize the risky, the uncertain areas of judgment and discernment. We unwittingly teach our students to avoid risk, and cover over rather than learn from failure. But all practitioners must learn to be engaged in a dialogue with practice. They must learn to navigate the particular nurse-patient relationship and the particular clinical trajectory. In clinical practice, post-hoc reasoning is often the best we can do, and we owe it to our patients to do it as well as possible. We owe it to our students to teach them how to learn from their clinical practice. For this, we must create a climate of trust and openness with our students and an acknowledgment of the inordinate difficulties of doing well in the thick of most clinical situations. We need to learn and teach that skillful ethical and clinical comportment is learned by getting it better and worse and learning as we go. We need to reconnect means and ends, and stop devaluing the "mere means" (Borgmann, 1984; Guignon, 1983).

Clinical practice and caring relationships are privileged ways of meeting the other, and in meeting the other we meet ourselves. We confront vulnerability and suffering, but also possibility and courage. It is impossible to "master" or formalize all clinical and relational learning. Clinical encounters, by their nature, are open and infinite, but we can become wiser and we can embrace the adventure of learning. As educators, this is the invitation to learning that we must give our students. With the invitation we must courageously confront our own limits to knowledge and certainty. We must give up our penchant for judging and evaluating and become more open to learning from our students and patients. An invitation to dialogue and learning can never flow only in one direction.

Chapter 13

IMPLICATIONS FOR NURSING ADMINISTRATION AND PRACTICE*

The central thesis of this work is that nursing is a socially embedded practice concerned with the promotion of the recovery and well-being of others. This practice encompasses knowledge of science and technology, but is guided by the goals, knowledge, and skills of caregiving. Nursing is a coherent, socially organized practice and is, therefore, more than a collection of tasks and techniques. Expert nursing practice requires reasoning well in particular clinical situations and developing trusting relationships with patients and families. For example, the advanced beginner nurse seeks assistance in interpreting subtle changes in the patient's condition because the identification of a trend downward, or a deviation from a range of "normal," is a set of distinctions learned over time by comparing many patients. In the observation of nurses at work, expert caring practices (e.g., attentiveness, care of the body, coaching patients and families about the foreign environment, and orienting and clarifying the patient's sense of situation) make a humane difference that sustains the level of trust required to submit to "intensive care"(Benner, Wrubel, Phillips, Chesla, & Tanner, 1995). In the case of the critically ill, stemming the tide of fear and panic is lifesaving, since distressed emotional states threaten already delicate physiological states.

We found that some expert nurses shared an ethos of following the body's lead and limiting the use of technology in order to restore the patient to their own bodily powers of recovery as soon as possible (Benner,

*The contributions of Richard V. Benner, Ph.D., to this chapter are gratefully acknowledged.

1994d). Although there is a "technological imperative" operating in critical care units, it is not entirely unopposed by a vision of placing the person in the best condition for self-repair and healing (Nightingale, 1860/ 1969). As one nurse pointed out when making a case to wean a premature infant, "If you are not helping with [the use of] technology, you are almost always causing harm." Learning to assess and manage technology is a crucial area of clinical learning and caring practice.

MANAGERIAL IMPLICATIONS

This research suggests several major implications for nursing management. The major points we will explicate may seem obvious, but they are consistently ignored in the developing organizational structures for nursing practice:

1.   The skill levels of clinicians need to be determined, recognized, rewarded, and utilized accordingly.

2.   Attention must be given to the distribution of skills of nurses for proper staffing of shifts and modes of care delivery, such as primary care or team nursing.

3.   The creation of "acute care hospitals" requires the identification of expert practitioners across all units and specialties where direct patient care occurs. Anything, whether staffing mix or patient-nurse ratio, that reduces the contact of the nurse with the patient or the continuity of care with a particular patient, flattens the practice of even the most expert nurse.

4.   High use of non-nursing personnel as a part of a patient care system is more difficult to manage and creates greater risk to patient safety than having a high number of advanced beginners. The introduction of more salary differential for the beginning and expert nurses could alleviate much of the need for cross-training of lesser educated personnel.

5.   Managers, particularly at the unit level, can promote the development of expertise in individual nurses and in groups of nurses by attending to the stages of skill acquisition.

Organizing Care According to Skill Levels

This research confirms in depth what was indicated by the research reported in *From Novice to Expert* (Benner, 1984a), that nurses, even those with many years of experience, practice at different skill levels. There are distinct skill levels among nurses, which translates directly into how patients are cared for. The view that "a nurse is a nurse" is quickly translated in an era of health care efficiency, productivity, and profitability into the stance that "anyone can do it." But as anyone who has studied the organizational literature knows, true productivity and profitability over the long term are based first and foremost on strong quality and reliability. Car manufacturers have learned this lesson (Pascale, 1990). And it is likely to be even more true in health care. While competent clinical nurses are highly skilled, the ability of the expert nurse to be proactive rather than reactive and to see and act on behalf of the patient before the formal indicators are clear, is such a leap in applied nursing that their performance must be recognized, rewarded, and provided the organizational support to operate effectively (Aikin, Smith, & Lake, 1994; Hartz et al., 1989).

In the past there has been a "quiet" recognition of differences in clinical skill among nurses. Most nurses know whom they would seek out to solve a difficult or uncertain clinical situation. This inherent understanding led to the development of clinical ladders which tried to identify these differences as something different from length of experience. The attempt to identify differences was based on a variety of indicators such as professional activities, educational and teaching activities, citizenship work, such as involvement in various hospital governance committees, or some formal instrument with a set of abstract criteria or behavioral statements used to judge the level of practice. Too often the result was a system which did not discriminate between the practice skills of nurses—a system in which many of the "best" nurses did not participate, because it trivialized their practice. We offer an alternative to these traditional clinical ladders based on part of the methodology of this research: the use of clinical narratives, combined with a peer review process. When the system for promotion and reward accurately identifies the skill level of the clinician, the clinical ladder system has integrity and the results of that system in identifying expertise gives confidence to others to learn from the judgment of those practitioners.

Staffing with a Blend of Skill Levels

The ability to identify skill levels among nursing personnel suggests the need for management to take into account the skill mix on any one shift. Historically, nurse managers have assigned a minimum number of "experienced" nurses to each shift. Staffing has also been based on acuity levels of patients. With the recent efforts to cut costs in highly competitive environments, hospitals have cut staff to a fixed patient-staff ratio, aiming at a minimal staff-to-patient ratio. With the shorter length of stays for patients and higher acuity levels, assigning a minimal number of expert nurses per shift to coach and extend the clinical judgment of less experienced nurses is a minimal response to this cost-cutting for patient safety.

Developing Expertise with Specific Patient Populations

Hospitalization is designed to provide attentive monitoring and care of unstable patient conditions. Recognizing deviations from the normal and responding promptly requires both knowing the patient (Tanner et al., 1993) and understanding the usual trajectories for specific patient conditions. Hospitals need some flexibility in moving staff to meet patient census fluctuations. This can best be done on a preplanned basis, where nurses float only to units related to the patient populations with which they are familiar and for which they have specialized orientation. It is also desirable to assign clinical resource nurses for the nurse working on a less familiar unit.

The Reliability Costs of Non-Nursing Personnel

Hiring narrowly trained non-nursing personnel to do assigned tasks has real limitations for the development of clinical expertise or for the safe care of highly unstable patients. Currently, salaries in nursing are compressed, with little difference between the beginning and expert nurses. Recognizing the importance of well-established teams in the development of expert nursing practice suggests graded salary differences for the advanced beginner, competent, proficient, and expert levels of practice. With advanced beginning nurses, clinical learning is cumulative and the investment in teaching and developing the nurse has long-term pay off. Since there is much local- and institution-specific knowledge that must be taught to the new employee, long-term costs for orientation of new employees can be decreased by hiring advanced beginner nurses at lower salaries but with the prospect of significantly increasing salaries with the development of clinical expertise. Such a strategy allows the hospital to retain excellent clinicians and reap the benefit of the large amount of orientation and staff development invested in the nurse.

Nurse managers need to find ways to assist nurses in developing continuous improvement in patient outcomes on specific units. To do this, nurses need aggregate data on common deviations from expected critical pathways, and on the occurrence of preventable complications. Developing shared distinctions about patient signs, symptoms, and responses to treatment requires continuity and good communication of clinical knowledge between nurses who have a broad and common knowledge base about the patient populations being cared for.

Developing Expertise and a Climate for Clinical Learning

Learning to recognize the different learning issues and the different possibilities for agency at different levels of skill offers the manager guidance for fostering the development of clinical expertise within a group of nurses. For example, nurses who consistently recognize early warnings of any number of clinical conditions can be assisted in articulating their clinical knowledge and encouraged to coach other nurses when the opportunity for clinical learning arrises. Since clinical knowledge is socially embedded and can be enhanced by dialogue and consensual validation of clinical assessments, highlighting clinical problem-solving and learning can greatly increase collective clinical learning. Augmenting informal exchanges by planned dialogues and presenting clinical exemplars can enhance this learning.

IMPLICATIONS FOR ORGANIZATIONAL DESIGN AND RE-ENGINEERING

We believe that designing nurses' work so that they have the continuity and context for developing trusting relationships and astute clinical judgments based on knowing their patients provides the safest, most humane, and most cost-effective care. Clearly, patients who are currently hospitalized are the sickest and most labile patients. Bureaucratic and engineering strategies (Champy, 1995) that break the tasks down into divisible units run the risk of being both more dangerous and more expensive in the long run. Micromanagement in the form of critical paths and case management that overrides professional judgment with individual patients threatens to be far more costly in terms of both efficiency and effectiveness. While aggregate data and critical pathways (generalized plans of patient care based upon normative patient care data) can serve as guidelines, they must not be slavishly followed, because such averages cannot replace attuned judgment. Some patients progress faster than expected, others much slower. Micromanagement that ignores the variation in patients and families by mindlessly following the norms blunts innovation and attuned variation. More important, arbitrarily following normative practice undermines the ethos of good practice, that is, the commitment to serve patients' and society's best interests (Hofman, 1994; Pellegrino, 1994; Sulmasy, 1992).

Developing teams with continuity and good information on repeated breakdowns and complications can create the possibility of group problem-solving and continuous improvement. Expert nursing practice can be served by collecting aggregate data on patient outcomes and identifying common recurring breakdowns with particular patient populations. But this aggregate can only serve to guide improvement at the individual patient level. In considering norms, concern for individual patients' well-being must not be violated. Managing knowledge workers, whose expertise must develop in the care of particular patients, using a static command-and-control approach blunts direct learning and guidance from those patients and limits the development and sharing of innovation and initiative in practice. Organizational design that overlooks the social embeddedness of knowledge, the nature of skilled know-how, and clinical and ethical judgment will be subintelligent. Wisdom and compassion cannot be replaced by information. But neither can they be sustained without good information and continuous attentiveness to patient care outcomes. Our organizational designs dare not succumb to cynicism and distrust of the desire and possibility of excellent practice sustained by practitioners who intend to do well by patients. The fact that health care practitioners do not always actualize their intent, or don't always have the patient's best interests foremost, need not fuel cynicism, nor motivate the care designed for the lowest common denominator. The fact that not all practitioners take up the ethos of advocating and serving the patient's best interests does not mean that we should abandon our efforts to design organizational structures and climates that reward good service and continuous improvement. At their best, nurses and physicians are knowledge workers whose practice is shaped by an evolving, living tradition of improving service to patients. Falling short of this goal is no excuse for abandoning the ethical vision of creating realistic organizational climates that promote rather than threaten this vision.

Expert clinical reasoning in transitions requires that practitioners develop and transmit their acquired skilled judgments and skilled ethical comportment to other practitioners. This does not mean that designing work should rigidly adhere to one type of delivery of health care. For example, it is doubtful that nurses at the advanced beginner stage should be given full "primary nurse" responsibilities, since they need access to expert nurses who also know their patients. Likewise, it is doubtful that any money can be saved by having lesser skilled workers provide care for the very ill. For example, in the case of premature infants, every intervention and handling of the infant should yield information about the infant's clinical condition, since there is so little lead time in recognizing crucial changes and handling the infant must be attuned to the infant's wake-sleep cycles. This care should be provided by expert nurses and coached family members.

Caring for acutely ill and vulnerable patients requires facing the anxiety of being responsible for another's life and well-being. Abstract institutional controls do not remove this responsibility. Aggregate morbidity and mortality studies do not capture the ethical demands faced by health care practitioners. We found in both narratives and field observations that in a patient resuscitation effort, everyone felt equally responsible. How could it be otherwise? This daily extremity must be acknowledged in organizational design, and in planning the most cost-effective skill mix. This is captured in the following exemplar from a competent nurse who was required to practice with too few experienced staff to cover the level of patients in her critical care unit. A long portion of the interview is used to convey both the voice and the tone of voice of the nurse:

Nurse 1:   I work 12-hour shifts, and I was scheduled to take over charge at 11:00, which was fine. Unfortunately, I was the only person on the schedule with any kind of experience. The other three nurses that were ICU nurses had less than a month of experience and I had three floats, and that was my staff. We had 11 patients, very high acuity. I believe we had 5 vents, a couple patients on Nipride, a 5150 (a psych hold), a couple fresh postops (new surgical patients) . . . So, it was very high acuity and I was not comfortable being the only person there with any experience. Nobody else was trained to go to codes, even. I mean, it was just me. They had given a regular staff person with experience an unscheduled day off, for some reason, staffing screwed up. An absent day, they just let her have the night off. So we had tried, at 7:00 when I came on, I knew that was the situation and we were trying to get C. to come back in. We told staffing we needed her to come back in, and they were arguing with us, saying, "Well, no, you have enough people. You're already overstaffed. We can't call her back in." We were talking with the house supervisor explaining to her what the situation was, and she's saying, "Well, your float nurses are real strong nurses, you know, we just can't do this." We ended up talking to the charge nurse of the intensive care unit, and she said, "Well, L., which is one of the new grads, is ACLS-certified and the other two are very familiar with the crash cart." And she was upset with us for being overstaffed. That was her response to the situation. Now, just as an aside, L., the one that was ACLS-certified, it was her second night ever, as working as a nurse on her own (laughter). Ever. So there was no support for me whatsoever.

Int.:   And for her.

Nurse 1:   For her, for anyone, you know. So I was pretty upset to be placed in that kind of jeopardy to begin with. I finished giving report and uh, I noticed, while I was giving report, I noticed this one particular patient kept coming off the monitor, so I finished at about 11:30 giving report on the two patients that I'd had from 7–11, and I went in there to put the guy back on the monitor, and he was in extreme respiratory distress. He was gone. He was becoming obtunded. He was diaphoretic. His pressure was dropping. You could hear him from the doorway, he was so wet. He went into frank pulmonary edema, acute pulmonary edema. So I asked the nurse that had been taking care of him, she also had been there for 12 hours—I said, "How long has he been breathing like this?" She says, "Well, I noticed, I went in there at 11:15 and I noticed he was breathing like that, but I didn't want to interrupt you while you were giving report." (laughter) That's what I said. Oh, God. I said, "Please, interrupt me. Please." So fortunately we had a real strong respiratory therapist on, this guy is real good, and he helped me suction patient and he suctioned the patient. Got pink frothy and we drew some gases on him and he was 43 and 43, so T. was bagging him while I called the doctor. T's wonderful. It was like, "Thank God," it was him. The doc says to me, "Well, give him 40 Lasix, start an aminophylline drip and draw gases in 2 hours and let me know if his PO2 is less than 60." So I said, "He'll be dead in 2 hours. He needs to be intubated right now." And so he says, "Well, okay, what was his PO2 again?" I said, "43." And he goes, "Oh, well, okay, call ER" So the ER doc came up and intubated him and, you know, fussed around with him a little bit and he was progressively deteriorating. I mean the man was just full out crashing.

Int.: What was his diagnosis?

Nurse 1: He was, I'm sorry, I didn't tell you. He was admitted with hepatitis and a GI bleed. And I, that's about really all I knew about him because I had been real busy my previous hours and I didn't really have a good feel for what was going on in the unit because I was so busy with my patients. So all I knew was what his diagnosis and that he was stable.

Int.: So now you're charge.

Nurse 1: So now I'm charge, right. I'm charge. I walk into this situation where this patient's crashing. The nurse that had him didn't have a clue. I mean, I can't believe that she knew that the man was in such respiratory distress and wouldn't come to me, so I have to believe that she just didn't have a handle on what was going on. You know, she just didn't comprehend that this patient was crashing.

Int.: Yeah, that's exactly right because you can't know it and ignore it.

Nurse 1: Right, and ignore it.

Int.: So she just didn't know it on some level.

Nurse 1: She had absolutely no idea that this man was so critical at this point. This guy is a full code. So, uh, the emergency room doctor called in the guy's doc, uh, he was a patient of Dr. X. who was on call, or Dr. Y. was on call for him. The on-call guy didn't really know him. He had just heard from J. that "Yeah, the patient's stable." You know, I mean, that's about all he'd heard. So he didn't really know the patient. And the guy's other primary, the GI primary doc was off call, and his on call didn't really know the patient. So the emergency room doctor convinced Dr. G. to come in and see this patient. He said, "Look, if you don't come in this man is going to die." I mean he was that bad. He was just crashing. So the cardiologist came in. We ended up putting lines in, starting dopamine, dah-dah-dah, the whole rigamarole that you go through when a patient's crashing. Well, I was the only one there that knew what to do. I mean I was the only one there. Nobody else knew where anything was. You know, the float nurses didn't know where anything was. They certainly didn't know what to anticipate, what would be happening, you know. They didn't, you know, they didn't know how to call x-ray even. They didn't know how to get the cardiology tech. I mean, they just didn't know what you need to do to go through these things that happen. And so I was the only person there that could deal with that. And still having to be responsible for the rest of the unit with these unstable patients.

Int.:   That nurse assigned to him really couldn't . . .

Nurse 1:   She, she sat and cowered in the corner. She was petrified. The poor thing was just petrified. She didn't know what the hell was going on. I mean, she just stayed out of the way, you know. I mean, she couldn't even, she was so scared, she couldn't even run and, you know, run to pharmacy and run dah-dah-dah. She couldn't, she just stayed out of the way. I mean, she was just in so far over her head.

Int.:   Now was she a new graduate?

Nurse 1:   No, actually, she works in the burn unit. I don't know why she was so out of her depth because, you know, they get some pretty critical patients down there. I don't know why she just wasn't with it at all. My three ICU nurses, you know the new grads, are so tunnel-vision, all they can see is their patients. I had to keep asking them, "Please watch the monitors. Please answer the phone." Repeatedly, repeatedly. "Watch the monitors." We had some patients in the back on this particular bank of monitors they kept, their heart rate would keep going down to like 47 and it would trigger the low heart alarm on the monitor, and this particular bank it'll keep alarming, and keep alarming until you push a reset button. And they would just let it go off, and let it go off. (laughter) And the way our unit is set up here are the monitors, over here, and then there's a walkway and then behind over here is where we prepare all our drugs, and at one point I was in the room hearing the monitors ding-ding-dinging, alarming, and so I thought, "Geez, I'll go out and see what's going on." And here was the nurse with her back to the monitors drawing up a medication and she never even once turned around to look at this monitor to see what was going on. You know, so they didn't even realize a patient was crashing. You know, they just had no clue as to what was going on. Thankfully the two other nurses, the float nurses from RCU [*Respiratory Care Unit*], they were wonderful. One of them did all the paperwork, the charge nurse stuff. She did my staffing and my census and my labs, and stuff like that. She took care of that. And the other one took over the burn unit nurse's other patient. But it was horrendous. I mean I had absolutely no support. If another patient had crashed, I don't know what would have happened. There was nothing. There was nothing there. You know, the patient lived. You know, he finally got semi-stable around 3:30–4:00, then at 4:30 I got an admission, a patient on a ventilator. You know. He was fairly stable, but still, you know, it's a lot to go through. Then at 5:30 we ended up having to push and drip a patient who went into V-tach [*ventricular tachycardia*], and it just so happens that the nurse that had that patient was the one that was ACLS certified, and she didn't even know how, she'd never done, she never pushed and dripped a patient. So she, she didn't know . . .

Int.:   What medication were you using?

Nurse 1:   Lidocaine. She didn't know how much Lidocaine to give, and then she was trying to figure out . . .

Nurse 2:   She would have been no good in a code.

Nurse 1:   She was trying to, yeah, she was trying to figure out the dosage like you do dopamine in mics per kilogram and so she didn't even have a clue, and that stuff's on ACLS. So it just sort of proved my point that what good is ACLS if you just, if you've never gone through a code? I mean, it's worthless. So, fortunately I made it through the night. But it was awful, you know, it was like the worst-case scenario happened, the patient crashed and I was left holding the bag.

Nurse 2:   Is your Charge Nurse usually supportive, or is she . . .

Nurse 1:   Uh, she's new. She started last December. She hasn't been here a year and I'd say the first three or four months she seemed pretty supportive and you know, I really think it's a difficult position to be in, you're torn between administration and you're torn between your nursing. And I think now with all the hospital's financial woes and so forth and contracts, she's sort of being pulled toward management and she's becoming less supportive of us, of our nursing staff. And uh, you know, I felt like her response that this one nurse was ACLS and the others knew the crash cart, and being angry that we were overstaffed, it was like slapping me in the face and telling me to go off, you know.

Int.:   But what happened afterwards? Did you get, did you have a conference with her?

Nurse 1:   Well, I filled out an ADO form and this morning . . .

Int.:   An ADO?

Nurse 1:   Assignment Despite Objection form from [*the professional nursing union*]. And I had a conference with her for this morning and I told her exactly, I called her on the carpet about her comments about being ACLS and I told her I felt that I had zero support from her and that indeed I felt like she slapped me in the face and so on and so forth. And she said, "Well, she didn't mean to be not supportive and she should have talked to me instead of the other nurse." Because I never actually spoke with her, and you know. And I guess she could tell by the expression on my face, she said, "I haven't made you feel better, have I?" I said, "No, you haven't." I said, "I don't know what will make me feel better about it." I said, " Yeah, maybe some time and distance so I can start focusing on how good I performed that night." And I told her, I said, "I would also like to hear that in the future we would be listened to when we say we need a staff member, we'll get that staff member regardless of what the numbers say." And she kind of said . . .

Nurse 2:   Will she ever come in herself?

Nurse 1:   She never has but, you know, she'll take patients on day shift.

Nurse 3:   It's my understanding that they're obligated to do that. That's what the charge nurse in CCU [*Coronary Care Unit*] says.

Nurse 2:   And we have a policy that says we have to have at least two certified people on the unit.

Nurse 3:   Oh, right, that too.

Nurse 1:   Yeah, so it was just a horrible situation and I told her, I also told her if I was ever placed in that kind of position again, she'd have my resignation in the morning. It wasn't worth it.

Nurse 2:   Turn around and leave you.

Nurse 1:   And I won't give her 2 weeks' notice. She'll have my resignation effective that day. I'll complete the assignment and that'll be that.

Nurse 2: When you have, how did those other nurses feel? Were they angry that they didn't have uh, a learning.

Nurse 1: Oh, absolutely. Oh, that's what else happened. Another patient pulled out his art line. The nurse told me about it after the fact. I thought, "Well, gee, I hope she knew what to do." 'Cause I don't know, I mean, these people, they don't even have a month under their belt, you know, they just don't. And yeah, they felt frustrated because I was so stressed, and they felt like they were of no help to me. You know. And I, being pretty new myself, and have been in that position of feeling helpless, I tried to make them feel like well, they were a help in the sense that at least I felt that they were competent to take care of their patients, and I didn't feel like I had to deal with this crash plus look over their shoulder and make sure that they were doing whatever. You know, that they were suctioning their patient or whatever. And I did kind of tell each of them that, you know, that they need to be more aware of the monitors. I mean, that's one thing that I think even being new that it's essential that you have to be, you have to keep the monitors, you have to pay attention to them. But I tried not to, you know, make them feel guilty for being new. 'Cause it's not their fault, you know, it's not their fault at all.

Int.: Think for a minute, just sort of imagine what the same scenario would have been like had you been well staffed. What would, just, this is one of those obvious questions, but answer it anyway.

Nurse 1: I think it would have sailed just fine. I think that if there had been even one other person with experience, that person could have at least called X-ray, called in the cardiology tech, anticipated that this patient would need lines and get all that going, and you know, run to the blood bank. That's another thing I omitted, we dropped an NG tube and he bled out like 800 of bright red blood and so he was bleeding again, and you know, and if nothing else some moral support, you know. Say, "W., you're doing great." Or, "Isn't this a tough night?" Or something.

Int.: Exactly.

Nurse 1: Some acknowledgement, some support.

Nurse 1: [*later in same interview*] Well, you know, I really think that patient had started going bad on p.m.'s and that nurse just didn't pick up on it. Not at all.

Int.: And was she fairly inexperienced?

Nurse 1: No.

Int.: No.

Nurse 1: She's an experienced burn unit nurse.

Int.: Okay.

Nurse 1: Which is why I don't understand how that happened. You know, but it happened. One of the patients, in fact, the patient that I'd had on p.m.'s, we had, I had to start him on Nipride and uh, he was not doing well on the Nipride. You know, his pressure really wasn't coming down. We were having to go up and up and up and up and up on the Nipride. He ended up coding and dying about noon the next day, and I really think had this not been going on that I might have been able to pick up some of the neuro [*neurological*] signs that were occurring, and they were occurring, you know, in retrospect, they were happening. His breathing pattern had changed somewhat, his level of consciousness decreased, and the nurse that had him just didn't have the experience to see that, you know. I don't know, I doubt that it would have changed the outcome . . .

Int.: Huh-huh.

Nurse 1: But perhaps . . .

Nurse 1: [*later in same interview*]: Well, it's 'cause you're responsible for these patient's lives, you know.

Int.: Yeah.

Nurse 1: I mean, I feel responsible that I wasn't available to pick up on these subtle signs, because that's what being in charge is all about. It's not, it's not about doing the paperwork, it's being responsible for the patients and your nurses, that's what it's all about, and I wasn't able to do that.

Nurse 1: [*later in same interview*]: Exactly, it was so dangerous. It was so dangerous.

Nurse 3: Oh, terrible.

Nurse 1: It was awful, awful.

Int.: Any of you have any other questions for W. on this situation?

Nurse 2: I saw her the night afterwards and she said you were still close to tears.

Nurse 1: I was. You know, I still sort of am, and probably because I had to speak with my Charge Nurse this morning about it and be firm, which is difficult with an authority figure, just to tell them that I'm not going to do this again. I felt shafted.

Int.: But you weathered that, didn't you? I mean . . .

Nurse 1: Oh, yeah. I'll never forget it.

Int.: Yeah, yeah.

Nurse 1: Yeah, it sticks with you.

The moral weight of the work itself cannot admit the logic of arbitrary, abstract cost controls that go by formula rather than the actual expertise level of the assigned nurses in the context of a particular patient mix. There is no way for the practicing nurse to delegate the responsibility for those lives she holds in her charge. It sticks with her. Here the requisite for professional judgment, and the limits of micromanagement that interferes with that judgment, is painfully clear.

TEAM BUILDING AND CLINICAL PROMOTION PROGRAMS

We recommend clinical promotion programs that foster the development and recognition of nursing expertise. While experience is required for the development of expertise, experience alone does not guarantee the development of expertise. We believe that it is possible for nurses to accurately evaluate one another's level of clinical expertise as outlined in this work and that such peer evaluation can foster the development of clinical expertise as well as recognize and reward extant nursing expertise. As hospital beds are reduced for cost savings, and nursing staffs are downsized, it is more important than ever to foster and retain the most expert nurses. This is best accomplished through peer review.

The research methods used in this study to identify levels of practice by examining clinical narratives and direct observation of practice can be adapted to develop clinical promotion programs. A number of hospitals have used this approach[1] that will be briefly described here.

First, a Clinical Development Program Committee is established and the best nurse clinicians are identified and asked to submit clinical exemplars that represent the best of their practice. These exemplars are used to describe the top level of clinical nursing practice. It is assumed that organizational demands, resources, and constraints set limits on the level of nursing that can be consistently practiced within a setting. Clinical and caring intents, knowledge, skills, and notions of good are identified in the narratives, and these characteristics are used to described the expert level of practice. With each descriptive area or domain, there are actual exemplars to illustrate what is being characterized as expert practice. This methodology captures a living and growing tradition of excellence. There is no assumption that the sampled practice will cover *all* possible areas of expertise; however, the Clinical Promotion Committee is charged with sampling and illustrating a good representative sampling of the best practice. Usually three levels (beginning, competent, and expert) are established to begin the program, because three levels can reliably be identified by most nurses using a narrative methodology. As the practice develops, additional levels can be added.

The program is given the charge to identify excellent practice. In the peer review committees, nurses are encouraged to develop concrete strategies for extending excellent practice and for removing impediments to the practice identified in the clinical narratives. The program is designed to reflect the understanding that clinical knowledge and ethical comportment are socially embedded and facilitated or hindered by organizational structures and processes that govern the practice.

The Clinical Promotion Committee develops a Promotion Portfolio prepared by the nurse seeking promotion. This Portfolio contains relevant evidence about the level of actual clinical practice. We recommend that the portfolio always contain at least three clinical narratives in addition to letters of support, examples of documentation of patient care, and other relevant evidence of level of practice. The backbone of the peer review process is based upon critically reading the clinical exemplars for the knowledge, skill, and notions of good evident in the nurse's narrative. The in-service education process of teaching nurses to develop clinical exemplars, and to critically evaluate them, is in itself a strategy for enhancing reflection on clinical reasoning in transitions.

THE USE OF NARRATIVES FOR PROMOTING CLINICAL LEARNING

The cumulative development of wisdom and improvement in a practice depends on dialogue and the possibility of sharing clinical knowledge gained about particular patients and their responses to therapy. This study supports the practice of having nurses present their narratives of clinical learning to one another in order to transmit and extend subtle clinical lessons learned. It suggests that bedside exchanges, illustrating nursing assessments of patients' conditions or care strategies, could enhance performance and clinical learning.

We recommend the use of clinical narratives as a powerful strategy for reflecting on practice and as a means for communicating a vision of excellent practice. Too often management is based on identifying performance deficits and correcting them. This is a necessary guiding and correcting task of management, but it is not sufficient, and can be demoralizing if strategies for recognizing and highlighting excellent practice never occur. Open forums for presenting clinical narratives, and organizational strategies for publishing narratives about clinical practice can do much to enrich the language for reflecting on expert clinical judgment and caring practices. These narratives are most effective when they are real, including the inevitable impediments that disrupt effective practice. The narratives should contain as much actual dialogue and realistic concerns as they occurred at the time as possible in order to allow for shared reflection on actual practice.

There are many organizational strategies for enhancing informal and formal dialogues about clinical learning, caring practices, and understandings gained about patient/family needs. It is clear from this research that interprofessional dialogue about clinical knowledge and clinical learning needs to be enhanced. We found that this exchange already occurs extensively between clinically expert physicians and nurses. The level of practice for physicians and nurses is interdependent, as demonstrated in Chapter 11. Because clinical knowledge requires practical reasoning in transitions, skill must be developed in presenting clinical observations and reasoning. Nurses and physicians can point to examples of successful communication about clinical judgments, as well as breakdown. Attending to the problems in communicating clinical judgments in doctors' rounds with patients and case presentations can help refine distinctions in clinical judgment (Pike, 1991).

A word of caution is in order. However, the use of first-person narratives in an organizational setting requires a climate of trust and an ethos of learning directly from practice. Narratives can reveal not only the strengths of the practice but also the impediments, blind spots, silences, and ignorance. Therefore, the narratives must be treated with openness and respect for the risks inherent in describing actual clinical experiences. We recommend that narratives be used for fostering clinical learning and the extension of clinical expertise. Therefore, managers and clinical educators, much like nurse educators in basic nursing education, should be taught to support and encourage the narrator in a process of identifying strengths, notions of good, silences, and areas for additional clinical learning. Clinical learning, by its nature, is open-ended. If an ethos is developed to support clinicians in clinical learning, then it will be safe to reveal the real struggles and risks inherent in clinical practice. The risky and demanding nature of the work requires support and openness rather than secrecy and cover-up (Benner & Wrubel, 1989). Thus, care must be taken to prevent using narratives to undermine the confidence and respect of a colleague.

Clinical narratives inevitably reveal institutional blocks to expert practice. Narrators and clinical coaches should be encouraged to read narratives for ideas of how to redesign care delivery to extend excellent practice and remove impediments to good practice. A clinical practice is necessarily housed in a spoken tradition of a community of practitioners. Therefore, team building and facilitation of the communication of hard-won clinical knowledge fosters organizational wisdom and continuous improvement of practice.

DEVELOPING AN ORGANIZATIONAL CLIMATE FOR CLINICAL LEARNING

Most educational programs within hospitals have emphasized orienting new employees, cross-training, and introducing new science and technology. While these educational activities will continue to require emphasis, they are not sufficient for developing clinical expertise for specific patient populations, because they do not focus on the development of clinical judgment. On one highly specialized pediatric unit in this study, a head nurse had rearranged her staffing pattern to allow for one expert nurse per shift to augment, educate, and enhance the clinical judgment of the practicing nurses. The following field observation note illustrates the weaving together of bits of experience and information now fragmented in this staff due to high staff turnover:

Observer Note: *The unit educator nurse, all the while I am observing, acts as a repository of quick information: How do you know when the bone marrow will be up for the bone marrow transplant? Should the float nurse go ahead and premedicate a patient who is supposed to go for surgery? What should be done with a morphine vial, unopened, not given, but signed out? Questions about IV lines. Much advice about who and when to call. Questions about disposal of toxic chemical IV bottles. The nurse educator told me which children she was most concerned about, as noted above, and needs to have in mind what she would do if she received an emergency admit. She showed me on the board what she would probably do. She would move a recovering open heart patient, who was doing well, to the step down unit. She would reassign patients to two of her best nurses who were doing a two-nurse-to-three-patient ratio, and she would have the float nurse admit the new patient. She discussed her strategies fluently, playing with different ideas in her mind. She mentioned that she did not know when the transport would arrive or whether that child would require a great deal of care.*

The amount of local specific clinical knowledge required to run any complex clinical unit with highly technical medical practice points up the effectiveness and efficiency of having a stable staff and an ongoing program of developing the local specific clinical knowledge within a group of caregivers. The "Unit Educator" is a temporary measure to shore up a fragmented staff, but some form of local clinical education is required on all units. Nurses who practice together with similar patient populations develop benchmarks and distinctions in patient recovery, in addition to shared wisdom about the hazards of the technology and strategies for managing it. This evolving clinical knowledge needs to be communicated and validated among staff. Breaking up seasoned clinical teams may be far more costly to the organization than has been recognized by the rampant practices of floating nurses and having only centralized staff development.

This research points up the importance of developing and selecting clinical preceptors. Engaged, committed preceptors instantiate the best of clinical practice, and should be selected for this culture-bearing role. Likewise, a poor selection of clinical preceptors can be extremely detrimental. Those who are selected as preceptors have the opportunity to put into language some of their clinical learning of which they may have little awareness. The learning process can be a two-way street, with the preceptor being exposed to the latest theoretical knowledge from the newcomer. And the act of teaching another can clarify tacit clinical expertise that the nurse has gained over time.

The use of clinical narratives on a unit can create concrete examples of excellent practice, in the midst of the contingencies of the particular unit. Orienting new staff members to unit logistics and organizational strategies, may require different preceptors than those selected to teach clinical judgment with particular patient populations. We found that advanced beginner nurses were actively evaluating the quality of clinical instructions and answers to their clinical questions. This is yet another informal side of learning clinical judgment. It is the beginning base for developing peer review.

In-service education should be designed to develop clinical knowledge across the stages of skill acquisition. More specific strategies for all of the skill levels have been elaborated in the earlier chapters. For example, the new graduate's assignment should be arranged so that on-the-spot consultation can occur when questions of interpretation of clinical data and patient trends occur (see Chapter 3). Staff development should be planned for the competent level nurse in order to support the ability to see changing relevance and begin to develop a more response-based practice. This means careful attention to the development of the newly graduated nurse, not just during the first 6 months or year of practice, but intermittently for the first 3 years. Well-timed coaching on how to cope with system failures and negotiate clinical knowledge can give the competent nurse new insights and strategies. Nursing narratives on recognizing changing relevance and the turning around of preconceptions of the clinical situation can be instructive for all levels of practitioners. Highlighting the clinical learning required to become more attuned to patient needs and changing relevance can reassure the proficient level nurse, who may perceive the change as a decrease in "organization." Competent level nurses can be helped to see this as a higher form of organization, one that is responsive to early warnings and unexpected changes. Expert clinicians should have the opportunity to discuss their ethical dilemmas and the experience of discovering the "unexpected" in patient situations. By giving language to clinical expertise, expert clinicians can take more active roles in designing the organizational structures and processes for improved patient care.

DESIGNING PATIENT CARE RECORDS FOR CLINICAL KNOWLEDGE DEVELOPMENT

Patient records and the requirements for documentation of work guide the beginner's practice, yet these documents have seldom been designed with guidance of clinical practice in mind. In the climate of the automated patient record, we recommend that the documentation be designed with both the patient and the practitioner in mind. Documentation can guide the nurse's clinical grasp of the patient and facilitate a presentation of the most salient patient information, or it can provide little evidence of clinical interpretations and concerns. With computerized charting it may be possible to relegate the most summary clinical information into the patient's permanent patient record, while keeping a working document of clinical concerns and clinical observations about the patient's responses and preferences. Critical care nurses talked about "fine-tuning" patients, and also gave information about patients' responses to antiarrhythmic and vasopressor drugs. This clinical information needs to be conveyed, even though it is a tentative, time-limited clinical judgment. Creating a climate for conveying clinical knowledge and giving language to one's clinical observations enhances everyone's expertise.

In the quest to only present "objective signs and symptoms" for official documents, clinicians omit important clinical observations and understandings. Qualitative distinctions about patients' conditions can become more refined over time only if these clinical distinctions are given language and compared between clinicians. Public dialogue creates the possibility of making recognizable clinical distinctions accessible to other clinicians. When clinical expertise is discovered, for example, the ability to recognize early warnings of sepsis in a patient, or the ability to discern when a patient is safely able to swallow without aspirating, these clinical skills should be demonstrated and illustrated by concrete examples. Often such clinical skills go unnoticed and are not communicated to other clinicians. Thus clinical dialogues that reflect clinical learning and questions could be communicated in less than permanent records as a way of enhancing the ability to make clinical distinctions and judgments. If the Respiratory Critical Care Unit has made great strides in weaning patients from respirators, this knowledge can be transmitted best by ongoing demonstrations and coaching by the Respiratory Critical Care Nurses to nurses on other units.

RE-ENGAGING CAREGIVERS

We can only speculate why nurses do not progress to a level of expert practice, but there is much in our organizational and cultural practices that cover over agency, skills of engagement, skilled know-how, and clinical judgment, as pointed out by Jane Rubin (see Chapter 7). In the quest to standardize and objectify decision making we must take care to attend to what cannot be standardized or objectified. We must clarify practical clinical reasoning in transitions. Providing concrete examples of engaged expert forms of nursing practice can rekindle a vision for nursing practice that is guided by the ethos of patient advocacy and caring practices. To the extent that nurses lose their learning curve through disengagement and disenchantment with nursing, consciousness-raising groups can be formed to address the sources of disengagement and disenchantment.

Sometimes the culture of a unit will develop that fosters disengagement and discourages patient involvement. This may be perpetuated by folk wisdom that care is too costly and that disengagement is the best protection against burnout (see Benner & Wrubel, 1989; Chapter 8). In-service education classes on developing the skills of involvement, healthy stress management, grief counseling, and focusing on caring for the caregiver can provide more effective ways of dealing with the stresses of caregiving (Benner & Wrubel, 1989). Positive team building that encourages direct assertive communication about problems, rather than divisive hidden criticism and undermining of colleagues' reputations, can do much to change the climate and mood of a unit to one of cooperation and affirmation. Nursing care is both intensive and extensive. No one nurse can accomplish "total" care for any patient or family. Cooperative teamwork and clear communication channels are required for passing on and developing cumulative wisdom about helping patients. This study points to the need to do studies of corporate levels of expertise and cultures of excellence in nursing practice. Clearly, there is a need for ways of improving the care of specific patient populations by systematically examining common patient trajectories and how these trajectories correspond with expected critical paths of recovery.

SUMMARY AND CONCLUSIONS

Organizational structures, processes, and climates set limits to the possibilities of expert nursing practice, just as the patient's condition and particular vulnerabilities guide the level of attentiveness and interventions required. Critical care units can exemplify this most acute care today, therapies are instantaneous and the patient's conditions are highly labile. Nurses are knowledge workers who must attend to reliability as well as efficiency. The margins for error are small. Most Americans are committed to the life-extending advances in medical technology, but the costs have become prohibitive. Many hospitals have responded by re-engineering strategies (Champy, 1995), reducing nursing staff, and training lesser educated workers to do tasks that do not require clinical judgement. This strategy may cut into the reliability and possibility for nurses to be attentive enough to patients to notice subtle changes, or to form trusting relationships that foster well-being and comfort. We found many examples where nurses who knew patients and families well were able to coach them in the transition from anticipating heroic recovery into preparing for death. Cost-cutting strategies that undermine astute clinical judgment and caring practices may be much more costly in terms of human lives and the overuse of prolonged, futile treatments. Money is probably best spent in providing the most expert nursing staff possible and providing organizational arrangements whereby nurses can be attentive to and know their patients (Tanner et al., 1993). These arrangements will probably be most conducive to reducing costly hospital stays to the minimum number of days possible.

NOTE

1. Richard Benner and his associates have developed a process for developing a clinical promotion program that identifies current levels of practice within an institution. This program fosters the growth of shared practice through the use of reflection on clinical narratives to describe levels of practice, give language to excellent practice, and to foster enhancement of clinical and ethical expertise.

BACKGROUND AND METHOD

The approach to understanding the practice of nurses in this project is hermeneutical phenomenology, a practice of interpretation and understanding of human concerns and practices. This approach attempts to capture everyday skills, habits, and practices by eliciting narratives about the everyday and by observing action in meaningful contexts. The particular hermeneutic tradition within which we worked derives from the phenomenological work of Heidegger (1926/1962) and Kierkegaard (1843/1985). Present-day interpreters of this existential phenomenology have articulated the philosophical underpinning of a hermeneutic approach and furthered the possibilities for its use in examining engaged practices. They include Dreyfus (1979, 1991a), Taylor, (1985a) and Rubin (1984). Benner (1994b) provides a full discussion of the ways in which this form of interpretation articulates with and is shaped by an existential philosophy and various strategies and processes for interpreting human concerns and action.

This study of clinical judgment and knowledge development was shaped by a preunderstanding of human action and engagement. We wish to point to our preunderstandings because they in every way directed our approach to the study of nursing practice, including the stance we took vis-à-vis the nurse informants; the mode of inquiry that we used to capture the nurses' concerns and action; and the approaches we used to interpret those narratives and recordings of that action. In what follows, we point out how our preunderstandings of human existence and activity structured the design of the study. A detailed discussion of how the study was conducted is accompanied by a commentary on why certain actions and choices were made. Throughout this discussion we describe how we attempted to maintain a) integrity in the data; b) openness in the research processes of collecting and interpreting data; c) dialogue with our preunderstandings of the practice and with current presentations of that practice in the literature; and d) rigor in presenting the interpretations so that they are bolstered by the textual evidence.

At base we understand that human lives are situated within meaningful activities, relationships, commitments, and involvements that set up both possibilities and constraints for living. Humans become situated within their worlds by being raised up and living within a complex of understandings about the world and ways of being and acting in the world in that particular time in history, in the culture, and in the family in which they find themselves. Being situated means that one is neither totally determined or constrained nor radically free in how one acts. Rather, one has situated possibilities, certain ways of seeing and responding that present themselves to the individual in certain situations, and certain ways of seeing and responding that are not available to that individual.

A second assumption is that the basic way that humans live in the world is in engaged, practical activity. Being fully and unreflectively involved in everyday action has been described as being in the ready-to-hand mode of existence (Dreyfus, 1991; Heidegger, 1926/1962). Despite the terms used, the intent is to capture the basic and predominant way humans live their lives, which is commonplace, or taken for granted and therefore difficult to describe. Engaged practical activity is the smooth way that one moves through a day: cooking breakfast, dressing children, and driving to work, all without deliberation or reflection on these actions. Additional ways that humans are involved in everyday activities are: standing back and thinking about how one's everyday activities, which is a more abstract, reflective mode of engagement (present at hand); and a middle ground of being disrupted, but still involved in one's activity, by an unexpected turn of the situation (unready-to-hand). The second mode of engagement is familiar but derivative of the first; an example is sitting down and reflecting on one's parenting after the children have been settled in bed. The third mode of engagement in everyday life is also common, but arises only when one's taken-for-granted expectations of a situation momentarily fail, when one's skills falter, or there is some breakdown in the smooth flow of the person acting within the situation. An example of the third form of involvement is when, while dressing a child for the day, a parent is startled to find that both pairs of the child's shoes are muddy and wet. Quickly, consciously reviewing the possibilities, the parent decides that slippers will suffice at the babysitter's that day, puts them on the child's feet, and re-enters the taken-for-granted flow of the morning.

A third assumption is that the way that humans are engaged in their worlds is set up and bounded by what matters to them. Concerns, or those things that matter to the person, set up how a person enters any situation, what is seen and unseen, and how the person acts. When one is wildly making final party arrangements and waiting for guests to arrive, the concern for readiness sets up a more acute awareness of the sounds of cars parking in front of the house. Similarly, what matters to an individual sets up their interest and involvement in each situation. For example, parents primarily concerned about equity and those primarily concerned about teaching generosity and flexibility will respond quite differently to a situation where their child is involved in an argument with a peer. Often concerns that cannot be directly expressed because they are not readily conscious and available show up in the actions and responses of the individual within situations.

These assumptions structured our study of nursing practice in several ways. First, we assumed that nurses, like all human beings, were situated within their practice, relying on background understandings which were not fully articulated, but operative nonetheless. These understandings pertain to the human beings in their care, the nature of nursing, the possibilities and constraints of treatments available, and the local settings in which they work. How nurses were situated in their practice would be most evident within practice with particular patients rather than in reflective accounts about practice in general. Consequently, the study was designed to capture practice with particular patients, within particular historical and social contexts rather than abstract constructs of nursing, classes of patients, or abstract systems of care. The study was designed to capture situatedness via close observations of direct practice with patients and via interviews about care of particular patients.

If the basic way of being in the world is engaged practical activity, then the method of study must try to access rather than cut off the structure of that involvement. One method of accessing involved activity is through thoughtful observation and discussion with the nurses about activity as it is in progress. This probably affords the greatest possibility of grasping ready-to-hand nursing practice, because the nurse informant is *in* the situation acting out his or her concerns and practices, while at the same time providing situated commentary on that action.

A second approach to accessing smooth flow or engaged activity is to ask nurses for full narratives about care of particular patients, which includes the context and history of the episode, the ways in which the situation presented itself and how it evolved over time, and the nurse's concerns and actions throughout the episode. The narrative form of expression seems to most closely match the structure of everyday living, and thus is the most apt form of expression to capture everyday involvements.

> It is because we all live out narratives in our lives, and because we understand our own lives in terms of the narratives we live out, that the form of narrative is appropriate for understanding the actions of others. Stories are lived before they are told- except in the case of fiction. (MacIntyre, quoted in Mishler, 1986, p. 68)

This study was structured primarily to elicit interpretive narratives of practice from nurses at different levels of experience. Adopting a narrative rather than the logico-scientific mode of inquiry, served the aims of this project in several ways. First, the narrative mode provides access to particular experience rather than to abstract or general constructions about that experience. Narratives allow the temporal unfolding of events to be captured in text and interpreted with that temporal structure intact, rather than deducing timeless processes about those events based on their external ordering. Within narrative, everyday language is encouraged, complete with multiple meaning, ambiguity, and nuance. The aim of the interpretive process is to make a clearing and offer one grasp of the meanings evident in this everyday language, rather than specifying the terms up front and constraining the storying within the investigation to those terms defined a priori. Setting out the terms in advance reduces the the complexity of the possible narrative. Narrative recognizes and makes a space for the person/ narrator to be present him or herself in the actions and relationships (White & Epston, 1990).

The third assumption, that humans move and act within situations according to their concerns or what matters to them, was additionally addressed by using a narrative structure for data. Concerns show up most forcefully in the actions taken by an individual in a particular situation. Within interviews, care was taken to elicit sufficient detail about all the possible interpretations of the situation the nurse could recall, as well as all of the possible courses of action considered, alongside her description of action taken. In eliciting such detail, it was possible to arrive at an interpretation of the concerns that were orienting the nurse within the situation. A good illustration of how narrative gives evidence of concerns in action is the contrast between the narratives of the advanced beginner and the expert regarding crisis situations. As was explicated in Chapter 3, advanced beginners' narratives were structured so that concerns about the nurses' performance had almost equal weight with the concern for the patient's trajectory. In contrast, expert nurses provided narratives in which they were driven by a concern to obtain the best grasp of the evolving patient situation, and anxiety about the self or one's performance ability was not in evidence.

Concerns can be partially explicated by most informants once they reflect on their experience. Thus, nurse informants were asked to describe the concerns that were salient in the situations they presented in narratives, as well as when they were being observed. Although these statements are helpful, in that they are the informants' retrospective or reflective interpretation about what was salient at that moment in time, the statements are most helpful when interpreted vis-a-vis their concrete actions within the situation.

Narrative Interviews

Given our concern for accessing situated practice with as much of the context and history intact, we encouraged the nurse informants to use a natural, narrative form to describe that practice. Small group interviews with nurses who had practiced for similar amounts of time and who were identified by their supervisors as practicing at similar levels of skill were the forum within which we elicited narratives of practice. Nurses were apprised of the nature of the interview before attending their first session, in that they were asked to complete written stories of care with particular patients. Additionally, nurses were asked to think about their recent practice prior to coming to the first interview, in order that specific instances of patient care might be more readily available for the telling.

Care was taken to make the tone of the interview that of an informal conversation between peers. Using everyday language, the interviewers asked nurses to tell stories of their practice in which they felt they made a difference, or that were memorable because the nurse learned something new. To achieve this informal tone, interviewers asked nurses to try to talk as if they were meeting with another nurse over coffee, or were talking with a roommate about something important that happened at work. We found it helpful to name examples of the types of stories that might come to mind; for example, "a situation where you felt you made a difference with a patient," or "where you felt that you really blew it, but learned from your experience." We found it unhelpful to ask for war stories, because that elicited unusual stories about grossly inequitable treatment of patients and nurses.

Narratives, rather than general abstract discussions of practice were used because:

> Narrative accounts of actual situations differ from questions about opinions, ideology or even what one does in general, because the speaker is engaged in remembering what occurred in the situation. Spoken accounts allow the speaker to give more details and include concerns and considerations that shape the person's experience and perception of the event. A story of an event is remembered in terms of the participant's concerns and understanding of the situation. Therefore, narrative accounts are meaningful accounts that point to what is perceived, worth noticing, and what concerned the storyteller. Narrative accounts of actual situations give a closer access to practice and practical knowledge than questions about beliefs, ideology, theory or generalized accounts of what people typically do in practice. Therefore, narratives can be used to examine discontinuities between theory and practice. (Benner, 1994b, p. 110)

At the start of each meeting, we as interviewers invited members of the group to take turns presenting stories. Each person in the room was asked to tell one or more stories, to actively listen, ask questions, and understand the story well before the group moved onto the next story. Nurses then took turns relating their narratives of patient care. The quality and tone of the interviews varied greatly, but in general we found that in the first of the three group interviews nurses were more reluctant or unfamiliar with the structure of narrating, and the process started slowly. We therefore spent time putting the nurses at ease, talking in general about their practice, and then helping the nurses move to stories about particular patients. If nurses continued to have difficulty identifying specific patient incidents, we asked about patients they had cared for recently or even that day. By the second and third interview, nurses were well-versed on what we were seeking, and were generally quite lively in relating particular patient incidents.

The aim of each interview was to understand each story as it unfolded. Once the nurses became versed in storytelling, their narratives were told in swift, condensed form. The task of the interviewer and group at that point was to retrace the story and fill in details about what happened and what was important to the nurse in terms of her concerns, understandings, and actions at each turn in the story. It was the role of the interviewer to allow nurses to tell their stories in personal, emotion-filled terms, and at the same time, to slow the pace of the interview so that the detail would not be lost to future interpretation. Nurses readily took up the role of co-interviewer, providing dynamic, insightful questions that led the narrator to fill in aspects of the narrative that might have been passed over in the excitement and action of the telling. Nurses became quite involved in their group participation, evidenced by the fact that they asked follow-up questions about a narrative in subsequent meetings or told parallel or counterinterest stories of their own in subsequent narratives.

A set of probes and questions for following up on and filling in narratives was developed by Benner at the inception of the project (see Appendix B). Interviewers used these probes as a general guide and orienting device within the interview. We reviewed these probes prior to each interview, and kept them close at hand during interviews, but inserted questions only as the interview flow allowed for it. There were interviews where the pacing of stories was quite rapid and interviewers did not have time to go back to each narrative and go through the detailed questions. Although these interviews are revealing because of the connections nurses made between stories they heard and subsequently told, these "thin" narratives that have not been filled in with detail and meaning are much less intelligible.

Small group interviews with the same participants were held on three separate occasions in order to derive multiple instances of practice from nurses at each level of practice, and to give nurses the opportunity to present instances from their practice that became salient in the course of the study as they listened to others' narratives. To complete the interpretive task of understanding skill development at many stages of nursing practice, the project required a large, varied and detailed set of narratives from nurses at each skill level. Narrative description and clarification are time-consuming processes, and commonly each nurse was able to present only one narrative per session. Thus, repeat interviews allowed us to hear multiple narratives from each nurse informant. In addition, both within interviews and between interviews, stories of particular patient situations triggered similar and contrasting stories from other nurses. In their responding narratives nurses evidenced their practical understanding and interpretation of the first story, in that they presented narratives that provided parallel or contrasting dialogue with the first. The similarities or differences of follow-up narratives were on multiple planes. Sometimes the narrative was about a similar work dilemma, such as working out the balance of power and decision making with other health professionals. Often the narrative evidenced a similar moral concern that was being worked out in the practice. For example, a narrative about the competing moral claims on the nurse by a gravely ill infant and his family who wishes to have "everything done for our baby" might precipitate a second story about a family locked in disagreement about pursuing heroic measures to maintain life. In presenting these comparison-and-contrast narratives, nurses offer a first level of interpretation of the original narrative and also point to practical engaged reasoning.

Interpretive work between interviews on the text of the preceding session also allowed the research team to enter the next session oriented to the particular nurse's practice and to the practice of nurses at that level of skill. New dialogue was then proposed by the research team about particular narratives that were puzzling or incomplete. Initial interpretations were offered by the research team and nurse-informants responded with both their own interpretations and further narratives that enriched the dialogue.

By bringing nurses who practiced at similar levels of practice into the same small groups, the natural form of narrative for that level of practice emerged. Nurses were encouraged to speak to each other in spontaneous terms and to resist speaking down or up to the interviewers. Nurses' natural ease in speaking to one another, as they would informally on their units, was readily captured in most interviews.

The risk of overstructuring or leading the nurse informants' narratives was resisted by staying close to the language and structure of the narratives that were already presented. Questions and interpretations were offered tentatively and in concrete terms immediately linked to practice, rather than in abstract, theoretical, power terms. In every encounter, effort was made to empower the informants to speak as experts on their practice, clarifying or correcting others' interpretations of their story and offering opportunities for counterinterpretations of their own. Interviewers modeled respectful listening and a stance of nonintrusion, particularly when the narrative was first being presented. Often, the story would be presented in shifting time frames, but by its conclusion, the temporal ordering of the complete story was clear. Only when the initial telling was complete would clarifying questions be initiated.

> In summary: Small group interviews achieve several purposes. (1) They create a natural communicative context for telling stories from practice, allowing peers to talk to one another as they ordinarily talk rather than translating their clinical world for the researchers. (2) They provide a rich basis for active listening where more than one listener is trying to understand the story. (3) Meanings of the stories can be enriched by stories triggered to counter, contrast or (address) similarity. . . . (4) Hearing other nurses' stories creates more of a work-like situation, creating a forum for thinking and talking about work situations that simulates a work environment. (Benner, 1994b, p. 109)

Observations of Nurses Engaged in Practice

In observing nurses in everyday practice, the aim is to further articulate the practices that nurses describe in the group interview narratives. In direct observation of a practice, there is a temporal immediacy and proximity to the exigencies of that practice that is less available in the narrative presentation. The context of the practice, which may be largely invisible to the practicing nurse because of its familiarity, stands out for an observer, particularly one who has not been fully assimilated into intensive care environments. Context includes the physical environment, the resources on hand and the tempo and energy in the surrounding unit, as well as the events that unfold prior to a particular incident in the nurse's practice. Smooth functioning in nursing practice is more evident in observation than in narratives because the background, self-evident nature of unproblematic practice is very hard for an engaged practitioner to describe. For example, in interviews, experts seldom mentioned their extraordinary monitoring of patients for new signs of instability that were a basic part of their everyday practice. However, when standing in the room with their patients, experts readily described their personal systems for monitoring drips or for working with cardiac monitors and alarms. Some nurses, for example, liked to set the alarms "tight" on particular patients, so that minor changes in the patient's cardiac status would be drawn to their attention. These differences in ease and manner with which nurses worked with the technologic surroundings in caring for patients were more evident in direct observation.

Forty-eight nurses at various levels of practice were repeatedly observed during their regular shifts in their assigned units for at least three observation periods. Nurses who were observed volunteered, or were invited by the research team to be a part of this additional data collection. The team asked to observe nurses who were good informants in interviews, as well as nurses who demonstrated a range of practice in their interview narratives from excellent to problematic, for each level of nursing practice in the sample. Each observation period lasted from 2–4 hours. With some groups, particularly the advanced beginners, there was some reluctance to volunteer or respond to the request to be observed. However, reassurance that the aim of observation was to understand, rather than judge their practice against a particular standard, seemed to dispel the anxiety and reluctance.

Care was taken to situate nurse observers so that the natural flow of practice was not impeded, but made more evident. The concern was to understand nurses' grasp of what they were encountering, the central concerns for the patient that were organizing their orientation to and work with the patient, the ways in which they reasoned or intuited the impact of their actions on the patient, and how emotional cues figured into their perceptions and actions.

Observations began with the practicing nurse reviewing her evaluation of the patient's overall status and history, her central concerns for the patient at that moment in time, her anticipation of what might happen in the next few hours, and her anticipated involvement in bringing that change about. This review was accomplished informally, often in piecemeal fashion as the nurse moved in and out of her required activities at the bedside. This review and other direct questions that were addressed to nurses intermittently throughout the observation were audiorecorded by the observers, who carried tape recorders unobtrusively in their pockets. After the brief review, practicing nurses were invited to describe changes in their grasp of what was happening with the patient, or changes in their concerns, or their anticipated movement with that patient at any time during the observation. Observers then stayed in the room, attending to the nurse's involvement with the patient and the flow of action in the room and the unit. Observers kept notes on salient aspects of this action and questioned the nurses about specific aspects of their involvement with the patient at quiet moments in the activity. Discussions of patient status or changes in that status were conducted out of the hearing of the patient or family. Observations were closed by a final review by practicing nurses of what had happened in the time that had elapsed, how they currently evaluated

the patient, their current concerns, and how they evaluated their own involvement in the care of that patient during the observation period.

Recording the events of the observation periods required an interweaving of the observers' impressions, emotions, observational notes, and the
actual recorded statements of the nurse describing the situation and her
practice. As soon as possible after the observation period, observers typed
their observational notes, so that the fullness of their impressions and
emotions might be captured. Observers then constructed texts that included
the transcribed statements of the nurse, the flow of events, and initial
experience-near interpretations of what had happened.

INTERPRETATION AND UNDERSTANDING

A text of this range and depth, which is grounded in the vital practice of
particular nurses within an equally vital profession, is multivocal. Although
the investigation was structured to generate a text which would address
the initial study aims and questions, the process of gathering and initially
analyzing the text generated additional, central lines of inquiry that we
knew must be pursued. This is always the case in interpretive projects
(Benner, 1994b). However, because of the size and complexity of this
dataset, we were particularly concerned that any effort at data organization and retrieval would keep the team in constant flexible contact with
the whole of the data and with meaningful subsets of data that would preserve the narrative structure of the practice that had been studied.

Interpretation of data occurred in several phases. In initially approaching the text, the research team was guided by the background frameworks
from which the project had been organized, that is, the Dreyfus Model of
Skill Acquisition (Dreyfus & Dreyfus with Athanasiou, 1986), Benner's
domains of nursing practice (1984a) and the concerns about the limits evident in the literature on clinical judgement (Tanner, 1987; 1993). Following in the hermeneutic tradition, however, the team purposefully worked
at remaining open to the many assertions made by the text about the content, concerns, and nature of the practice.

Care was taken in maintaining the fidelity of recorded and written text.
For interviews, the first review was comprised of listening to the tape and
correcting errors in the transcribed text, by a member of the team who had
conducted the interview. Shifts in meaning that might be introduced by
small errors in transcription were therefore eliminated. In addition, speaker
identifiers could consistently be applied to the various participants in the
group interviews, a process that proved important in groups where the

participants demonstrated clear distinctions in their practice that were important to the analysis.

The process of data interpretation involved the independent and then consensual interpretation of all aspects of text, including the interviews, and observational session recordings. Individuals read and interpreted interviews, attending most carefully to the narratives of practice contained within each interview, but also taking note of important themes in the general discussion portions of the text. Next the team met to discuss interpretations in an effort to work out the most completely nuanced yet coherent understanding of the text.

Because there were multiple readers approaching the text, multiple insights about a particular narrative, that were often additive, would come to light in the process of group discussion. In addition, conflicting or incompatible interpretations were worked out within the group by relying on thoughtful rereading of text for evidence about the interpretation that most matched the overall story presented by the participant.

The Process of Interpretation

When studying the everyday, lived experience of nurses engaged in the practice of nursing, understanding proceeds unevenly. Using care to examine the best available record or "fixing" of the practice, the narrative descriptions provided by nurses allow one the possibility of an improved grasp and eventual articulation of that practice. The basic unit of text that was considered throughout the interpretation was the story about a particular patient. The context of that story was also considered, including where it arose in the course of an interview and what stories preceded and followed it, as well as the larger context of the story, the nurse's practice.

As noted by Benner (1994b) the early leaps in understanding often occur when encountering a particularly vibrant example of practice that stands out from other examples when one is considering the whole text of an interview or a group of interviews. Part of the work of interpretation is puzzling through, with close attention to the text, how and why this particular instance of practice stands apart, catches the attention, or disrupts some taken-for-granted grasp of how nurses are involved in their work. These vibrant examples are paradigm cases, defined as strong instances of particular patterns of concerns, ways of being in the world, or ways of working out a practice. Paradigm cases benefit the interpreter because within the narrative account lies the possibility of understanding in a new way the whole of a nurse's concerns, practical knowledge, forms of engagement, and forms of reasoning in action within the practice.

In this study, paradigm cases were of two types. The first were those strong examples of nursing care that stood out for our research team as being new or puzzling or as illustrating aspects of nursing that we recognized as important but largely unarticulated. Often paradigm cases, or strong examples of practice that substantially shifted our interpretation of practice, were full vibrant stories about care of a particular patient that extended over time and involved many points of learning for the nurse as well. Smaller stories, which contained narrative about a particular patient on a particular shift or portion of a shift, also served as powerful paradigms that allowed the team to recognize a new pattern of involvement in the practice. Identification of narratives that were paradigmatic was almost always a shared experience. That is, individual team members worked out their initial personal interpretations of an interview and then came together with some general agreement about which narratives stood out, and which might be approached as particularly telling or informative. There were also instances where only one interpreter grasped a narrative as being significant, and in the group interpretive session laid out for the group the ways in which the narrative shed new light on a problem or concern that we had been pursuing. Because members of the team entered the project with divergent backgrounds, skills, and understandings of nursing practice, they had different possibilities for seeing the significance of various texts.

Narratives that provided paradigmatic shifts in understanding often did so on many fronts. For example, one detailed narrative provided by an expert nurse about her care over several months of an extremely fragile, ventilator-dependent elderly gentleman illuminated for the team, in a new way, what it meant to know a patient's physiologic rhythms (Tanner et al., 1993). The same narrative dramatically enriched our understanding of the demands involved and the skill demonstrated by the nurse in working with a family when a patient's prognosis is ambiguous but extremely guarded for a period of months. Therefore, the narrative was paradigmatic on at least two levels: for knowing a patient and for understanding family care.

The prior instance illustrates the second form of paradigm case encountered in this study: stories about patients that nurses identified as important because they changed or reoriented the nurse's practice. In the example mentioned above, the nurse herself identified care of this patient to be a paradigmatic experience, in that the gentleman helped her integrate into her practice a concern for holistically working with a patient's possibilities despite external evidence of limitations. Narratives that nurses identified as paradigmatic to their practice were attended to carefully for what they might show generally about experiential learning within a practice, about advances in nursing skill via practice itself, and specifically for the new practice possibilities recognized by the nurse in telling the narrative.

In studying a paradigmatic narrative, the aim is to understand the situation within the practical lived world of the participant, with all of its constraints, realities, and possibilities. The aim is not to identify abstract structures within action or basic social processes that underlie the action. Rather than making a theoretical move away from the action-in-context described in the narrative, the interpreter tries to enter into a dialogue with the narrative, and to understand it through the concerns of the interpreter, but also to grasp the concerns and action of the narrator.

While considerable attention was paid to narratives that result in paradigmatic shifts in understanding, all of the narratives and discussions by nurses captured in interviews and observations contributed to the further articulation and understanding of the practice. Each narrative offers further understanding of some aspect of practice. Some narratives provide important background about the contextual requisites of the practice; some illuminate aspects of practice with particular patient populations, or with patients at particular junctures in the illness trajectory. A rigorous examination of a text requires that all narratives be examined for what they make clear. Examination of only the most vibrant or paradigmatic cases would leave the interpretive project with a biased and thin understanding of the whole of the practice that the nurses gave us access to with their narratives. Rigor in the interpretive process also requires that interpreters listen for and make sense of silences, or stories that we expected to hear and did not.

Analysis of all narratives, particularly those that are not paradigm cases, is called an examination of exemplars. Benner clarifies that:

> Exemplars substitute for "operational" definitions in interpretive research because they allow the researcher to demonstrate intents and concerns within contexts and situations where the "objective" attributes of the situation might be quite different. . . . Each exemplar may add nuances and qualitative distinctions that were unavailable in previous exemplars. A range of exemplars allows one to establish a cultural field of relationships and distinctions. (Benner, 1994b, p. 117)

Most of the interpretive analysis in this project occurred via analysis of exemplars. It is through the thoughtful taking up of example after example of practice that the story gets filled in, that understanding is deepened, that qualitative distinctions about practice are grasped, and that the interpreter becomes more and more grounded in the range of possibilities for involvement in the practice under study. Collection of exemplars that contribute to the understanding of an aspect of practice is never complete, in that the possibilities for how that aspect gets worked out can never be fully articulated for all time. There can be, however, a fairly complete explication of what a particular text, which is bounded, has to say about that aspect of practice. Interpreters attain the best grasp they can in articulating the text that has been fixed, prior to publicly presenting their interpretations.

A third level of interpretive analysis is the identification and working out of themes in the text. This process is integrally involved in the same readings of text that bring forth the identification of paradigm cases and the dialogue with the text about exemplars. Thematic analysis is made possible by the accretion of understanding of the phenomena that occurs via the engagement of the interpreter with the text, and the working out of understanding that occurs via reading and writing about portions of that text. Thematic analysis is the attempt to articulate the broader understandings that arise from constant comparison and reading side by side of different paradigm cases and exemplars. Examples of themes that have been articulated in this project are clinical world, clinical agency, perceptual grasp (Benner, Tanner, & Chesla, 1992) and what it means to know a patient (Tanner et al., 1993).

As Benner (1994b) notes, we do not assume that a text will be completely coherent and rational, nor do we assume that there will be a complete match between participants' ideas about their practice and their actual demonstrations of practice. Rather, we assume that the text contains inconsistencies and conundrums, and that the task of interpretation is to bring to light the most coherent and complete story possible. Inconsistencies and unanswered puzzles must be acknowledged. When presenting themes about the text, it is important to specify the paradigmatic narratives that evidence those themes as well as the multiple exemplars that demonstrate variation in those themes.

The Role of Observations in the Interpretive Process

Observations of practice with nurses and observational notes from those sessions served several important purposes in the overall interpretive project. Observational sessions filled in the context of the practice that was described in the narrative sessions, kept the research team grounded in the unstated realities of the practice setting, and provided a better access to practice that was everyday, mundane, and routine as well as practice that was expert, intuitive, and ineffable. Despite our concerted effort to capture the context of the narrative provided by nurses in the small group interviews, the incredible press of the situation that exists in most hospital and critical care settings is difficult to capture in words, particularly for one who already works smoothly within that environment. Time spent in units with practicing nurses highlighted for the research team the noisy, busy, and stressful situations in which the participants typically worked.

It is hard to imagine the temporality of a unit where activities and time are divided into 5-minute segments. Within this context the narratives were worked out, and yet nurses filtered from their stories these contextual distractions and strains. At most, nurses might note that the unit was really busy that shift, or that it had been a particularly trying week on the unit because of multiple patient deaths. Attempting to do focused observations in these contexts helped the research team appreciate the press of the situation and how it might impede the nurses' intended practice.

Observations served to help the research team appreciate the context of practice in both data collection and interpretation. Most observations were conducted concurrent with the narrative interviews, and thus insights gained in observational sessions could be checked in the following interviews. Aspects of practice that were observed but not mentioned in the interview could be questioned, because of the researchers' heightened awareness of this fuller practice gained during observations. Interpretation of interview text was also moderated by the observational experience in units. Having observed closely the mundane or the exemplary but ineffable practice of nurses brought the interpreter to a closer understanding of the lived practice and allowed her to imaginatively fill in some of the gaps in the story. Recent and ongoing contact with the lived experience of nurses' practice helped us to avoid errors of theoretically abstracting from the narrative, or making idealized or overly critical interpretations of the action described.

Finally, the observation and the fixing of observations in notes contributed to the overall interpretive project by presenting paradigmatic examples of practice for each level of practice that were not apparent in the narratives. For example, in advanced beginner observations, the practice and pervasiveness of delegating up the line of authority became evident. Although advanced beginners described for us their reliance on more experienced staff for treatment decisions, the ways in which they delegated the assessment and management of complex situations were only apparent in the observations. Another example was expert nurses' capacity to establish a climate for care amidst the tumult of the ICU. This capacity to establish a tone of calm attentiveness to the patient that was more powerful than the noise, activity, and anxiety that prevailed on the unit was a skill of working with a context rather than working directly with a patient and thus nurses didn't talk about it. Only in observations was the skill recognized.

Observational notes and interpretations proved essential in understanding nurses whose work lacked a narrative structure (see Chapter 7). In interviews, these nurses posed significant dilemmas for interpretation, because the stories that they presented didn't cohere and their memories of even recent patient care situations seemed partial. In this text, observational notes of nurses' practice proved essential to understanding the nature of their relationship to their practice, and the particular breakdowns and possibilities of this practice.

Naming Versus Coding the Text

Efforts to organize the text for further analysis and discussion of particular lines of inquiry were attempted after interpretation had been completed on the text from nurses at all levels of practice from one entire hospital (approximately one sixth of the total text.) From the background theoretical frameworks for the project, pilot work (Benner & Tanner, 1987) and from these early interpretive summary notes, descriptive names were developed and broadly defined for aspects of text viewed as salient to the study questions. These names were then used to mark various aspects of text for future retrieval. Examples of broad inclusive names that were generated include "MD-Relations" for any text that referred to practice that was qualified or shaped by the nurse-physician interaction; "Notion of the Good" for text that addressed nurses' concerns (stated or enacted) about the ends of their work; and "Family" for any text that included nurses' concerns about or care of patients' families. These names were then used to systematically mark all of the text in the research project for subsequent retrieval using the software program Ethnograph (Seidel, 1987). Because the lines of inquiry for the study were multiple and overlapping, most text received multiple names. In addition, narratives of practice were preserved intact, marking the entire narrative as a piece which then also received numerous content names.

The process of establishing the names with which we would mark text was dialogical with the text and with members of the team. In developing these names we attempted to capture the major lines of inquiry that would be taken up with the text and that would allow various groups of interpreters access to portions of the text most suitable to their questions. Several iterations of the names were developed before settling on a list that adequately addressed the major lines of inquiry as we understood them early in the project. Throughout the project, the team continually discussed the meanings that were captured by various names. A few names had to be changed and added later in the project to adequately address the new understandings we had gained. There was always the understanding that new lines of inquiry might become important and that interpretation for that inquiry would require a return to a whole text (Benner, 1984a). Also, for many members of the team, working out interpretations required a return to the full interviews from which retrieved text was drawn. Therefore, the naming was always recognized as an essential but imperfect tool for gaining access to portions of text.

We wish to distinguish our efforts to name text for future retrieval from what is commonly defined as "coding" in various forms of qualitative research. The marking of text with names conducted in this project was qualitatively different from many forms of coding in terms of its guiding aims, how the team was involved with the text, and who participated in the naming process. Qualitative coding (Miles & Huberman, 1984) typically involves coding some aspects of subjects' beliefs or actions which are singled out for study and then operationally defined. The aim in such coding is the recognition of similar abstract forms of such action or belief in all participants. In rigorous coding, any well trained coder, even one who is marginally involved in the research, can complete the abstract coding task. At the extreme, researchers test their coders for inter-rater reliability, a clear indication that they are asking coders to be objective and distant from the text and to follow set rules or criteria for recognizing the action of interest. In such an endeavor, coders are not interpreting but scoring a text in that they systematically distance themselves from the text, notice only what the recognition "rules" require them to notice, and are in error if they become personally involved or engaged with the levels of meaning in the text.

In contrast, the aim of *naming* text is to capture examples of patterns of meaning in action, including salient context, that are evident in the text. In this effort, the names are used to mark text with related qualities of meaning for future retrieval, but the names never replace the text (Packer, 1989). A stance of involvement with the text was asked of all who participated in marking text. At base, those who helped mark the text understood the central aims of the project, were familiar with nursing practice, and were oriented, via concrete examples to the patterns of meaning, that the names were used to mark. In the process of naming text, each member of the team was encouraged to confront the text, to consider the adequacy of the list of names and to interpretively respond, in terms of marginal notes and feedback to the team, about the meanings that they encountered.

Guidelines for naming text addressed multiple interpretive concerns. First, all aspects of narrative and related discussion were marked together, so that the narrative structure of the action could be accessed during any subsequent search. This addressed the concern that the team have open and ready access to action and its context. We were concerned that the person working out the interpretation, rather than the person doing the initial marking of the text, learn the borders, diversity, and contrast cases in each pattern of meaning, and thus text was marked to include all of these under a particular name. Given our understanding that any portion of text, including narratives and theoretical discussions, can inform multiple questions that might be put to the text, multiple names were applied to many portions of text.

The overriding concern in naming text was to provide order for retrieval of text for future interpretation. Therefore, considerable care was taken to teach project staff who were marking text to recognize stories that contained elements of what we were concerned about in a particular name. However, we were not concerned about inter-rater reliability per se, because the text marked was still to be interpreted. If errors or misunderstandings were introduced in marking text, the person retrieving the text for that particular name could work through the puzzle about which text informed or did not inform that analysis. Text that was important to a particular theme, but was somehow omitted, was often recalled by members of the team who knew the whole text. In addition, complete hard copies of all interviews were available and frequently consulted during intensive interpretation.

In practice, the strategies established for training and guiding those who marked text worked well, but better for some meanings than for others. It is now apparent that our names represent patterns of meaning and action that are distinct in how readily they are apprehended, in their complexity, and in how deeply interpretive the name itself actually is. Some of our names, such as "Family," required only an appreciation that the family was being cared for, or should have been considered in care if they were not, and were fairly faithfully recorded. Recognizing levels of practice required a fairly full grasp of the Dreyfus model of skill acquisition and the evolving understanding of levels of practice that was developed in the course of the study. Finally there were names, such as "Social embeddedness of nursing knowledge" that the team had initially glimpsed as essential to an understanding of the practice, but did not have a well-rounded grasp of when text marking proceeded. Even with such names, we learned by the way that various project staff marked text that they believed evidenced that pattern. Understandings and misunderstandings of what the social embeddedness of knowledge might be within particular text eventually helped the team to sort out the content and borders of this particular theme.

EVALUATING THE INTERPRETIVE ACCOUNT

Discussing the credibility of an interpretive account proves difficult in a scientific environment that is so thoroughly oriented to the rational-empirical concerns of reliability and validity. Even when interpretive scientists attempt to reorient the discussion of evaluation to the interpretive project, they do so in reaction or response to these empirical concerns. Sandelowski (1986) in nursing and Guba and Lincoln (1981) in education suggest parallel concepts in qualitative research that address the empirical concerns for internal and external validity, reliability and objectivity. In taking up the argument in this way, these authors diminish rather than highlight the differences in the interpretive and empirical projects. They also set up the argument in such a way that the interpretive project is always a lesser cousin, not quite as good as, the solidly situated empirical project.

The basic problem seems to be the lack of an alternative truth theory that matches the appeal of the correspondence theory of truth. The attraction of seeking an account of the way things "really" are via objective procedures which can be evaluated via interpretation-free standards holds tremendous appeal because it provides the illusion of solidity and security and removes one from the anxiety about having no irrefutable standards (Bernstein, 1983; Taylor, 1985a). It also displaces the responsibility for the outcome of the research from the investigator to the procedures within the research project.

This project was conducted with the understanding that the most adequate interpretive account is one that addresses the practical concerns that motivated the inquiry in the first place (van Manen, 1990). We acknowledge that there is no correct, all-inclusive, undisputed account of clinical knowledge and skill development in nursing that can stand for all time. We also acknowledge that there are multiple pathways to accessing understanding and explanation of these nursing concerns. Acknowledging these things does not leave us, however, in a position of total subjectivity and relativism. Rather, there is the possibility of an account that is coherent, well interpreted, and systematically and rigorously worked out via the available points of access to nursing practice and that derives from a careful orientation of the researcher to the lived experience of the nurse-in-context. The powers of understanding are enhanced by multiple dialogues with the text and by dialogues among multiple researchers engaged in interpreting the text (Packer & Addison, 1989; Taylor, 1985a).

Throughout the detailed discussion of the methods of study employed in this project we have attempted to address our concerns for rigor. In what follows, we outline some overriding concerns that have not been previously addressed. The discussion considers the way in which this project was conducted to address: a) our concern to orient ourselves to nursing practice in a way that allowed us to uncover the practice in new ways; b) attentiveness to the ways in which the text was generated and interpreted; c) care and deliberation in how the interpretations were presented; and d) the protection of and respect for the nurse informants and their stories.

In hermeneutic investigation, there is always a concern to enter the hermeneutic circle in the "right" way, which means a way that is shaped by one's early grasp of the phenomenon, but at the same time respects the possibilities of the phenomenon showing itself in new ways.

We must show the entity or, more precisely, let it show itself, not forcing
our perspective on it. And we must do this in a way that respects the way it
shows itself. (Packer & Addison, 1989, p. 278)

Efforts to orient this investigation to the practice of nurses, and in particular to their clinical judgments and skill development, included a systematic and thorough examining of the field for knowledge and understanding of these two concerns (Benner, 1984a; Benner & Wrubel, 1989;
Tanner, 1987). Based on this prior work and early grasp of the practice, the
study was designed to access the everyday practice of nurses via narrative accounts and participant observation.

Considerable attention was paid to how the textual accounts of nursing
practice were elicited. From the first point of contact with the nurses on the
units to the final interview, we communicated to nurses that we were interested in seeing the full range of their practice, but that our concern was
to understand, from the inside, the possibilities and constraints of that practice, rather than to establish standards by which the practice would be evaluated. Subjects in the study included nurses from the very beginning period
of practice to the most advanced practitioner that our practical wisdom
about the practice allowed us to access. In addition, we attempted to include
nurses who were experienced but not expert in practice, so that the alternative accounts of how practice progresses over time might be accessed. Narratives of positive, meaningful, and exemplary practice, as well as practice
that went awry, were elicited. Observations of practice focused on the exemplary, the mundane, and the breakdowns in practice.

Interviewers were always grounded in the study and/or the practice of
critical care nursing. Our concern to enter the circle in the right way meant
that everyone involved in the study was well versed in central research
questions and understood the lines of inquiry that guided the work; not so
that other lines of inquiry would be cut off, but so that the probes within
the interview would help the nurses tell us about their experiences in ways
that addressed the central guiding questions.

This was not a data collection effort that could be, or was, parceled out
to research assistants who had been trained in a data collection "procedure." Rather, teams of nurses who were, by virtue of their professional
affiliation, already familiar with the concerns and practices of those being
studied conducted all interviews. A cadre of nurses who had experience
in the practice of critical care nursing were involved so that the nuances of
the nurses' practice would not be missed, either in the interviews or the
observations. Finally, nurses familiar with the reflexivity, fluidity, and
openness of an interpretive interview were involved.

Care in interpretation of texts was taken by completing multiple readings of each particular text, as well as having multiple readers for texts

addressing different lines of interpretation. Respect for the claims that the text made on us as researchers and for its multiple accounts about different aspects of practice made textual interpretation arduous. However, in the process of working out multiple and intersecting lines of inquiry (for example, the interpretation of clinical judgment and expert practice) the text was considered repeatedly in both detailed and overview readings. Consequently, various members of the team knew intimately vast sections of the text, and the central investigators became familiar with the entire text. Within the team, a commitment to using the text as the basis for working out puzzles or disagreements in interpretation kept us constantly in dialogue with the interviews and observational notes themselves, rather than with our abstractions about these texts.

Presentation of interpretations was guided by a concern for presenting the clearest textual evidence available for the interpretations offered. Our intention was to give the reader access to the descriptions of practice provided by the nurses, as well as to some of our observational understandings.

Finally, our concerns regarding the nurse informants were to demonstrate respect for their practice, to systematically and rigorously consider all the points of access that they gave us to their practice, and to protect their confidentiality. The protocol for study was approved by the institutional review boards from the universities in which we worked as well as by boards in the various hospitals from which informants were recruited. Informants' privacy was protected by having all narratives and observational notes identified by code numbers for both the informants and the hospitals. Identifying information about the nurse or about specific patients was carefully monitored and deleted or altered in written presentations of the work. Once nurses were recruited to the study, there was no additional communication with their supervisor nurses about their practice. Nurses who participated in the observational portion of data collection were clearly evident as study participants to their peers, but again, specifics of their practice were held in confidence from any other staff or supervisors on the units.

SUMMARY

In this chapter we described the conceptualization, design and conduct of this study in sufficient detail that readers might appreciate and evaluate the process as well as the findings from the project. Our intent was to allow readers to understand our philosophical and practical pre-understandings about studying nursing practice and clinical judgment so that they might weigh our approach along with our findings. We believe that a basic grasp of the philosophical and methodological tradition in which we work is essential to understanding the work as a whole. We detailed the concerns that organized our approaches to design, data collection and interpretation because we view these as integral to the readers' understanding of what actually occurred. Throughout the discussion of the project, we addressed issues in rigor and judgment about the choices that were made, in an attempt to allow readers to see major decision points and processes that led to this book.

DESCRIPTION OF NURSE INFORMANTS

TABLE B.1 Experience in Years by Group

	Advanced beginner			Intermediate			Experienced			Proficient		
	X	S	Md	X	S	Md	X	S	Md	X	S	Md
Years since basic nursing education	.83	.7	.5	5.4	5.3	4.2	12.1	4.3	11.8	12.75	4.7	11.6
Years since BSN	.72	.41	.5	4.3	2.8	3.9	10.2	4.7	9.5	8.0	5.8	9.0
Years in current unit	.50	.26	.44	2.1	0.8	1.9	7.5	4.0	7.0	7.6	4.6	7.0

TABLE B.2 Principal Area of Practice by Group

	Advanced beginner		Intermediate		Experienced		Proficient		Total	
	N	%	N	%	N	%	N	%	N	%*
Children's ICUs										
PICU	3	12.5	3	9.1	2	4.7	2	8	10	7.7
NICU	2	8.3	5	15.2	11	25.6	8	32	26	20
Subtotal	5	20.8	8	24.3	13	30.3	10	40	36	27.7
Adult ICUs										
SICU	7	29.	7	21.2	5	11.6	3	12	22	16.9
CCU	0	0	9	27.3	10	23.0	1	4	20	15.4
MICU	3	12.5	4	12.1	3	7.0	6	24	16	12.3
ICU	2	8.3	3	9.1	10	23.3	5	20	20	15.4
Subtotal	12	50	23	69.6	28	65.1	15	60	78	60.0
Floor	7	29.2	0	0	0	0	0	0	7	5.4
Other			2	6.1	2	4.7			4	3.1
Missing									5	3.8
Total	24		33		43		25		130	100

Note: Percentages do not total 100 because of rounding numbers.

BACKGROUND QUESTIONS FOR INTERVIEWS AND OBSERVATIONS

I. GUIDELINES FOR COLLECTION OF DATA ON DIMENSIONS OF EXPERTISE

The following are interview and data collection guidelines that will be used in researching the nine dimensions of expertise.

Dimension 1:   *Differences in kinds of unstructured problem identification. Content (and issues) selected for examples of optimal and suboptimal performances.*

Data sources: Narrative account of clinical episodes.

Dimension 2:   *Awareness and use of strategies to handle "changing relevance" as the problem unfolds.*

Data sources: Narrative account plus the following interview probes:

     1.   Through the course of this incident, did you come to see the situation in a different way?
     2.   What were your priorities during the situation?
     3.   Did your priorities change during this clinical episode? If so, how?

4. Did your focus on major concerns change over the course of this clinical situation? How?

5. Can you think of any generalizations you were making from your prior work with patients that you used with this clinical problem?

Dimension 3:   *Expectations and "sets" evident in clinical performance.*

Data sources: Narrative accounts and participant observation with the following probes:

1. What were your major expectations in this clinical situation?
2. Where do you think those expectations came from?
3. Did anything take you by surprise in this clinical situation?
4. What were you watching out for in this clinical situation (were they looking for the unlikely or dangerous situation?)
5. Do you think your perspectives on patient care have changed since coming to this patient care unit?

Dimension 4:   *The role of rules, principles, guidelines, and maxims at different levels of skill acquisition.*

Data sources: Narrative account, participant observation plus the following interview probes:

1. Would you have done _____ (fill in with specific action) with any patient with this particular problem?
2. Can you identify any rules, guidelines, or principles that were guiding your behavior in this clinical situation?
3. What guidelines would you give another nurse for handling this situation?
4. How would your advice change if you were talking to a beginner? To an expert?
5. What were the do's and don'ts that you were concerned about in this case?
6. Maxims are brief descriptions of skilled practice. Can you identify any maxims in your own or other practices. (This will be asked of nurses in the small group interviews.)
7. Tricks of the trade or rules of thumb: Nurses will be asked to describe some of these during participant observation, and in small group interviews.

Dimension 5:   *The use of relevant clinical population comparisons that demon-strate the ability to recognize similarity in the particular case with an appropriate group of similar patient problems.*

Data sources: Narrative account, participant observation plus the follow-ing probes:

1.   Had you worked with patients with similar problems before?
2.   Did any particular prior cases come to mind when work-ing with this patient?
3.   What led you to identify this _____ (name specific clinical assessment) as the problem?
4.   What were you ruling out in this situation?
5.   Were you drawing on your reading or a lecture about this problem?

Dimension 6:   *The use of analytic versus instance-oriented strategies.*

Data sources: Narrative accounts; fund of memorable paradigm cases; questions on Dimensions 4 and 5.

1.   In looking at what you did in this situation, would you say that you were guided more by past experience with similar cases or by what you have learned by books? Lectures? Please describe.
2.   Did you reason out what to do in this case?

Dimension 7:   *The role of hunches or understanding without obvious rational explanation in problem identification and intervention.*

Data sources: Narrative accounts and participant observation, plus the following interview probes for participant observation:

Introduction: First could you tell me something about this patient? (Inter-viewer will get as narrative a description as possible.)

1.   What are all the hunches you have about this patient and what is wrong with him/her, based on what you know about him/her?

Probes: Who is this patient?
What is his problem?
What are you most concerned about?

2.   Based on these hunches, what will you be looking for in the clinical situation?

3.   Are you going to (or did you) do anything on the basis of the hunch?

4.   What do you think your hunch is based on?

Probes: Have you had prior experience with this type of situation? Does this case bring to mind any other cases?
What do you think is giving you this reading of the situation? How do you account for this hunch?

5.   Do you have any physical or emotional sensations associated with your hunch? Please describe.

6.   How certain do you feel about this hunch?

7.   Do you often have hunches in your practice? Do you remember when they began? Around what issues do you have hunches?

8.   Do any past hunches you have had stand out in your mind? Please describe.

Probe: For example, have you ever had a sense that a patient was deteriorating before you had any objective data, such as vital sign changes, to back up your assessment? Please tell me about it.

Dimension 8:   *Differences in the fund of memorable "paradigm cases," cases that stand out as teaching a new clinical understanding or recognitional ability.*

Data sources: Narrative accounts; homework assignment to be given at time of first interview (see "Guidelines for Recording Paradigm Cases").

Dimension 9:   *Characterization of the nature of the task along the dimensions identified by Hammond (1984: Intuitive, analytical and quasi-rational).*

Data sources: Narrative accounts and participant observation.

1.   Analytical (cannot be done intuitively), for example, reading EKGs.

2.   Quasi-rational, for example, judging electrolyte and fluid replacement.

3. Intuitive, for example, early warning signal recognition; patient's readiness to learn; perceptual recognitional skills; graded qualitative distinctions.

II. GUIDELINES FOR STUDYING PERSONAL APPROACHES AND SITUATIONS THAT FACILITATE AND HINDER LEARNING FROM EXPERIENCE

The following questions were used in the narrative interviews and in participant observation:

1. When you proceed through your work these days, on any given week, would you say that you feel that you are learning something?
2. Please describe one of those incidents.
3. From whom do you learn most?
4. Are you often surprised in your work by what happens with a patient?
5. What forums have been most instrumental for your learning?
6. What do you think would facilitate your learning more from your clinical experience?
7. What are some of the obstacles that exist to your learning more from your clinical experience, that you are aware of?

III. GUIDELINES FOR DATA COLLECTION ON CHARACTERISTICS OF BEGINNING, INTERMEDIATE, AND EXPERT CLINICAL PERFORMANCE: MONITORING AND FOLLOW-UP STRATEGIES

The following questions and probes were used in interviews and participant observation to fill out the narratives of patient care being described.

1. Do you have some self-checks that you routinely use to avoid omissions or errors?

2. Do you regularly use these "self-checks," or only in particular situations?

3. What kinds of reminders do you use for yourself when taking care of a complicated patient?

4. How often are you able to find out what impact or outcomes your nursing interventions had on your patient? Is this a problem for you? (If so, please describe.)

5. Do you routinely talk about patients with nurse colleagues? With others?

6. Do you ever find out how patients on your unit do after they leave your unit? (Probe for kinds and sources of follow-up information.)

IV. INTERVIEW AND OBSERVATION GUIDELINES FOR IDENTIFYING LEVELS OF PROBLEM ENGAGEMENT AND EMOTIONAL INVOLVEMENT

A. *Problem Engagement*

1. Are you aware of times in your practice where you lose a sense of time and awareness of what is going on around you? Please describe any instances of this that come to mind. How often would you say that you have these experiences in your practice? How would you characterize your performance during these periods? Are there characteristic situations in which you lose awareness?

2. Are there times in your practice that you would describe as being disengaged from what you are doing? Please describe. How often would you say that you have these experiences in your practice? What is your practice like during these instances? Are there any characteristic reasons why you might be disengaged?

3. In terms of involvement and engagement in what you are doing, have you noticed any regular differences in this area as it is connected to your skill in a particular area? For example, do you notice that as you become more proficient with a complex skill; do you notice that you are more absorbed or less absorbed? Please describe.

4. At what level of absorption in the problem do you think your practice is best?

B. *Emotional Involvement*

We expect that you are emotionally involved in different ways with your patients at different times.

1. Do you regard a particular level of involvement as optimal for patient care/performance? Please describe as fully as possible.
2. What gradations of involvement are you aware of?
    a. Let's consider when you are very involved. Do you even realize this is happening when you are involved, or is it only after the incident?
    b. Do you notice any changes or differences in your performance when you are very involved? Please describe.
3. Does it make a difference in your practice if you are very involved with a patient, versus clearly not involved? Can you give any specific examples?
4. Please give an example of when you thought your emotional involvement got in the way of your clinical performance.
5. Now, can you give an example of when your emotional involvement with the patient improved your nursing care?
6. Do you find that you are easily distracted when you are giving patient care? Please describe.

REFERENCES
AND BIBLIOGRAPHY

Ackerlund, B. M., & Norberg, A. (1985). An ethical analysis of double bind conflicts as experienced by care workers feeding severely demented patients. *International Journal of Nursing Studies, 22*, 207–216.

Aiken, L. H., Smith, H. L., & Lake, E. T. (1994). Lower medicare mortality among a set of hospitals known for good nursing care. *Medical Care, 32*, 771–787.

Aristotle. (1953). Nicomachean ethics (J. K. Thomson, Trans.) as *The Ethics of Aristotle*. New York: Penguin.

Ashley, J. (1976). *Hospitals, paternalism and the role of the nurse*. New York: Teachers College Press.

Ashley, J. (1980). Power in a structured misogyny. *Advances in Nursing Science, 2*(3), 3–14.

Association of Academic Health Centers (1989). The supply and education of nurses (Policy Paper No. 1). Washington, DC: Author.

Baggs, J. G. (1989). Intensive care unit use and collaboration between nurses and physicians. *Heart and Lung, 18*, 332–338.

Baggs, J. G., & Schmitt, M. H. (1988). Collaboration between nurses and physicians. *Image: The Journal of Nursing Scholarship, 20*, 145–149.

Barnard, D. (1988). "Ship? What ship? I thought I was going to the doctor!" Patient-centered perspectives on the health care team. In N. M. P. King, L. R. Churchill, & A. W. Cross (Eds.), *The physician as captain of the ship: A critical reappraisal* (pp. 89–111). Boston: D. Reidel Publishing Company.

Barnett, G. O. The computer and clinical judgment. *New England Journal of Medicine, 307*, 493–494.

Belenky, M. F., Clinchy, B. M., Goldberger, N. R., & Tarule, J. M. (1986). *Women's ways of knowing*. New York: Basic Books.

Bellah, R. N., Madsen, R., Sullivan, W. M., Swindler, A., & Tipton, S. M. (1985). *Habits of the heart*. Berkeley, CA: University of California Press.

Bellinger, S. R., & McCloskey, J. C. (1992). Are preceptors for orientation of new nurses effective? *Journal of Professional Nursing, 8*, 321–327.

Benner, P. (1974). In Kramer, M. *Reality Shock: Why nurses leave nursing*. St. Louis, MO: Mosby.

Benner, P. (1982). From novice to expert. *American Journal of Nursing, 82*, 402–407.

Benner, P. (1983). Uncovering the knowledge embedded in practice. *Image: The Journal of Nursing Scholarship, 15*(2), 36–41.

Benner, P. (1984a). *From novice to expert: Excellence and power in clinical nursing practice*. Menlo Park, CA: Addison-Wesley.

Benner, P. (1984b). *Stress and satisfaction on the job: Work meanings and coping of mid-career men*. New York: Praeger.

Benner, P. (1985). Quality of life: A phenomenological perspective on explanation, prediction, and understanding in nursing science. *Advances in Nursing Science, 8*, 1–14.

Benner, P. (1989, December). *Nursing as a caring profession*. Working paper presented at the meeting of the American Academy of Nursing, Kansas City, MO.

Benner, P. (1990). The moral dimensions of caring. In J. Stephenson (Ed.), *Care, research and state of the art* (pp. 5–17). Kansas City: American Academy of Nursing.

Benner, P. (1993). The quest for control and the possibilities of care. In H. L. Dreyfus & M. Zimmerman (Eds.), *Applied Heidegger*. (Book manuscript in progress). University of California, Berkeley.

Benner, P. (1994a). Discovering challenges to ethical theory in experience-based narratives of nurses' everyday ethical comportment. In J. F. Monagle & D. C. Thomasina (Eds.), *Health care ethics: Critical issues* (pp. 401–411). Gaithersburg, MD: Aspen.

Benner, P. (1994b). The tradition and skill of interpretive phenomenology in studying health, illness, and caring practices. In P. Benner (Ed.), *Interpretive phenomenology: Embodiment, caring and ethics in health and illness* (pp. 99–127). Newbury Park, CA: Sage.

Benner, P. (1994c). Caring as a way of knowing and not knowing. In S. Phillips & P. Benner (Eds.), *The crisis of care: Affirming and restoring caring practices in the helping professions* (pp. 42–62). Washington, DC: Georgetown University Press.

Benner, P. (1994d). The role of articulation in understanding practice and experience as sources of knowledge. In J. Tully & D. M. Weinstock

(Eds.), *Philosophy in a time of pluralism: Perspectives on the philosophy of Charles Taylor* (pp. 136–155). Cambridge: Cambridge University Press.

Benner, P., & Benner, R. V. (1979). *The new nurse's work entry: A troubled sponsorship*. New York: Tiresias.

Benner, P., & Gordon, S. (in press). The knowledge and skill embedded in caregiving. In S. Gordon, P. Benner, & N. Noddings (Eds.), *The care voice and beyond*. Philadelphia: University of Pennsylvania Press.

Benner, P., Hooper, P., & Stannard, D. (1995). *Nursing therapeutics in critical care: Caring practices linked to treatment*. Unpublished manuscript, University of California, San Francisco.

Benner, P., Janson-Bjerklie, S., Ferketich, S., & Becker, G. (1994). Moral dimensions of living with a chronic illness: Autonomy, responsibility and the limits of control. In P. Benner (Ed.), *Interpretive phenomenology: Embodiment, caring and ethics* (pp. 225–254). Thousand Oaks, CA: Sage.

Benner, P., & Tanner, C. (1987). Clinical judgment: How expert nurses use intuition. *American Journal of Nursing, 87*, 23–31.

Benner, P., Tanner, C., & Chesla, C. (1992). From beginner to expert: Gaining a differentiated clinical world in critical care nursing. *Advances in Nursing Science, 14*, 13–28.

Benner, P., & Wrubel, J. (1982). Clinical knowledge development: The value of perceptual awareness. *Nurse Educator, 7*, 11–17.

Benner, P., & Wrubel, J. (1989). *The primacy of caring: Stress and coping in health and illness*. Menlo Park, CA: Addison-Wesley.

Benner, P., Wrubel, J., Phillips, S., Chesla, C., & Tanner, C. (1995). Critical caring: The knowledge and skill embedded in helping. Unpublished manuscript. University of California, San Francisco.

Bernstein, R. (1983). *Beyond objectivism and relativism: Science, hermeneutics and praxis*. Philadelphia: University of Pennsylvania Press.

Bevis, E., & Watson, J. (1989). *Toward a caring curriculum: A new pedagogy for nursing*. New York: National League for Nursing.

Bishop, A. H., & Scudder, J. R., Jr. (1990). *The practical, moral and personal sense of nursing: A phenomenological philosophy of practice*. Albany, NY: State University of New York Press.

Bishop, A. H., & Scudder, J. R., Jr. (1991). *Nursing: The practice of caring*. New York: National League for Nursing.

Borgmann, A. (1984). *Technology and the character of contemporary life*. Chicago: University of Chicago Press.

Bordieu, P. (1972/1977). *Outline of a theory of practice*. (R. Nice, trans.). Cambridge, UK: Cambridge University Press.

Bordieu, P. (1980/1990). *The logic of practice*. (R. Nice, trans.). Stanford, CA: Stanford University Press.

Boyer, E. (1990). *Scholarship reconsidered: Priorities for the American professoriate*. Princeton, NJ: Carnegie Foundation for the Advancement of Teaching.

Brasler, M. E. (1993). Predictors of clinical performance of new graduate nurses participating in preceptor orientation programs. *Journal of Continuing Education in Nursing, 24*, 158–165.

Brown, L. (1986). The experience of care: Patient perspectives. *Topics in Clinical Nursing, 8*, 56–62.

Bruner, J. (1986). *Actual minds, possible worlds*. Cambridge, MA: Harvard University Press.

Burnard, P. (1987). Towards an epistemological basis for experiential learning in nurse education. *Journal of Advanced Nursing, 12*, 189–193.

Burnard, P. (1989). The "sixth sense." *Nursing Times, 85*, 52–53.

Callahan, S. (1988). The role of emotion in ethical decision making. *Hastings Center Report 18*(3), 9–14.

Callahan, D. (1993). *The troubled dream of life, living with mortality*. New York: Simon and Schuster.

Campbell-Heider, N., & Pollock, D. (1987). Barriers to physician-nurse collegiality: An anthropological perspective. *Social Science and Medicine, 25*, 421–425.

Cassel, E. J. (1989). *The nature of suffering and the goals of medicine*. Oxford: Oxford University Press.

Champy, J. (1995) *Reengineering management*. New York: Harper Business.

Chesla, C. A. (1990). *Care of the family in critical care*. Unpublished manuscript. University of California, San Francisco.

Chesla, C. A. (In press). Reconciling technologic and family care in critical care nursing practice. *Image, The Journal of Nursing Scholarship*.

Clarke, M. (1986). Action and reflection: Practice and theory in nursing. *Journal of Advanced Nursing, 11*, 3–11.

Clift, R. T., Houston, W. R., & Pugach, M. C. (Eds.). (1990). *Encouraging reflective practice in education*. New York: Teachers College Press.

Coles, R. (1989). *The call of stories*. Boston: Houghton Mifflin.

Corcoran, S. (1986). Planning by expert and novice nurses in cases of varying complexity. *Research in Nursing and Health, 9*, 155–162.

Corcoran, S. A., Narayan, S., & Moreland, H. (1988). "Thinking aloud" as a strategy to improve clinical decision making. *Heart & Lung, 17*, 463–468.

Corcoran, S. A., & Tanner, C. A. (1988). Implications of research on clinical judgment for teaching. In *Curriculum revolution: A mandate for change*. New York: National League for Nursing.

Corless, I. B. (1982). Physicians and nurses: Roles and responsibilities in caring for the critically ill patient. *Law, Medicine and Health Care, 10*, 72–76.

Damrosch, S. P., Sullivan, P. A., & Haldeman, L. L. (1987). How nurses get their way: Power strategies in nursing. *Journal of Advanced Nursing,* 13, 284–290.

Darbyshire, P. (1987, January 28). Doctors and nurses: The burden of history. *Nursing Times,* pp. 32–34.

Davis, B. G. (1972). Clinical expertise as a function of educational preparation. *Nursing Research,* 21, 530–534.

Davis, B. G. (1974). Effect of levels of nursing education on patient care replication. *Nursing Research,* 23, 150–155.

del Bueno, D. J. (1990). Experience, education, and nurses' ability to make clinical judgments. *Nursing and Health Care,* 11, 290–294.

Descartes, R. (1641/1960). *Meditations on first philosophy.* (L. J. Lafleur, trans.). Indianapolis: Bobbs-Merrill.

Dewey, J. (1904). The relation of theory to practice in education. In C. A. McMurry (Ed.), *Third yearbook of the National Society for the Scientific Study of Education* (pp. 9–30). Chicago: University of Chicago Press.

Dewey, J. (1973). Experience and thinking. In J. J. McDermott (Ed.), *The philosophy of John Dewey* (Vol. 2, pp. 494–506). New York: Putnam's. (Original work published 1916.)

Dewey, J. (1922). *Human nature and conduct: An introduction to social psychology* (pp. 177–178). London: George Allen and Unwin.

Dewey, J. (1960). *Theory of the moral life.* New York: Holt, Rinehart and Winston.

Diekelmann, N. L. (1989). The nursing curriculum: Lived experiences of students. In *Curriculum revolution: Reconceptualizating nursing education* (pp. 25–42). New York: National League for Nursing Press.

Diekelmann, N. (1991). The emancipatory power of the narrative. In *Curriculum revolution: Community building and activism* (pp. 41–62). New York: National League for Nursing Press.

Diekelmann, N. L. (1992). Learning-as-testing: A Heideggerian hermeneutical analysis of the lived experience of students and teachers in nursing. *Advances in Nursing Science,* 14(3), 72–83.

Diekelmann, N. (1993). Behavioral pedagogy: A Heideggerian hermeneutical analysis of the lived experiences of students and teachers in baccalaureate nursing education. *Journal of Nursing Education,* 32(6), 245–250.

Dreyfus, H. L. (1979). *What computers can't do: The limits of artificial intelligence.* (Rev. ed.). New York: Harper & Row.

Dreyfus, H. L. (1991a). *Being-in-the-world, a commentary on Heidegger's* Being and Time, Division I. Cambridge, MA: The MIT Press.

Dreyfus, H. L. (1991b). Towards a phenomenology of ethical expertise. *Human Studies,* 14, 229–250.

Dreyfus, H. L., & Dreyfus, S. E., with Athanasiou, T. (1986). *Mind over machine, the power of human intuition and expertise in the era of the computer.* New York: The Free Press.

Dreyfus, S. E. (1982). Formal models vs. human situational understanding: Inherent limitations on the modeling of business expertise. *Office, Technology and People, 1,* 133–55.

Dworkin, G. (1978). Moral autonomy. In T. Engelhardt & D. Callahan (Eds.), *Morals, science and sociality* (pp.156–170). Hastings-on-Hudson, NY: Hastings Center.

Dyck, B., & Benner, P. (1989). In silence and tears. *American Journal of Nursing, 89,* 824–825.

Edgerton, R. (1993). A new intellectual adventure [Editorial]. *Change, 25*(6), 4–5.

Ehrenreich, B., & English, D. (1973). *Witches, midwives and nurses: A history of women healers.* Old Westbury, NY: The Feminist Press.

English, I. (1993). Intuition as a function of the expert nurse: A critique of Benner's novice to expert model. *Journal of Advanced Nursing, 18,* 387–393.

Eubanks, P. (1991). Quality improvement: Key to Changing Nurse-MD Relations. *Hospitals, 65* (8), 26–30.

Fagin, C. M. (1992). Collaboration between nurses and physicians: No longer a choice. *Academic Medicine, 67,* 295–303.

Field, P. A. (1987). The impact of nursing theory on the clinical decision making process. *Journal of Advanced Nursing, 12,* 563–571.

Fisher, J. A., & Connelly, C. D. (1989). Retaining graduate nurses: A staff development challenge. *Journal of Nursing Staff Development, 5,* 6–10.

Fleming, M. H. (1991). The therapist with a three-track mind. *American Journal of Occupational Therapy, 45,* 1007–1014.

Fonteyn, M. E. (1991). Implications of clinical reasoning studies for critical care nursing. *Focus on Critical Care, 18,* 322–327.

Ford, J. S., & Profetto-McGrath, J. (1994). A model for critical thinking within the context of curriculum as praxis. *Journal of Nursing Education, 33*(8), 341–344.

Freire, P. (1970). *Pedagogy of the oppressed* (M. Ramos, Trans.) New York: The Continuum Publishing Corp.

Gadamer, H. (1975). *Truth and method.* (G. Barden & J. Cumming, Trans.) New York: Seabury.

Gadow, S. (1988). Covenant without cure: Letting go and holding on in chronic illness. In J. Watson & M. A. Ray (Eds.), *The ethics of care and the ethics of cure: Synthesis in chronicity* (pp. 5–14). New York: National League for Nursing.

Gadow, S. (1991). Clinical subjectivity: Advocacy with silent patients. *Nursing Clinics of North America, 24,* 535–541.

Gardner, H. (1985). *The mind's new science: A history of cognitive revolution.* New York: Basic Books.

Giles, P. F., & Moran, V. (1989). Preceptor program evaluation demonstrates improved orientation. *Journal of Nursing Staff Development*, 5, 17–24.

Gilligan, C. (1982). *In a different voice: Psychological theory and women's development*. Cambridge, MA: Harvard University Press.

Gilligan, C. (1986). On In a Different Voice: An interdisciplinary forum. *Signs: Journal of Women in Culture and Society, 11*, 327.

Gordon, S., Benner, P., & Noddings, N. (In press) *The care voice and beyond*. Philadelphia, PA: University of Pennsylvania Press.

Gortner, S. R. (1958). Ethical inquiry. *Annual Review of Nursing Research, 3*, 193–214.

Grobe, S. J., Drew, J. A., & Fonteyn, M. E. (1991). A descriptive analysis of experienced nurses' clinical reasoning during a planning task. *Research in Nursing and Health, 14*, 305–314.

Guba, E. G., & Lincoln, Y. S. (1981). *Effective evaluation*. San Francisco: Jossey-Bass.

Guest, K. A. (1993). APACHE III and assessment of severity of illness. In J. B. Hall, G. A. Schmidt, & L. D. H. Wood (Eds.), *Principles of critical care: Companion handbook*. New York, NY: McGraw-Hill.

Guignon, C. B. (1983). *Heidegger and the problem of knowledge*. Indianapolis, IN: Hackett Publishing Co.

Habermas, J. (1982). A reply to my critics. In J. B. Thompson & D. Held (Eds.), *Habermas Critical Debates* (pp. 253–258). Cambridge, MA: MIT Press.

Habermas, J. (1992). *Moral consciousness and communicative action* (C. Lenhardt & W. Nicholson, Trans). Cambridge, MA: MIT Press.

Hall, J. B., Schmidt, G. A., & Wood, L. D. H. (1993). *Principles of critical care*. New York: McGraw-Hill.

Hamilton, E. M., Murray, M. K., Lindholm, L. H., & Meyers, R. E. (1989). Effects of mentoring on job satisfaction, leadership behaviors, and job retention of new graduate nurses. *Journal of Nursing Staff Development, 5*, 159–165.

Hartshorn, J. C. (1992). Characteristics of critical care nursing internship programs. *Journal of Nursing Staff Development, 8*, 218–223.

Hartz, A., Krakauer, H., Kuhn, E., Young, M., Jacobsen, S., Gay, G., Muenz, L., Katzoff, M., Bailey, R., & Rimm, A. (1989). Hospital characteristics and mortality rates. *The New England Journal of Medicine, 321* (25), 1720–1725.

Hauerwas, S. (1981). *A community of character*. Notre Dame: University of Notre Dame Press.

Heidegger, M. (1926/1962). *Being and time*. (J. Macquarrie & E. Robinson, Trans.). New York: Harper and Row.

Heidegger, M. (1975/1982). *The basic problems of phenomenology* (A. Hofstadter, Trans.). Bloomington, IN: Indiana University Press.

Henry, S. B. (1991). Effect of level of patient acuity on clinical decision making of critical care nurses with varying levels of knowledge and experience. *Heart and Lung: Journal of Critical Care, 20*, 478–485.

Hofman, P. B. (1994). Ethical issues in managed care. *Healthcare Executive, 9*(2), 40.

Hooper, P. L. (1995). *Expert titration of multiple vasoactive drugs in post-cardiac surgical patients: An interpretive study of clinical judgment and perceptual acuity.* Unpublished doctoral dissertation. University of California, San Francisco.

Hughes, A. (1988). When nurse knows best: Some aspects of nurse/doctor interaction in a casualty department. *Sociology of Health and Illness, 10*, 1–22.

Huston, C., & Marquis, B. (1987). Use of management and ethical case studies to improve decision-making skills of senior nursing students. *Journal of Nursing Education, 26*, 210–212.

Hutchings, P. (1993a). Windows on practice. *Change, 25*, 14–22.

Hutchings, P. (1993b). *Using cases to improve college teaching.* Washington, DC: American Association for Higher Education.

Itano, J. K. (1989). A comparison of the clinical judgment process in experienced registered nurses and student nurses. *Journal of Nursing Education, 28*, 120–126.

Jenny, J., & Logan, J. (1992). Knowing the patient. One aspect of clinical knowledge. *Image: The Journal of Nursing Scholarship, 24*, 254–258.

Jenks, J. M. (1993). The pattern of personal knowing in nurse decision making. *Journal of Nursing Education, 32*, 399–405.

Jones, J. A. (1989). The verbal protocol: A research technique for nursing. *Journal of Advanced Nursing, 14*, 1062–1070.

Jonsen, A., & Toulmin, S. (1988). *The abuse of casuistry.* Berkeley, CA: University of California Press.

Josselson, R., & Lieblich, L. (Eds). (1993). *The narrative study of lives.* Newbury Park, CA: Sage.

Kalisch, B. J. (1975). Of half gods and mortals: Aesculapian authority. *Nursing Outlook, 23*, 22–28.

Kalisch, B. J., & Kalisch, P. (1977). An analysis of the sources of physician-nurse conflict. *Journal of Nursing Administration, 7*, 51–57.

Kant, I. (1781/1963). *Critique of pure reason* (N. K. Smith, trans.). New York: St. Martin's Press.

Katefian, S. (1988). Moral reasoning and ethical practice. *Annual Review of Nursing Research, 6*, 173–195.

Katzman, E. M., & Roberts, J. I. (1988). Nurse-physician conflicts as barriers to the enactment of nursing roles. *Western Journal of Nursing Research, 10*, 576–590.

Keddy, B., Jones-Gillis, M. Jacobs, P., Burton, H., & Rogers, M. (1986). The doctor-nurse relationship: An historical perspective. *Journal of Advanced Nursing, 11,* 745–753.

Kerwin, A. (1993). None too solid: Medical ignorance. *Knowledge: Creation, diffusion, utilization, 15,* 166–185.

Kierkegaard, S. (1848/1962). *The present age.* (A. Dru, Transl.). New York: Harper and Row.

Kierkegaard, S. (1843/1985). *Fear and trembling.* (A. Hanney, Trans.). New York: Penguin.

Kintgen-Andrews, J. (1991). Critical thinking and nursing education: Perplexities and insights. *Journal of Nursing Education, 30,* 152–157.

Kleinman, A., Eisenberg, L., & Good, B. (1978). Culture, illness and care: Clinical lessons from anthropologic and cross-cultural research. *Annals of Internal Medicine, 88,* 251–258.

Kleinman, A. (1988). *The illness narratives: Suffering, healing and the human condition.* New York: Basic Books.

Knaus, W. A., Draper, E. A., Wagner, D. P., & Zimmerman, J. E. (1986). An evaluation of outcome from intensive care in major medical centers. *Annals of Internal Medicine, 104,* 410–418.

Koenig, B. (1988). The technological imperative. In M. Lock & D. Gordon (Eds.), *Biomedicine examined.* Boston, MA: Kluwer.

Koerner, B. L., Cohen, J. R., & Armstrong, D. M. (1985). Collaborative practice and patient satisfaction. *Evaluation and the health professions, 8,* 299–321.

Koerner, B. L., Cohen, J. R., & Armstrong, D. M. (1986). Professional behavior in a collaborative practice. *Journal of Nursing Administration, 16,* 39–44.

Kohlberg, L. (1981). *The philosophy of moral development: Moral stages and the idea of justice. Essays on Moral Development,* Vol. 1. San Francisco: Harper & Row.

Kohlberg, L. (1984). *The nature and validity of moral stages. Essays on Moral Development,* Vol. 2. San Francisco: Harper & Row.

Kramer, M. (1974). *Reality shock.* St. Louis: C. V. Mosby.

Kuhn, T. (1970). *The structure of scientific revolutions* (2nd ed.). Chicago: University of Chicago Press.

Kuhn, T. (1991). The natural and the human sciences. In D. R. Hiley, J. F. Bohman, & R. Shusterman (Eds.), *The interpretive turn* (pp. 17–24). Ithaca, NY: Cornell University Press.

Lave, J., & Wenger, E. (1991). *Situated learning: Legitimate peripheral participation.* New York: Cambridge University Press.

Leners, D. W. (1993). Nursing intuition: The deep connection. In D. A. Gaut (Ed.), *A global agenda for caring* (pp. 223–240). New York: National League for Nursing.

Leonard, V. W. (1989). A Heideggerian phenomenologic perspective on the concept of a person. *Advances in Nursing Science, 11*(4), 40–55.

Leonard, V. (1993). *Stress and coping in the transition to parenthood of first-time mothers with career commitments: An interpretive study.* Unpublished doctoral dissertation. University of California, San Francisco.

Leonard, V. W. (1994). A Heideggerian phenomenological perspective on the concept of person. In P. Benner (Ed.), *Interpretive phenomenology: Embodiment, caring and ethics* (pp. 225–254). Thousand Oaks, CA: Sage.

Lieb, R. (1978). Power, powerlessness and potential—nurses' role within the health care delivery system. *Image: The Journal of Nursing Scholarship, 10,* 75–83.

Lock, M., & Gordon, D. R. (Eds). (1988). *Biomedicine examined.* Dordrecht, The Netherlands: Kluwer Press.

Logstrup, K. E. (1956/1971). *The ethical demand* (T. I. Jensen, Trans.). Philadelphia, PA: Fortress Press.

Lovell, M. C. (1981). Silent but perfect "partners": Medicine's use and abuse of women. *Advances in Nursing Science, 3,* 25–40.

Lovell, M. C. (1982). Daddy's little girl: The lethal effects of paternalism in nursing. In J. Juff (Ed.), *Socialization, sexism and stereotyping: Women's issues in nursing* (pp. 210–220). St. Louis: The C.V. Mosby Company.

Lowenberg, J. S. (1989). *Caring and responsibility.* Philadelphia: University of Pennsylvania Press.

Lysaught, J. (1986). Retrospect and prospect in joint practice. In J. E. Steel (Ed.), *Issues in collaborative practice* (pp. 15–33). Orlando: Grune & Stratton.

MacIntyre, A. (1981). *After virtue.* Notre Dame, IN: University of Notre Dame Press.

MacIntyre, A. (1984). *After virtue.* Second edition. Notre Dame, IN: University of Notre Dame Press.

MacLeod, M. (1993). On knowing the patient: Experiences of nurses undertaking care. In A. Radley (Ed.), *Worlds of illness: Biographical and cultural perspectives on health and disease* (pp. 38–56). London: Routledge.

Magnan, M. A., & Benner, P. (1989). Listening with care. *American Journal of Nursing, 89,* 219–221.

Mandelbaum, M. (1955). *The phenomenology of moral experience.* New York: The Free Press.

Martinsen, K. (1989). Omsorg, sykepleie og medisin. Historisk-filosofiske essays [Caring, nursing and medicine historical–philosophical essays]. Oslo: Tano.

Mattingly, C. (1991a). The narrative nature of clinical reasoning. *American Journal of Occupational Therapy, 45,* 998–1005.

Mattingly, C. (1991b). What is clinical reasoning? *American Journal of Occupational Therapy, 45,* 979–988.

May, W. F. (1988). Adversarialism in America and the professions. In C. H.

Reynolds & R. V. Norman (Eds.), *Community in America* (pp. 185–201). Berkeley: University of California Press.

May, C. (1991). Affective neutrality and involvement in nurse-patient relationships: Perceptions of appropriate behavior among nurses in acute medical and surgical wards. *Journal of Advanced Nursing, 16,* 552–558.

McGrath, B. J., & Princeton, J. C. (1987). Evaluation of a clinical preceptor program for new graduates—Eight years later. *Journal of Continuing Education in Nursing, 18,* 133–136.

McLain, B. R. (1988). Collaborative practice: A critical theory perspective. *Research in Nursing and Health, 11,* 391–398.

Mechanic, D., & Aiken, L. (1982). A cooperative agenda for medicine and nursing. *New England Journal of Medicine, 307,* 747–750.

Merleau-Ponty, M. (1962). *Phenomenology of perception.* (C. Smith, Trans.). London: Routledge and Kegan Paul.

Miles, M. B., & Huberman, A. M. (1984). *Qualitative data analysis: A sourcebook of new methods.* Newbury Park, CA: Sage.

Miller, R. A., Harry M. D., Pople, E., Jr., & Myers, J. D. (1982). INTERNIST-1, an experimental computer-based diagnostic consultant for general internal medicine. *The New England Journal of Medicine, 307,* 468–476.

Mishler, E. G. (1986). *Research interviewing: Context and narrative.* Cambridge, MA: Harvard University Press.

Mitchell, P. H., Armstrong, S., Simpson, T., & Lentz, M. (1989). American Association of Critical Care Nurses Demonstration Project: Profile of excellence in critical care nursing. *Heart and Lung, 18,* 219–237.

Mohr, W. L., & Mohr, H. (1983). *Quality circles: Changing images of people at work.* Reading, MA: Addison-Wesley.

Murphy, J. M., & Gilligan, C. (1980). Moral development in late adolescence and adulthood: A critique and reconstruction of Kohlberg's theory. *Human Development, 80,* 79.

National League for Nursing. (1988). *Curriculum revolution: Mandate for change.* New York: National League for Nursing Press.

National League for Nursing. (1989). *Curriculum revolution: Reconceptualizing nursing education.* New York: National League for Nursing Press.

National League for Nursing. (1990). *Curriculum revolution: Redefining the student-teacher relationship.* New York: National League for Nursing Press.

National League for Nursing. (1991). *Curriculum revolution: Community building and activism.* New York: National League for Nursing Press.

National League for Nursing. (1993). *A vision for nursing education.* New York: Author.

Nightingale, F., (1969) *Notes on nursing: What it is and what it is not.* (Philadelphia: J.B. Lippincott. (Original work published 1860.)

Packer, M. (1989). Analytic hermeneutics and the study of morality in action. In W. Kurtines & J. Gewirtz (Eds.), *Handbook of moral behavior and development* (pp. 262–280). Hillsdale, NJ: Erlbaum.

Packer, M. J., & Addison, R. B. (1989). *Entering the circle: Hermeneutic investigation in psychology.* Albany, NY: SUNY Press.

Palmer, P. J. (1966). *To know as we are known: A spirituality of education.* New York: Harper & Row.

Palmer, P. J. (1993). Good talk about teaching. *Change, 25,* 8–13.

Pascale, R. T. (1990) *Managing on the edge.* New York: Simon and Schuster.

Pellegrino, E. D. (1994) Ethics. *Journal of the American Medical Association, 271,* 1668–1670.

Perry, W. B. (1968). *Forms of intellectual and ethical development in the college years; a scheme.* New York: Holt, Rinehart & Winston. As cited in J. M. Murphy & C. Gilligan (1980). Moral development in late adolescence and adulthood: A critique and reconstruction of Kohlberg's theory. *Human Development, 23*(2), 77–104.

Pew Health Professions Commission. (1991). *Healthy America: Practitioners for 2005: An agenda for action for U.S. health professional schools.* Durham, NC: Author.

Phillips, S., & Benner, P. (1994). *The crisis of care: Affirming and restoring caring practices.* Washington, DC: Georgetown University Press.

Piaget, J. (1960). *The moral judgment of the child.* (M. Gahain, Trans.). Glencoe, IL: The Free Press. (Original work published 1935)

Pike, A. (1991). Moral outrage and moral discourse in nurse-physician collaboration. *Journal of Professional Nursing, 7,* 351–363.

Plato. *The dialogues of Plato* (1937). (B. Jowett, Trans.). New York: Random House.

Plunkett, E. J., & Olivieri, R. J. (1989). A strategy for introducing diagnostic reasoning: Hypothesis testing using a simulation approach. *Nurse Educator, 14,* 27–31.

Polanyi, M. (1958/1962). *Personal knowledge: Towards a post-critical philosophy.* New York: Harper and Row.

Polkinghorne, D. E. (1988). *Narrative knowing and the human sciences.* Albany, NY: SUNY Press.

Powell, J. H. (1989). The reflective practitioner in nursing. *Journal of Advanced Nursing, 14,* 824–832.

Prescott, P. A., & Bowen, S. A. (1985). Physician-nurse relationships. *Annals of Internal Medicine, 103,* 127–133.

Prescott, P. A., Dennis, K. E., & Jacox, A. K. (1987). Clinical decision making of staff nurses. *Image: The Journal of Nursing Scholarship, 19,* 56–62.

Pyles, S. H., & Stern, P. N. (1983). Discovery of nursing gestalt in critical care nursing: The importance of the gray gorilla syndrome. *Image: The Journal of Nursing Scholarship, 15,* 42–45.

Reverby, S. (1976). Health: Women's work. In D. Kotelchuck (Ed.). *Prognosis negative: Crisis in the health care system* (pp. 170–183). New York: Vintage Books.

Reverby, S. (1987). *Ordered to care: The dilemma of American nursing: 1850–1945.* Cambridge: Cambridge University Press.

Rew, L. (1988). Intuition in decision making. *Image: The Journal of Nursing Scholarship, 20,* 150–155.

Rew, L. (1991). Intuition in psychiatric-mental health nursing. *Journal of Child and Adolescent Psychiatric and Mental Health Nursing, 4,* 110–115.

Rew, L., & Barrows, E. M. (1987). Intuition: A neglected hallmark of nursing knowledge. *Advances in Nursing Science, 10,* 49–62.

Roberts, S. J. (1983). Oppressed group behavior: Implications for nursing. *Advances in Nursing Science, 5,* 21–30.

Rubin, J. (1984). *Too much of nothing: Modern culture, the self and salvation in Kierkegaard's thought.* Unpublished doctoral dissertation, University of California, Berkeley.

Ruddick, S. (1989). *Maternal thinking: Toward a politics of peace.* Boston: Beacon.

Sandel, M. (1982). *Liberalism and the limits of justice.* London: Cambridge University Press.

Sandelowski, M. (1986). The problem of rigor in qualitative research. *Advances in Nursing Science, 8*(3), 27–37.

Saylor, C. R. (1990). Reflection and professional education: Art, science and competency. *Nurse Educator, 15,* 8–11.

Scherubel, J., & Carlson, B. (1991). Nurses' use of cues in the critically ill. *Heart and Lung: Journal of Critical Care, 20,* 302–306.

Schmitt, M. L., & Williams, T. F. (1985). Nurse-physician collaboration and outcomes for patients [Letter to the editor]. *Annals of Internal Medicine, 103,* 956.

Schon, D. A. (1983). *The reflective practitioner: How professionals think in action.* New York: Basic Books.

Schon, D. A. (1987). *Educating the reflective practitioner.* San Francisco, CA: Jossey-Bass.

Schraeder, B. D., & Fischer, D. K. (1987). Using intuitive knowledge in the neonatal intensive care nursery. *Holistic Nursing Practice, 1,* 45–51.

Schwartz, K. B. (1991). Clinical reasoning and new ideas on intelligence: Implications for teaching and learning. *American Journal of Occupational Therapy, 45,* 1033–37.

Seidel, J. (1987). *The Ethnograph.* Boulder: Qualis Research Associates.

Seyffert, O. (1956). *Dictionary of Classical Antiquities.* New York: Meridian Books.

Shamian, J., & Inhaber, R. (1985). The concept and practice of preceptorship in contemporary nursing: A review of pertinent literature. *International Journal of Nursing Studies, 22,* 79–88.

Shils, E. (1981). *Tradition.* Chicago: University of Chicago Press.

Shulman, L. S. (1993). Teaching as community property. *Change, 25,* 6–7.

Smoyak, S. (1987). Nurses and doctors: Redefining roles. *Nursing Times,* 35–37.

Spoth, R., & Konewko, P. (1987). Intensive care staff stressors and life event changes across multiple settings and work units. *Heart and Lung, 16,* 278–284.

Stein, L. I. (1967). The doctor-nurse game. *Archives of General Psychiatry, 16,* 699–703.

Stein, L. I., Watts, D. T., & Howell, T. (1990). The doctor-nurse game revisited. *New England Journal of Medicine, 322,* 546–549.

Stevens, B. J. (1984). Nurse-physician relations: A perspective from nursing. *Bulletin of the New York Academy of Medicine, 60,* 799–806.

Sulmasy, D. P. (1992). Physicians, cost control, and ethics. *Annals of Internal Medicine, 116,* 920–926.

Stotland, E. (1969). *The psychology of hope.* San Francisco: Jossey-Bass.

Tanner, C. (1987). Teaching clinical judgment. In J. Fitzpatrick & R. Taunton (Eds.), *Annual review of nursing research* (Vol. 5) (pp. 153–173). New York: Wiley.

Tanner, C. (1989). Using knowledge in clinical judgment. In C. Tanner & C. Lindeman (Eds.), *Using nursing research* (pp. 19–34). New York: National League for Nursing.

Tanner, C. (1993). Rethinking clinical judgment. In N. Diekelmann & M. Rather (Eds.), *Transforming RN education* (pp. 15–41). New York: National League for Nursing.

Tanner, C. A. (1993). Conversations on teaching [Editorial]. *Journal of Nursing Education, 32,* 291–292.

Tanner, C. A., Benner, P., Chesla, C., & Gordon, D. (1993). The phenomenology of knowing a patient. *Image: The Journal of Nursing Scholarship, 25,* 273–280.

Tanner, C. A., Padrick, K. P., Westfall, U. E., & Putzier, D. J. (1987). Diagnostic reasoning strategies of nurses and nursing students. *Nursing Research, 36,* 358–363.

Taylor, C. (1985a). *Philosophical Papers* (Vols. I & II). Cambridge, MA: University of Cambridge Press.

Taylor, C. (1985b). What is Human Agency? In Charles Taylor, *Human Agency and Language: Philosophical Papers 1* (pp. 15–44). Cambridge, Cambridge University Press.

Taylor, C. (1985c). Social theory as practice. In C. Taylor, *Philosophical Papers, Vol. 1* (pp. 42–57). Cambridge, MA: Cambridge University Press.

Taylor, C. (1989). *Sources of the self.* Cambridge, MA: Harvard University Press.

Taylor, C. (1991). *The ethics of authenticity.* Cambridge, MA: Harvard University Press.

Taylor, C. (1993). Explanation and practical reason. In M. C. Nussbaum & A. Sen (Eds.), *The quality of life.* Oxford: Clarendon Press.

Thiele, J. E., Holloway, J., Murphy, D., Pendarvis, J., & Stucky, M. (1991). Perceived and actual decision making by novice baccalaureate students. *Western Journal of Nursing Research, 13,* 616–626.

Thomstad, B., Cunningham, N., & Kaplan, B. (1976). Changing the rules of the doctor-nurse game. *Nursing Outlook, 23,* 422–427.

Urden, L. D. (1989). Knowledge development in clinical practice. *Journal of Continuing Education in Nursing, 20,* 18–22.

van Manen, M. (1990). *Researching lived experience: Human science for an action sensitive pedagogy.* Ontario: Althouse.

van Manen, M. (1991). *The tact of teaching: The meaning of pedagogical thoughtfulness.* Albany, NY: SUNY Press.

Verhonick, P. J., Nichols, G. A., Glor, B. A. K., & McCarthy, R. T. (1968). I came, I saw, I responded: Nursing observation and action survey. *Nursing Research, 17,* 38–44.

Vetlesen, A. J. (1994). *Perception, empathy and judgment—an inquiry into the preconditions of moral performance.* University Park, PA: University of Pennsylvania Press.

Walters, K. S. (1990). Critical thinking, rationality and the Vulcanization of Students. *Journal of Higher Education, 61,* 448–467.

Wandel, J. C., & Pike, A. W. (1991). Moral outrage and moral discourse in nurse-physician collaboration. *Journal of Professional Nursing, 7,* 351–363.

Webster, D. (1985). Medical students' views of the nurse. *Nursing Research, 34,* 313–317.

Weiss, S. J. (1982). The health care team: Changing perceptions of roles and responsibilities in caring for the critically ill patient. In A. E. Doudera & J. D.Peters (Eds.), *Legal and ethical aspects of treating critically and terminally ill patients* (pp. 253–266). Ann Arbor, MI: AUPHA Press.

Weiss, S. J. (1983). Role differentiation between nurse and physician: Implications for nursing. *Nursing Research, 32,* 133–139.

Weiss, S. J. (1985). The influence of discourse on collaboration among nurses, physicians and consumers. *Research in Nursing and Health, 8,* 49–59.

Weiss, S. J., & Davis, H. P. (1985). Validity and reliability of the collaborative practice scales. *Nursing Research, 34,* 299–306.

Weiss, S. J., & Remen, N. (1983). Self-limiting patterns of nursing behavior within a tripartite context involving consumers and physicians. *Western Journal of Nursing Research, 5,* 77–89.

Westcott, M. R. (1968). *Toward a contemporary psychology of intuition.* New York: Holt, Rinehart & Winston.

Whitbeck, C. (1983). A different reality: Feminist ontology. In *Beyond domination, new perspectives on women and philosophy* (pp. 64–88). Totowa, NJ: Rowman & Allenheld.

White, M., & Epston, D. (1990). *Narrative means to therapeutic ends.* New York: W. W. Norton.

Wros, P. (1994). The ethical context of nursing care of dying patients in critical care. In P. Benner (Ed.), *Interpretive phenomenology, embodiment, caring and ethics in health and illness* (pp. 255–277). Thousand Oaks, CA: Sage.

Wrubel, J. *Personal meanings and coping processes: A hermeneutical study of personal background meanings and interpersonal concerns and their relation to stress appraisal and coping.* Unpublished doctoral dissertation, University of California, San Francisco.

Wrubel, J., Benner, P., & Lazarus, R. S. (1981). Social competence from the perspective of stress and coping. In J. D. Wine & M. D. Smye (Eds.), *Social competence* (pp. 61–99). New York: Guilford Press.

Young, C. E. (1987). Intuition and nursing process. *Holistic Nursing Practice, 1,* 52–62.

Yu, V. L., et al. (1979). Antimicrobial selection by a computer. *Journal of the American Medical Association, 242,* 1279–1282.

Zagarell, S. A. (1988). Narrative of community: The identification of a genre. *Signs: Journal of Women in Culture and Society, 13,* 498–527.

INDEX

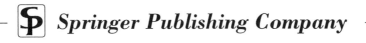
Springer Publishing Company

ADVANCED PRACTICE NURSING
A Guide to Professional Development

Mariah Snyder, PhD, RN, FAAN and
Michaelene Mirr, PhD, RN

This textbook is written for nurses preparing for the advanced practice role which encompasses nurse practitioners, clinical nurse specialists, nurse midwives, and nurse anesthetists. The book provides an overview of this evolving field, including issues such as reimbursement, prescriptive privileges, and licensure. It describes clinical skills common to all APNs, such as advanced clinical decision-making, client education and advocacy, collaboration and consultation skills, and case management. Important professional skills such as research, writing for publication, and independent practice are also addressed.

Partial Contents:

I: The Dimensions of Advanced Practice Nursing. Characteristics of the Advanced Practice Nurse, *M. Snyder and M. Yen* • Evolution of the Advanced Practice Nurse Role, *M. Mirr and M. Snyder* • Advanced Practice Within a Nursing Paradigm, *M. Snyder*

II: Clinical Issues. Clinical Decision-Making, *S. Corcoran-Perry and S. Narayan* • Developing Clinical Protocols and Guidelines for APN Practice, *C. Hilgart and M. H. Karl* • Client Advocacy, *M.L. Nelson* • Client Education, *R. Kisting-Sparks*

III: Professional Issues. Collaboration, *M. Kyle* • Consultation in Advanced Practice Nursing, *D.R. Monicken* • The Advanced Practice Nurse as a Change Agent, *H.E. Hansen* • Professional Communication: Publishing and Public Speaking, *M. Snyder* • Research, *K. Hampton and M. Snyder*

Springer Series on Advanced Practice Nursing
1995   312pp   0-8261-8850-8   *hardcover*

536 Broadway, New York, NY 10012-3955 • (212) 431-4370 • Fax (212) 941-7842

S *Springer Publishing Company*

A VIRGINIA HENDERSON READER
Excellence in Nursing

Edward J. Halloran, RN, PhD, FAAN, Editor
Foreword by Angela McBride, PhD, RN, FAAN

This book provides a sampling of Virginia Henderson's classic writings in patient care, nursing education, nursing research, and nursing's role in the larger health care system. Ms. Henderson was an early advocate of autonomy for nurses and the importance of nursing scholarship—her writings have much to say to today's nurses.

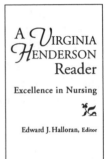

Partial Contents:

I: Patient Care. Excellence in Nursing • The Essence of Nursing in High Technology • The Art and Science of Health Assessment • The Importance of Observation

II: Nursing Education. Preparation for Specialized Nursing Graduate Programs • Nursing Process —Is the Title Right? • The Nature of Nursing

III: Nursing Research. Research in Nursing Practice—When? • An Overview of Nursing Research • We've "Come A Long Way" But What of the Direction? • Basis for Selection of Method: Research as a Means of Improving Nursing Practice

IV: Nursing in Society. Nursing as an Aspect of Health Care • Nursing as a Constant Factor in Health Services

1995   424pp   0-8261-8830-3   hardcover

536 Broadway, New York, NY 10012-3955 • (212) 431-4370 • Fax (212) 941-7842

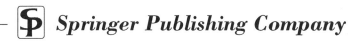

Springer Publishing Company

ANNUAL REVIEW OF NURSING RESEARCH, Volume 13
Focus on Key Social and Health Issues

Joyce J. Fitzpatrick, PhD
Joanne Stevenson, PhD, Editors

The newest volume in this landmark series reviews research on key social and health issues relevant to nursing, such as child sexual abuse, case management, feminism in nursing, and quality of life with HIV infection.

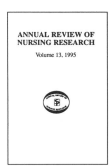

Contents:

Research on Nursing Practice. Quality of Life and the Spectrum of HIV Infection, *W. L. Holzemer and H. Skodol Wilson* • Physical Health of Homeless Adults, *A. M. Lindsey* • Child Sexual Abuse: Initial Effects, *S. J. Kelley* • The Neurobehavioral Effects of Childhood Lead Exposure, *H. vonKoss Krowchuk*

Research on Nursing Care Delivery. Case Management, *G. S. Lamb* • Technology and Home Care, *C.E. Smith* • The Nursing Minimum Data Set, *P. Ryan and C. Delaney* • Pediatric Hospice Nursing, *I.M. Martinson*

Research on Nursing Education. Faculty Practice: Interest, Issues, and Impact, *P. H. Walker*

Research on the Profession of Nursing. The Professionalization of Nurse Practitioners, *B. Bullough* • Feminism and Nursing, *P. Chinn*

Other Research. Health Risk Behaviors in Hispanic Women: Adolescent Pregnancy, Sexually Transmitted Disease, and Substance Abuse, *S. Torres and A. M. Villarruel*

1995   360pp   0-8261-8232-1   hardcover

536 Broadway, New York, NY 10012-3955 • (212) 431-4370 • Fax (212) 941-7842

Springer Publishing Company

A videotape companion...

FROM BEGINNER TO EXPERT
Clinical Knowledge in Critical Care Nursing

Patricia Benner, RN, PhD, FAAN
Christine A. Tanner, RN, PhD, FAAN
Catherine Chesla, RN, DNSc

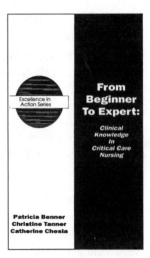

This videotape highlights and expands the information in the book *Expertise in Nursing Practice: Caring, Clinical Judgement, and Ethics* by Patricia Benner, RN, PhD, FAAN, Christine A. Tanner, RN, PhD, FAAN and Catherine Chesla, RN, DNSc. Enhancing the book with a roundtable discussion by the authors, the videotape also provides "action" footage of clinical incidents that illustrates the stages of clinical skill acquisition and the components of expert practice. An invaluable educational tool, the videotape supplements textbook learning with practical, hands-on demonstrations of clinical skill applications in real-life situations. Excellent for classroom use.

*Distributed by Springer Publishing Company for the
Fuld Institute for Technology in Nursing
1992   VHS format 0-8261-8701-3
(VHS PAL 0-8261-8702-1)*

536 Broadway, New York, NY 10012-3955 • (212) 431-4370 • Fax (212) 941-7842